AF681293

DENTAL SCIENCE, MATERIALS AND TECHNOLOGY

CLINICAL DENTISTRY

DENTAL SCIENCE, MATERIALS AND TECHNOLOGY

Additional books in this series can be found on Nova's website under the Series tab.

Additional E-books in this series can be found on Nova's website under the E-books tab.

DENTAL SCIENCE, MATERIALS AND TECHNOLOGY

CLINICAL DENTISTRY

SCARDINA GIUSEPPE ALESSANDRO
EDITOR

Nova Science Publishers, Inc.
New York

Copyright © 2011 by Nova Science Publishers, Inc.

All rights reserved. No part of this book may be reproduced, stored in a retrieval system or transmitted in any form or by any means: electronic, electrostatic, magnetic, tape, mechanical photocopying, recording or otherwise without the written permission of the Publisher.

For permission to use material from this book please contact us:
Telephone 631-231-7269; Fax 631-231-8175
Web Site: http://www.novapublishers.com

NOTICE TO THE READER

The Publisher has taken reasonable care in the preparation of this book, but makes no expressed or implied warranty of any kind and assumes no responsibility for any errors or omissions. No liability is assumed for incidental or consequential damages in connection with or arising out of information contained in this book. The Publisher shall not be liable for any special, consequential, or exemplary damages resulting, in whole or in part, from the readers' use of, or reliance upon, this material. Any parts of this book based on government reports are so indicated and copyright is claimed for those parts to the extent applicable to compilations of such works.

Independent verification should be sought for any data, advice or recommendations contained in this book. In addition, no responsibility is assumed by the publisher for any injury and/or damage to persons or property arising from any methods, products, instructions, ideas or otherwise contained in this publication.

This publication is designed to provide accurate and authoritative information with regard to the subject matter covered herein. It is sold with the clear understanding that the Publisher is not engaged in rendering legal or any other professional services. If legal or any other expert assistance is required, the services of a competent person should be sought. FROM A DECLARATION OF PARTICIPANTS JOINTLY ADOPTED BY A COMMITTEE OF THE AMERICAN BAR ASSOCIATION AND A COMMITTEE OF PUBLISHERS.

Additional color graphics may be available in the e-book version of this book.

LIBRARY OF CONGRESS CATALOGING-IN-PUBLICATION DATA
Clinical dentistry / editor, Scardina Giuseppe Alessandro.
p. ; cm.
Includes bibliographical references and index.
ISBN 978-1-61122-354-5 (hardcover : alk. paper)
1. Dentistry. I. Alessandro, Scardina Giuseppe.
[DNLM: 1. Dental Care. 2. Dentistry--methods. WU 29]
RK51.C563 210
617.6--dc22
2010038637

Published by Nova Science Publishers, Inc. † New York

D
C6162
2011

OCLC#667609232

CONTENTS

7-18-2011 B135.69

PREFACE

This book presents comprehensive coverage of new techniques, important developments, and innovative ideas in all fields of clinical dentistry. Topics discussed herein include indirect composite restoration in the posterior region; fissure sealings with resin modified glass-ionomer cement; craniofacial anthropometry; oral cavity overinfection during non-surgical cancer therapies; numb chin syndrome; and the growing need for collaboration between dentistry and medicine.

Chapter 1 - The dental profession is unique among the various types of health care providers since in most instances, only the dental practitioner is responsible for the diagnosis process, determination of treatment options, and performing the chosen treatment. Variations have been found among dental practitioners regarding diagnosis and treatment in the various fields of dentistry. This article reviews the educational factors influencing the clinical decision making and treatment planning in the dental practice. As a part of the first issue of the new *International Journal of Clinical Dentistry,* it is believed that continuing education, exchange of opinions as well as clinical research in a multidisciplinary forum for publications from all fields of oral medicine is of utmost importance to bridge basic and clinical sciences, promoting the exchange of information and the advancement of oral medicine for the benefit of patients.

Chapter 2 - The recent emergence of highly pathogenic H5N1 strains and the occurrence of human cases of H5N1 infection have prompted predictions of a pandemic-scale avian influenza viral infection among humans. Highly pathogenic H5N1 avian influenza viruses have become endemic among birds throughout the world, owing to the rapid carriage of H5N1 by migrating birds around the globe. In a relatively short period of time, H5N1 has acquired the ability to infect more mammalian species with fatal outcomes than any other influenza virus. So far, H5N1 has spread to more than 12 countries and its mortality rate reportedly exceeds 50%. It is difficult to predict when, whether, or which type of H5N1 influenza A virus will acquire efficient human-to-human transmission and lead to a pandemic, and the most important public health strategy at present therefore is to prevent the spread of the virus through the education of both health care workers and the general public. In this review, the authors summarize the current knowledge in H5N1 virology, its historical and epidemiological background, and clinical and hospital management strategies including those appertaining to dentistry.

Chapter 3 - *Purpose:* To evaluate the clinical performance of two self-etching adhesives and one total-etch adhesive in Class V carious lesions.

Methods: Two self-etching primers, 'Clearfil SE bond' and 'Hybrid Bond' and one total etch adhesive, 'Admira bond', were placed in 244 Class V carious lesions. Restorations were evaluated at base line, one and two year using USPHS criteria.

Results: No loss of restorations was recorded after one and two year for all materials. There was no significant difference between the base line and two-year results for Admira bond and Clearfil SE bond restorations. In contrast, restorations of Hybrid bond showed significant deterioration in marginal adaptation and cavosurface marginal discoloration after two years. No significant differences were found between Admira bond and Clearfil SE bond at each recall period.

Clinical Significance: Total-etch adhesive (Admira bond) and two-step self-etch adhesive (Clearfil SE Bond) when placed in Class V carious lesions showed excellent clinical performance after two years. In contrast, one step self-etch adhesive (Hybrid Bond) showed significant deterioration with regard to the marginal adaptation and marginal discoloration.

Chapter 4 - The site-specific nature of the volumetric features and enzymatic profile of gingival crevicular fluid (GCF): Analysis of myeloperoxidase (MPO) activity at distinct sampling sites.

Purpose: Further clarification of the biodynamics and the site-specific nature of gingival crevicular fluid (GCF), in terms of volume and content, may serve both for a better understanding of periodontal pathogenesis and developing reliable diagnostic tools. Thus, the aim of the present study was to analyze, on a site-specific basis, the potential variances in GCF volume and its myeloperoxidase (MPO) content and the relationship of these two measures with the clinical periodontal status.

Methods: At a total of 719 sites, representing either clinical periodontal health (n=175), or gingivitis (n=308), or periodontitis (n=236), clinical parameters were recorded, GCF samples were obtained and MPO activity was spectrophotometrically determined. Statistical analyses considered the comparison of the three periodontal conditions, multi-rooted or single-rooted teeth, and mesio-buccal (MB) and disto-buccal (DB) sites, and the correlations among the clinical parameters, GCF volume and MPO activity.

Results: There were clear differences between all site-analysis and analysis of distinct sites. For all sites clinical parameters, GCF volume, and GCF MPO activity generally presented with a disease-related spectrum; healthy<gingivitis<periodontitis ($p<0.05$). However, differences in GCF volume and MPO profile between multi-rooted and single-rooted sites and between MB and DB sites were observed ($p<0.05$). Site–specific differences were also observed regarding the presence/absence of GCF and MPO and correlations.

Clinical Significance: The site-specific nature of periodontal diseases and the apparent variances in both the GCF volume and its enzymatic profile at the individual sites needs to be taken into account for a precise GCF-methodology and also for the correct interpretation of the GCF-related data.

Chapter 5 - *Aim:* A retrospective study was undertaken to assess causes of maxillofacial trauma in Recife, Pernambuco, Brazil.

Method: A review of 126 patients with maxillofacial injuries aged 1 and 18 years old seen and treated at the Hospital da Restauração between January and December 2006 was conducted and were analyzed according to age, sex, etiology, site of fracture, dentoalveolar trauma and alcohol abuse. Analysis was made in Epi Info using the Chi-square and Fisher's Exact Tests.

Results: It was found that maxillofacial injuries were most frequent in males (69%) and in the 11-18 year age group (50.8%). Falls (34.1%) and pedestrian accidents (19%) were the most common aetiological factor. The most common facial fracture was mandible (40%), followed by the zygomatic-orbital complex (23.1%). A positive association between the presence of facial fracture and age (P=0.000) and alcohol consumption was strongly associated with facial fracture (P = .008). Dentoalveolar injuries were present in 14.3% of patients.

Conclusion: The incidence of facial fractures in children is higher than previously reported elsewhere. There were most common in male patients, mainly due to falls and pedestrian accidents. Therefore, strategies to prevent pedestrian related accidents need to be identified, evaluated, and implemented.

Chapter 6 - *Objectives:* Techniques relying on the use of II generation laboratory composites to carry out indirect restorations ensure long-lasting and predictable results also in posterior teeth. The evolution of restorative materials and adhesive systems improved chemical-physical characteristics of resins (resistance to stress and to wear, hardness) and allowed to perform bonded restorations that respect the biologic and aesthetic principles.

Methods: We have clinically evaluated different types of indirect composite restorations (inlay, onlay and overlay) performed to treat carious lesions in posterior teeth.

After analyzing occlusion and structural factors, the treatment plan included the cavity preparation and, if necessary, a preliminary build-up with a nano-hybrid composite (Filtek Supreme, 3M ESPE). After cavity preparation, indirect composite restorations were fabricated using post-polymerized laboratory composite (Sinfony, 3M ESPE). The following cementation procedure was carried out with the same adhesive system and composite resin used in the preliminary build-up step.

Results: According to our clinical evaluation, the operative protocols applied have proved to be efficient, versatile and simple to perform, providing effective solutions for all the analyzed cases. The technique we have standardized allowed to obtain satisfactory results both for functional and aesthetic aspects.

Conclusion: indirect composite restorations allow maximum preservation of sound dental structure, better plaque control, good marginal seal and high resistance of the tooth-restoration complex, because of the homogeneous biomechanical properties of the different parts of the restoration.

Chapter 7 - The aim of the present study was to evaluate retention and clinical success rate of a resin modified glass ionomer cement (compomer) fissure sealant in comparison to a bis-GMA sealant. Three hundred and fifty-two fissure sealings (Helioseal or Ionosit Seal) were placed in 1st and 2nd permanent molars of 95 patients using a split-mouth design. The subjects were five to 15 years old. All 352 sealed teeth could be included in the final analysis. The mean observation time was 3.16 (SD 0.5) years. Over the entire observation period, 90.4% of the bis-GMA based sealants (6.8% partial loss, 2.8% complete loss) and 5.1% of the resin modified glass ionomer sealants (18.1% partial loss, 76.8% complete loss) remained intact. Established caries was found in ten occlusal surfaces sealed with resin modified glass ionomer and in two cases when the bis-GMA sealer was used. In one case each, caries developed after partial loss, whereas in all the other cases complete loss was preceding caries. The caries frequency was not statistically significantly different between the materials (Fisher's exact test, p=0.35). With "established caries" as failure criteria, the three-year survival rate was 96.7% for the resin modified glass ionomer sealants and 99.5% for the bis-

GMA sealants (Kaplan-Meier analysis). Log-rank analysis showed a statistically significant difference between the materials (p=0.02). From a clinical point of view, however, it can be concluded that a resin modified glass ionomer sealer is as effective in caries prevention as a bis-GMA sealer after three years.

Chapter 8 - *Purpose:* Since the ultraviolet (UV) component of a light can brighten a fluorescent material like human teeth, a color difference between tooth and a non-fluorescent esthetic material would be more apparent when viewed under the UV included light. The purpose of this study was to evaluate the fluorescence of simulatedly layered all-ceramic materials at a clinically relevant thickness with a color-measuring spectrophotometer.

Methods: Seven all-ceramic core materials of Vita A2-corresponding shade, one sintering ceramic and one alloy core as references, were prepared in clinically relevant thicknesses (0.4 to 0.8 mm). A2- and A3-corresponding shades of each recommended veneer ceramic were fabricated so that the thickness of the layered specimens was 1.5 mm. Color and spectral reflectance of layered ceramics were measured over a white background according to the CIELAB color scale. An UV filter of the spectrophotometer was inserted or removed to exclude or include the UV component of illuminant D65 to determine the fluorescence. Seven specimens were made for each group and each specimen was measured three times. Difference in color (ΔE*ab-FL) and color coordinates by the fluorescence was calculated. From the spectral reflectance values, subtraction spectrum by the inclusion and the exclusion of the UV component was calculated. Three-way ANOVA was performed for the differences in color and color coordinates with the fixed factors of the type of core, the type of veneer and the shade of the veneer (α=0.05).

Results: ΔE*ab-FL was 0.6 to 4.3 for the A2-veneer layered ceramics and 0.4 to 2.1 for the A3-veneer layered ceramics. Differences in color and color coordinates were significantly influenced by the three factors ($p<0.05$).

Chapter 9 - *Purpose:* The aim of this review is to elucidate the relationship of micro-mechanical interlocking and chemical bonding of self-etching adhesives at the resin-tooth hard tissues interfaces.

Methods: Instrumental analysis is widely used for detection of surface chemistry. Electron microscopy is used to analyze the interfaces between adhesives and tooth surface. This paper critically reviews the recent research on the interaction of the self-etching primers/adhesives and some carboxylic acids with tooth hard tissues/ hydroxyapatite, and the interfaces of resin-tooth hard tissues.

Clinical Significance: Some self-etching adhesives have been proven to provide chemical bonding to hydroxyapatite. Thus, self-etching adhesives possess a high possibility to form a tight micro-mechanical interlocking at the tooth hard tissue-resin interfaces. However, the clinical performance of the self-etching adhesives such as bond durability, marginal adaptation, and sealing capacity or the potential to reduce post-operative hyper-sensitivity depends on the individual self-etching adhesive system used, the operator's/dentist's clinical technique, the chemical stability of the adhesive system itself and its chemical bonding to tooth hard tissues.

Chapter 10 - The aim of this study was to assess the prevalence of apical lucencies in a German population, radiographed between 1989 -1991 ("Group 1990") and 1999 - 2001 ("Group 2000").

Twelve hundred and forty-seven panoramic images were evaluated by two observers which were calibrated prior to evaluation. Numbers of endodontic treatments, apical lucencies, and quality of root fillings were registered. Relations between apical status and quality of root canal filling as well as quality and presence of coronal seal were statistically calculated with χ^2 test.

In group 1990, 5.2% of all teeth were endodontically treated (ET); 41.2% of these showed apical lucencies. In group 2000, 5.8% were ET and 49.1% showed apical lucencies. The quality of root fillings had decreased within ten years. In group 1990, the quality of coronal seal had no significant impact on the radiological status of apices, whereas in group 2000, unacceptable coronal fillings were significantly more often associated with apical lesions. The presence of a coronal filling and a good root filling had in both groups a significant positive impact on the apical status of ET teeth.

Chapter 11 - *Purpose:* To study age and gender differences regarding xerostomia in 50- and 60- year-old subjects. It was hypothesized that the prevalence would be higher in women and among older subjects.

Methods: Identical questionnaires were sent to all subjects born in 1942 and 1952 living in two Swedish counties (N=17138). The final response rate was 72.8 %. Responses regarding day- and nighttime xerostomia were analyzed.

Results: The prevalence of "often dry mouth" ranged from 6.9 % in 50 year old men to 16.0 % in 60-year-old women. Xerostomia was more common at age 60 compared to 50 and more common in women compared to men. Approximately twice as many subjects perceived "often dry mouth" at nighttime compared to daytime. Logistic regression showed that xerostomia was associated to impaired general and oral health. The hypothesis that xerostomia was higher in women and among the older subjects was confirmed.

Clinical significance: The dramatic increase of self-reported xerostomia between age 50 and 60, especially among women, needs to be considered in the management of this age group.

Chapter 12 - *Purpose:* This study was aimed to analyze the anthropometric measurements of parents who have a child with nonsyndromic orofacial cleft to determine deviations in craniofacial morphology.

Methods: Measurements (total of nine) characterizing head and face were taken from parents who have children with clefts and healthy Latvia residents as controls. As a reference group we have used established standards of North American whites.

Results: Statistical analysis showed significant differences ($p<0.05$) between the cleft parents, controls, and the reference group for four measurements in males and for six measurements in females. This suggests that craniofacial morphology in parents of children with clefts is distinctive from that observed in healthy individuals.

Clinical significance: Anthropometry could be useful in clinical practice as objective approach to evaluate changes in the craniofacial region.

Chapter 13 - Fusion is currently defined as a developmental anomaly that occurs due to an union of two or more adjacent teeth during morphodifferentiation of the dental germs. The present case reports the endodontic treatment of a fused maxillary lateral incisor and supernumerary tooth. A 12-year-old girl had an excessively large anterior tooth. The endodontic therapy was carried out, so the patient could receive a surgical therapy to remove the supernumerary tooth and orthodontic treatment to correct the malocclusion. Electronic apex locator, rotary instrumentation and thermo-mechanical obturation were used under the direct view of a dental operating microscope.

Chapter 14 - Success in endodonitc treatment based on diagnosis, treatment plan, debridement,sterilization and obturation. In an early radiographic study of success and failure, Ingle indicated nearly 60% of treatment failures were due to incomplete obturation . In reality, creating a fluid-tight apical, lateral and coronal seal is necessary to prevent recontamination and long-term clinical success.

Several root filling materials and techniques have been developed with purpose of obtaining a tight root canal seal. Most techniques employ a core material and sealer, and a wide variety of root canal sealers are available for obturation of the root canal system.

Over all many studies on the obturation of root canals indicated that most fillings do not completely fill the root canal systems.

Lateral and vertical compaction is two common methods for obturation. There are many studies about stress generation with in the canal form these two methods, and their sealing ability.

Mendoza et al. compared sealing ability of two different obturation techniques, they concluded that warm vertical compaction, provide better apical seal in canine teeth of dogs compared to heated lateral techniques, with fewer complications.

Many studies showed that thermafil obturators achieved seals comparable to lateral compaction.

Gernhardt et al. evaluated lateral and vertical condensation and thermafil and presented that thermafil and warm vertical condensation achieved seals with low dye penetration.

Reader et al. evaluated filling of the lateral and main canals using root canal obturation techniques, they found that flow of gutta and sealer was more in vertical and lateral techniques respectively. Yared compared the quality of coronal seal between these two techniques after removing coronal gutta and found better seal with vertical condensation independently of gutta removal technique. In addition Taylor et al showed removal of smear layer and the use of AH26 and and vertical condensation obturation; reduce coronal leakage.

Jayalatha et al compared sealing ability of three different root canal sealers (seal apex AH26 and ZnOE) and showed that AH26 has the maximum sealing ability followed by seal apex and ZnOE.

Suprabha and colleagues evaluated the apical leakage of AH26/silverfree and Tubliseal using methylene blue penetration and showed superior sealing ability of AH26(18).

Studies had shown more sealing ability of resin based sealers like AH26 or AH plus versus ZnOE or Ca (OH) 2 based sealers.

Some investigation have shown that sealing ability of Ca(OH)2 based sealers is more than AH26 and less than ZnOE sealers.

The aim of this study was to compare apical sealing ability of AH26 Apexit, pure ZnOE using lateral and vertical condensation.

Chapter 15 - *Background:* Recently, the study has shown negative correlation between the severity of the periodontal disease and sCD14 levels. However there are no reports correlating the levels of sCD14 in health, disease and after treatment of periodontitis. The present study was designed to explore further in understanding the role played by sCD14 in the pathogenesis of periodontal disease and also to gain insight into the levels of sCD14 in health, disease and after treatment of periodontitis affected individuals.

Methods: Age (29-39yrs) and sex matched (30 males and 30 females) sixty subjects were recruited and divided into 4 groups consisting of 20 subjects in each group based on clinical attachment loss (CAL) and radiological parameters (bone loss); healthy (group I), gingivitis (group II), periodontitis (group III) and after treatment of group III (groupIV) and GCF was collected. The sCD14 levels were determined by ELISA. Results were analyzed statistically.

Results: The sCD14 was detected in all 60 subjects tested for and values varied greatly among the subjects within the group. The mean concentration of sCD14 in GCF was observed to be highest in group I i.e., 1652.50 pg/μl (900-2300pg/μl) and lowest in group III i.e., 828.70 pg/ μl (213-1400 pg/ μl). The mean sCD14 concentrations of group II (1019.35 pg/μl ± 243.06) and group IV (1172.7 pg/μl ± 216.93) fell between the highest and lowest values. This suggests negative correlation between CAL and GCF sCD14 concentrations.

Conclusions: Currently, as our data shows inverse relationship between the levels of sCD14 and the clinical parameters like CAL and GI scores, which indicate the inflammatory conditions of the periodontal tissue, we speculate that sCD14 could be used as an inflammatory biomarker. However carefully controlled longitudinal, population-based studies are needed to verify this possibility.

Chapter 16 - *Introduction.* Oral mucositis represents one of the most frequent acute side effects during cancer therapies (chemotherapy and/or radiotherapy). It has been hypothesized that microbial (bacteria, fungi) overinfection of oral mucosa may enhance intensity and duration of mucositis. For this reason, a lot of studies have been performed in order to evaluate the efficacy of oral cavity bacterial decontamination and/or prevention and treatment of oral candidiasis.

Patients and methods. A comprehensive search of MEDLINE up to December 2007 (with no language restriction) was performed. "Mucositis", "Chemotherapy" and "Radiotherapy" were the key words used.

Results. Sixty clinical studies matched the key words listed above. Most papers were focused on oral cavity bacterial decontamination and prevention and/or treatment of oral candidiasis. Recent international guidelines and critical reviews of literature were also considered.

Conclusion. Available literature data do not support the use of preventive bacterial decontamination of oral cavity by antimicrobial agents. On the contrary, some evidences exist that prophylaxis of oral candidiasis with antimicotic agents (like fluconazole) could to be efficacious to reduce the impact of oral mucositis but further larger randomized trials are needed.

Chapter 17 - As the saying goes, "beauty is in the eye of the beholder." Oral esthetics is part art and part science. The enhancement of a person's smile culminates in the individualization of the general rules governing dental esthetics to that person. Every patient is different, and yet a nice smile is the result of several components coming together in an orderly fashion. Knowing the general guidelines that make a smile appealing and tailoring them to the individual patient gives that smile uniqueness.

The esthetic zone has been defined as the area encompassed by the upper and lower lip. It is the harmonious relationship between the dentition (premolar to premolar), the periodontium (gingival line) and the lips that will make or break a smile.

Chapter 18 - *Purpose:* To evaluate the clinical performance of a self-etching adhesive in Class V carious lesions with and without acid etching procedures.

Methods: A total of 183 Class V carious cavities with incisal margins in enamel and gingival margins in cementum were selected and restored with Futurabond NR self-etch adhesive and resin composite Grandio. Restorations were made using three different techniques; after etching of the enamel, after etching the whole cavity for 20 seconds and without acid etching (control). The restorations were evaluated at baseline, and every year up to 4 years using USPHS criteria.

Results: No loss of restorations was recorded after four year for all the three restorative techniques. There was no significant difference between the baseline and 4-year results for any of the tested technique. However, restorations made after acid etching showed less marginal discoloration at the enamel margins.

Chapter 19 - *Purpose* The numb chin syndrome is a mental nerve neuropathy that origins in the absence of a mandibular lesion or a dental cause. In most occasions it can be the first symptom of a malignancy. *Methods* We present a series of four oncologic patients that were complaining of oral and facial numbness associated with neuralgia. All subjects underwent neurological and dental examinations. Computed tomography, magnetic resonance imaging and bone scan were also carried out. Neoplastic neurological involvement was suspected and the analysis of the cerebrospinal fluid was performed.

Results The neurological examination, combined with the radiological features and the cerebrospinal fluid analysis confirmed the diagnoses of numb chin syndrome associated with carcinomatous meningitis.

Chapter 20 - *Purpose:* Gingival fenestration is a rare pathological entity, scarcely described in the literature. The purpose of this paper is to report a case of a tooth with a gingival fenestration which was successfully treated by the periodontal plastic surgical procedure with excellent aesthetic results.

Methods: A 27 year old male patient reported with a "Gingival fenestration" which persisted after a periapical surgery and apicectomy. The lesion was successfully treated using a modified free gingival graft with successful aesthetic and functional outcome. The hypothesis for the formation of such isolated gingival defect have been proposed.

Results: The aesthetic result obtained by the surgical procedure was successfully maintained during the one year follow up period.

Chapter 21 - Nowadays hygiene and asepsis took an important place in all the medical fields and particularly in Dentistry, because the "hand of the dentist" can constitute a important source of infection. So, one basic measure of infection control, supposes a careful hand washing and the use of gloves which form a physical barrier and protect the Health Care Workers from occupational exposure to blood and saliva.

Our study carried out with the University Dental Clinic of Monastir (Tunisia) aims to evaluate knowledge in dental practice and to investigate their attitudes and practices toward the use of the gloves. It consists of a survey by auto-administrated questionnaire managed to a sample of 106 dental practitioners including 16 teachers, 26 trainees and 64 dental students.

Findings revealed that about 78.3% of dentists wore gloves, 21.7% wore masks and 2% wore protective eyeglasses. The students have a minimum necessary knowledge about gloves use but do not have a correct practice while the other practitioners have the good knowledge and the good practical attitudes.

Our study shows an important need to improve the students' behaviour with respect of occupational hygiene and safety conditions in order to reduce occupational blood exposure hazards.

Chapter 22 - There is a bilateral relationship between oral health and general health and, without doubt, interdisciplinary management increases the efficiency of diagnosis and treatment, reduces complications and unnecessary treatment, and improves the quality of care and quality of life. Dental and medical professionals have always been in close cooperation particularly for the provision of comprehensive care for patients with specific needs; however, there seems to be a need for further improvement of the collaboration between the two health disciplines. Immunocompromised patients may well serve as a good example of the growing need for such an improved treatment alliance between the two health disciplines for provision of efficient care for special in-need groups, because of the increasing number of immunocompromised patients, particularly the bone marrow or solid organ transplant candidates and recipients, and due to the many areas of interface between dentistry and medicine regarding these patients, Recent advances in both disciplines are also likely to provide new opportunities for dental and medical professionals to provide comprehensive care for many of the immunocompromised patients. Further, an active team approach may enable both health professionals to significantly increase their part of contribution to the improvement of general health, oral health, well being, and quality of life of this specific patient category.

All of these chapters were previously published in *International Journal of Clinical Dentistry,* Volume 1, Issues 1-4.

In: Clinical Dentistry
Editor: Scardina Giuseppe Alessandro

ISBN: 978-1-61122-354-5
© 2011 Nova Science Publishers, Inc.

Chapter 1

CLINICAL DECISION MAKING IN THE EVIDENCE-BASED PRACTICE ERA[1]

Yehuda Zadik[§] and Liran Levin[*]

[§]Zrifin Central Dental Clinic, and The Center for Health Promotion and Preventive Medicine, Medical Corps, Israel Defense Forces, Jerusalem, Israel
[*]Department of Oral Rehabilitation
The Maurice and Gabriela Goldschleger School of Dental Medicine, Tel-Aviv University, Tel-Aviv, and Unit of Periodontology, Department of Oral and Dental Sciences, Rambam Medical Center, Haifa, Israel

ABSTRACT

The dental profession is unique among the various types of health care providers since in most instances, only the dental practitioner is responsible for the diagnosis process, determination of treatment options, and performing the chosen treatment. Variations have been found among dental practitioners regarding diagnosis and treatment in the various fields of dentistry. This article reviews the educational factors influencing the clinical decision making and treatment planning in the dental practice. As a part of the first issue of the new *International Journal of Clinical Dentistry,* we believe that continuing education, exchange of opinions as well as clinical research in a multidisciplinary forum for publications from all fields of oral medicine is of utmost importance to bridge basic and clinical sciences, promoting the exchange of information and the advancement of oral medicine for the benefit of patients.

---

[1] A version of this book was also published as a chapter in *International Journal of Clinical Dentistry, Volume 1, Issue1*, published by Nova Science Publishers, Inc. It was submitted for appropriate modifications in an effort to encourage wider dissemination of research.

[*] Address for Correspondence: Dr. Liran Levin, Department of Oral Rehabilitation, The Maurice and Gabriela Goldschleger, School of Dental Medicine, Tel Aviv University, Tel Aviv, Israel, Fax: +972-3-6409250, Email: liranl@post.tau.ac.il

Keywords: decision making, treatment planning, education, evidence based medicine, evidence based dentistry, dental research, continuing education.

INTRODUCTION

The dental profession is unique among the various types of health care providers. In most instances, only the dental practitioner is responsible for the diagnosis process, determination of treatment options, and performing the chosen treatment. Variations have been found among dental practitioners regarding diagnosis and treatment of dental caries lesions, [1-6] peri-apical lesions [5-14], third-molars [5, 15-18] and mal-occlusions [19,20], as well as differences in antibiotic prescription habits after endodontics [5, 6, 21] and extractions [5, 6, 22].

This article reviews the educational factors influencing the clinical decision making and treatment planning in the dental practice. As a part of the first issue of the new *International Journal of Clinical Dentistry,* we believe that continuing education, exchange of opinions as well as clinical research in a multidisciplinary forum for publications from all fields of oral medicine is of utmost importance to bridge basic and clinical sciences, promoting the exchange of information and the advancement of oral medicine for the benefit of patients. Other factors, such as financial (e.g., practitioners-to-patients ratio, available resources and reimbursement systems) as well as patient-dependent factors (e.g., dental caries risk, systemic health, compliance and age) are beyond the scope of this present article.

UNDERGRADUATE EDUCATION

In a series of recent studies we have published, a significant influence of graduation place (country) was demonstrated [5, 6, 18]. We have presented several clinical dilemmas in restorative dentistry, endodontics, third molar exodontia and post-operative antibiotic prescription to young dental surgeons (less than 10 years from graduation) who practiced in the same environment (military dental clinics) at the time the study took place. When the participating dentists were divided according the countries of dental graduation, several treatment plans were significantly common in some groups [6, 18]. This observation has importance for health authorities, which must keep in mind that foreign-trained dentists may have clinical philosophies that differ from the local common practice [23, 24]. When further dividing the dentists that graduated in Israel according the dental school, we revealed an influence of the school on their clinical decision making [5].

Similarly, Aryanpour et al. found that 'school-effect' provides an explanation for the disagreement among European practitioners regarding peri-apical disease treatment decisions [9]. In our developing 'global village' and the sophisticated communication ways and global accessed databases all over the world, we believe that throughout the years, those differences will have to disappear or at least diminish. Providing an international comprehensive coverage of new techniques, important developments, and innovative ideas in all fields of clinical dentistry will probably help in achieving this task.

Guidelines

The purpose of clinical guidelines is to limit inappropriate variation in clinical practice by outlining evidence-based practice [25]. van der Sanden et al. studied the effect of guideline on general dentists' decision making regarding third molar surgery in the Nederland. A group of dental surgeons were introduced to evidences-based third molar guidelines. The guidelines were found to improve dentists' knowledge on the current philosophies regarding third molar management and improved decision making in simulated cases. However, no clinical effect was demonstrated as there was no statistically significant difference between the groups in guideline-consistent patient referral rates (to surgical teeth removal) at the post-test assessment [26]. It seems that other influencing factors (e.g., culture, patients' preferences) played major role in this non-evidence-based decision making process [18].

Maybe the most wide-spread dental guidelines are the American Heart Association (AHA) recommendations for prevention of dental-related infective endocarditis [27]. Despite the potential harmful consequences of endocarditis and the acceptance of the guidelines as the standard of treatment both in clinical and legal aspects [28], several studies revealed inadequate compliance to the guidelines by dentists. For example, Epstein et al. described over-medication of 'antibiotic prophylaxis' before all dental procedures in patients with history of rheumatic fever or any heart murmur, nevertheless, only two-thirds of same cohort of British-Colombian dentists prescribed pre-operative antibiotics in case of extraction of impacted tooth in a prosthetic heart valve (high-risk for endocarditis) patient [29]. Both practices were violation of the AHA guidelines [30].

Palmer et al. reported an association between dentists' awareness of guidelines for use of antibiotics in the dental setting and their place of practice [31]. In a questionnaire regarding knowledge of the use of antibiotics, English dentists had a higher average score than their Scottish counterparts. It has been suggested that prescription of antibiotics is influenced by undergraduate and postgraduate education, publication and advertising [32, 33].

Post-Graduate Education

With the rapidly changing dental methodologies, techniques and philosophies in our era of innovations, the importance of post-graduate education of the practicing dentist can not be over-estimated. In many fields, the dental knowledge of the graduated dental practitioner is out-of-date and expires within a short time. Post-graduation education has several methods: reading of scientific journals, courses, seminars and professional meetings. Generally, it was reported that as much as the chosen educational method utilizes more passive involvement (e.g. large conventions), its influence might be less effective and unlikely to result in behavior change [34].

An essential aim of the *Journal* is to publish original scientific articles and invited reviews that provide an international readership with up-to-date results of basic and clinical studies in the field of oral and maxillofacial science and medicine. The *Journal* will also elucidate the relevance of these results for modern practices. By providing state-of-the-art reports, studies, information regarding new instruments and diagnostic equipment, as well as modern therapeutic drugs and devices our aim is to present the dental practitioner with an imperative educational tool. This will, hopefully, lead our profession to better worldwide practice.

Peer-review meeting is another reported method for self-appraisal and continuing education among dental practitioners. Peer-review meetings bring together practitioners from several different types of practice and experiences and accelerate exchange of views [34].

Palmer et al. examined the antibiotic prescription habits of English dentists and the influence of group meeting with an expert. The authors collected antibiotic prescription from 175 dentists. The participant dentists were then divided to 8 to 10 dentists groups. Each group meet with an oral microbiologist and discussed on the principles of appropriate prescribing, both therapeutically and prophylactically, based on the recently published guidelines and evidences. The authors collected the antibiotic prescriptions in the six-week post intervention and revealed a favorable reduction of 42.5% of prescribe antibiotics [32].

Clinical debates, opinions and research reports, can lead to a more rational and appropriate overall dental practice.

Specialization

Specialization is a unique form of post-graduate education. The certified specialist, who trained several years in a supervised program, has to be familiar with the current relevant literature, thus it is supposed that he or she would make clinical decisions on the basis of scientific evidences. Several studies compared the decision making and treatment planning of dental specialists (from different dental fields) and of general dental practitioners.

Review of the literature indicates that there is no consensus about peri-apical diagnosis and treatment decisions among practitioners. In one study in which 12 general dental practitioners (GDPs) were compared with 12 endodontic postgraduate students, GDPs decided re-treatment more often [10]. The opposite was found in a Swedish study involving 20 GDPs and 20 endodontists [13]. In a study conducted by Molven et al. that included one oral surgeon, one endodontist and an oral radiologist, the latter participant recommended more patients for re-treatment [8]. Reit and Hollander found consensus among practitioners for only 27% of pathologic patients and 37% of the healthy patients in a study involving 3 endodontists and 3 oral radiologists [7]. When Molven examined consensus among an oral surgeon and an endodontist, a 63% rate of agreement was found, and 94% rate of agreement after joint evaluation of the two practitioners [8].

Surprisingly, Epstein et al. reported of significant less prescription of pre-operative antibiotics among certified dental specialists in comparison to general practitioners in patients with prosthetic heart valves before scaling/root planning, periodontal surgery and tooth extraction, as indicated from the AHA recommendations for prevention of infective endocarditis [29].

Nevertheless, a sample of American general dental practitioners, orthodontists and pediatric dentists strongly agreed in evaluation of orthodontic treatment needs [19].

Here, again, the part of post graduation and post specialization updating and continues learning can not be over-estimated.

Conclusions

Continuing education should play a lifetime role in ones professional career in order to provide our patients with the best treatment available.

The current world-wide dental practice facing several revolutions: the dental implant revolution, the aesthetic revolution and the minimally invasive-conservative revolution. However, it seems that the *evidence-based practice* revolution has a special importance since it has a relevance to all dental fields and affects everyday clinical decisions [35]. Our universal goal should be promoting the exchange of information and the advancement of oral medicine for the benefit of patients worldwide.

References

[1] Bader JD, Shugars DA. Agreement among dentists' recommendations for restorative treatment. *J. Dent. Res*. 1993;72:891-6.

[2] Mejare I, Sundberg H, Espelid I, et al. Caries assessment and restorative treatment thresholds reported by Swedish dentists. *Acta Odontol. Scand*. 1999;57:149-54.

[3] Espelid I, Tveit AB, Mejare I, et al. Restorative treatment decisions on occlusal caries in Scandinavia. *Acta Odontol. Scand*. 2001;59:21-7.

[4] Tan PL, Evans RW, Morgan MV. Caries, bitewings, and treatment decisions. *Aust. Dent. J.* 2002;47:138-41.

[5] Zadik Y, Levin L. Decision making of Hebrew University and Tel Aviv University Dental Schools graduates in everyday dentistry: Is there a difference? *J. Isr. Dent. Assoc*. 2006;23:19-23.

[6] Zadik Y, Levin L. Clinical decision-making in restorative dentistry, endodontics and antibiotic prescription. *J. Dent. Educ*. 2008;72:81-6.

[7] Reit C, Hollender L. Radiographic evaluation of endodontic therapy and the influence of observer variation. *Scand. J. Dent. Res*. 1983;91:205-12.

[8] Molven O, Halse A, Grung B. Observer strategy and the radiographic classification of healing after endodontic surgery. Int J Oral Maxillofac Surg 1987;16:432-9.

[9] Aryanpour S, Van Nieuwenhuysen JP, D'Hoore W. Endodontic retreatment decisions: no consensus. *Int. Endod. J.* 2000;33:208-18.

[10] Pagonis TC, Fong CD, Hasselgren G. Retreatment decisions - a comparison between general practitioners and endodontic postgraduates. *J. Endod*. 2000;26: 240-1.

[11] Kvist T. Endodontic retreatment. Aspects of decision making and clinical outcome. *Swed. Dent. J.* 2001;144:S1-57.

[12] Heinikainen M, Vehkalahti M, Murtomaa H. Retreatment in endodontics: treatment decisions by general practitioners and dental teachers in Finland. *Int. Dent. J.* 2002;52:119-24.

[13] Rawski AA, Brehmer B, Knutsson K, et al. The major factors that influence endodontic retreatment decisions. S*wed. Dent. J.* 2003;27:23-9.

[14] Kvist T, Heden G, Reit C. Endodontic retreatment strategies used by general dental practitioners. *Oral Surg., Oral Med., Oral Pathol., Oral Radiol., Endod*. 2004; 97:502-7.

[15] Knutsson K, Lysell L, Rohlin M. Dentists' judgment strategies on prophylactic removal of mandibular third molars. *J. Dent. Res*. 2000;79:1989-95.
[16] Knutsson K, Lysell L, Rohlin M, et al. Comparison of decisions regarding prophylactic removal of mandibular third molars in Sweden and Wales. *Br. Dent. J.* 2001;190:198-202.
[17] Knutsson K, Lysell L, Rohlin M. Dentists' decisions on prophylactic removal of mandibular third molars: a 10-year follow-up study. *Community Dent. Oral Epidemiol.* 2001;29:308-14.
[18] Zadik Y, Levin L. Decision making of Israeli, East-European, and Latin American dental school graduates in third molar surgery: Is there a difference? *J. Oral Maxillof Surg*. 2007;65:658-62.
[19] Berk NW, Bush HD, Cavalier J, et al. Perception of orthodontic treatment need: opinion comparisons of orthodontists, pediatric dentists, and general practitioners. *J. Orthod.* 2002;29:287-91.
[20] Richmond S, Daniels CP. International comparisons of professional assessments in orthodontics: Part 1-Treatment need. *Am. J. Orthod. Dentofacial. Orthop.* 1998; 113:180-5.
[21] Yingling NM, Byrne BE, Hartwell GR. Antibiotic use by members of the American Association of Endodontists in the year 2000: report of a national survey. *J. Endod.* 2002;28:396-404.
[22] Piecuch JF, Arzadon J, Lieblich SE. Prophylactic antibiotics for third molar surgery. *J. Oral Maxillofac. Surg.* 1995;53:53-60.
[23] Rubin MK. Foreign-trained dentists - a problem in licensure. *NY State Dent. J.* 1982;48:704.
[24] Zadik Y, Proter N, Dinte AF, et al. Professional absorption of foreign-trained dentists in Israel: licensure, employment and language. *J. Isr. Dent. Assoc.* 2008; in press.
[25] Bonetti D. Guideline improved dentists' knowledge but not their clinical decision-making skills. *Evid. Based Dent.* 2006;7:8.
[26] van der Sanden WJM, Mettes DG, Plasschaert AJM, et al. Effectiveness of clinical practice guideline implementation on lower third molar management in improving clinical decision-making: a randomized controlled trial. *Eur. J. Oral Sci.* 2005; 113:349–354.
[27] Wilson W, Taubert KA, Gewitz M, et al. Prevention of infective endocarditis: guidelines from the American Heart Association. *Circulation* 2007;116:1736-54.
[28] Tzukert AA, Leviner E, Benoliel R, et al. Analysis of the American Heart Association's recommendations for the prevention of infective endocarditis. *Oral Surg. Oral Med. Oral Pathol.* 1986;62: 276-9.
[29] Epstein JB, Chong S, Le ND. A survey of antibiotic use in dentistry. *J. Am. Dent. Assoc.* 2000;131:1600-9.
[30] Dajani AS, Taubert KA, Wilson W, et al. Prevention of bacterial endocarditis. Recommendations by the American Heart Association. *Circulation*. 1997;96:358-66.
[31] Palmer NO, Martin MV, Pealing R, et al. Antibiotic prescribing knowledge of National Health Service general dental practitioners in England and Scotland. *J. Antimicrob. Chemother.* 2001;47:233-7.
[32] Palmer NA, Dailey YM, Martin MV. Can audit improve antibiotic prescribing in general dental practice? *Br. Dent. J.* 2001;191:253-5.

[33] Palmer NA, Dailey YM. General dental practitioners' experiences of a collaborative clinical audit on antibiotic prescribing: a qualitative study. *Br. Dent. J.* 2002;193:46-9.

[34] Maidment Y. A comparison of the perceived effects on Scottish general dental practitioners of peer review and other continuing professional development. *Br. Dent. J.* 2006;200:581-4.

[35] Sackett DL, Rosenberg WM, Gray JA, et al. Evidence based medicine: what it is and what it isn't. *Br. Med. J.* 1996;312:71-2.

In: Clinical Dentistry
Editor: Scardina Giuseppe Alessandro

ISBN: 978-1-61122-354-5
© 2011 Nova Science Publishers, Inc.

Chapter 2

AN OVERVIEW OF H5N1 INFECTION AND ITS IMPLICATIONS FOR DENTISTRY[1]

C. J. Seneviratne and L. P. Samaranayake#*
Oral BioSciences, Faculty of Dentistry,
The University of Hong Kong, Hong Kong

ABSTRACT

The recent emergence of highly pathogenic H5N1 strains and the occurrence of human cases of H5N1 infection have prompted predictions of a pandemic-scale avian influenza viral infection among humans. Highly pathogenic H5N1 avian influenza viruses have become endemic among birds throughout the world, owing to the rapid carriage of H5N1 by migrating birds around the globe. In a relatively short period of time, H5N1 has acquired the ability to infect more mammalian species with fatal outcomes than any other influenza virus. So far, H5N1 has spread to more than 12 countries and its mortality rate reportedly exceeds 50%. It is difficult to predict when, whether, or which type of H5N1 influenza A virus will acquire efficient human-to-human transmission and lead to a pandemic, and the most important public health strategy at present therefore is to prevent the spread of the virus through the education of both health care workers and the general public. In this review, we summarize the current knowledge in H5N1 virology, its historical and epidemiological background, and clinical and hospital management strategies including those appertaining to dentistry.

---

[1] A version of this book was also published as a chapter in *International Journal of Clinical Dentistry, Volume 1, Issue1*, published by Nova Science Publishers, Inc. It was submitted for appropriate modifications in an effort to encourage wider dissemination of research.

* Dr. Chaminda Jayampath Seneviratne BDS, MPhil Oral BioSciences, Faculty of Dentistry, University of Hong Kong, The Prince Philip Dental Hospital, 34, Hospital Rd, Hong Kong SAR, People's Republic of China. Phone: (852) 64064916 Fax: (852) 25476133. jaya@hku.hk

Prof. Lakshaman P Samaranayake, Hon DSc, BDS (Sri Lanka), DDS (Glasgow), MRCPath (UK), FRCPath (UK), MIBiol, Cbiol (UK), FDSRCSE (Hon), FHKCPath, FHKAM (Dental Surgery), FHKAM (Pathology), FCDSHK. Dean Chair Professor of Oral Microbiology Faculty of Dentistry,The University of Hong Kong, The Prince Philip Dental Hospital, 34, Hospital Rd, Hong Kong SAR, People's Republic of China. Phone: (852) 2859 0480 Fax: (852) 25476133. E-mail: lakshman@hku.hk

Introduction

The recent emergence of highly pathogenic H5N1 strains and human cases of H5N1 infection have prompted a global public health focus on predictions of pandemic-scale avian influenza viral infections, or "bird flu" as it is widely known. Although H5N1 avian influenza has so far not progressed to a pandemic level, past experiences with influenza pandemics and global surveillance indicate that the process has probably already been initiated. Early and alarming signs of human-to-human spread of H5N1 are appearing, although this mode of transmission has yet to be conclusively proven. When the H1N1 strain of influenza A caused pandemic-scale influenza in 1918, more than 40 million human lives were lost. Compared with the 2% mortality rate of H1N1, H5N1 is highly pathogenic, and its reported mortality rate of nearly 50% indicates the weight of the devastating event we are heading for [1]. It has been predicted that at least 2-7 million deaths could occur during a pandemic-scale H5N1 outbreak.

Aquatic birds are natural reservoirs of influenza viruses [2-4]. Birds can transmit influenza viruses directly to individual humans, but human-to-human transmission appears to be rare. However, if the virus acquired human-to-human transmission through genetic mutations, it could readily spread and cause lethal damage to multiple human hosts. In fact, all three major pandemic-scale influenza outbreaks in the past century occurred owing to the emergence of new avian influenza A viral strains that acquired human-to-human transmissibility.

It has been confirmed that the H5N1 virus has crossed the species barrier and possesses the ability to infect humans [5]. Furthermore, ever since H5N1 emerged in Hong Kong in 1997, increasingly virulent strains have developed that have had increasing mortality among humans, different antigenic properties, and different internal gene constellations, as well as an expanding host range. It is a matter of time that the virus will genetically reassort into a strain that is capable of human-to-human transmission. The worrying fact is that there are already reports that H5N1 has acquired this ability in isolated cases, although this is yet to be confirmed. In addition to the potential public health hazard, a large-scale influenza A H5N1 outbreak could cause severe economic losses. Therefore, the WHO has urged increased global surveillance of H5N1 and better preparation to face a possible pandemic. In this review, we outline the characteristics of the H5N1 virus; its historical, epidemiological, and clinical features; laboratory diagnosis of H5N1 infection; clinical and hospital management strategies; and infection control procedures particularly appertaining to dental practice.

Virology

Influenza A viruses occur naturally in wild waterfowl, which have historically carried these viruses in a "low-pathogenic" form and in an evolutionary equilibrium, without showing signs of disease [3]. Influenza A viruses replicate in the intestines of infected birds and are mainly transmitted to other birds by the fecal-oral route. Ponds used by migratory birds as a resting site play an important role in viral transmission. On occasion, the viruses infect other bird species with high pathogenicity. Infection among domestic birds such as chickens and turkeys sometimes result in large epidemics with high mortality [6]. These viruses are also sporadically transmitted to humans.

All influenza viruses belong to the family of Orthomyxoviridae and are classified into three genera (A, B, and C), on the basis of their internal protein antigens such as nucleoproteins and matrix proteins [6-9]. They are negative-stranded RNA viruses whose genome is composed of eight segments encoding up to 10 proteins. Influenza B and C viruses are not divided into subtypes, whereas influenza A virus has two subtypes, depending on its two envelope glycoproteins that protrude from the outer surface—namely, hemagglutinin (HA) and neuraminidase (NA). Influenza A is the most virulent of three types and is associated with severe disease in humans.

To date, 16 HA and 9 NA subtypes have been identified and used in the nomenclature of influenza A viruses [7, 9]. The letters H and N denote HA and NA, respectively, and are followed by the subtype number. The nomenclature of influenza virus strains is given as "type/animal/place of isolation/sequential number/year of isolation (subtype)". For instance, the first H5N1 virus that was isolated, from geese in China in 1996, was named A/Goose/Guangdong/1/96 (H5N1). No animal species is indicated in the designation of human isolates [6].

Antigenic changes in influenza viruses occur by two processes: "antigenic drift" and "antigenic shift". Antigenic drift consists of minor changes due to point mutations within the influenza virus at the HA or NA site, resulting in new strains after combination of different HAs and NAs. Although strains generated by antigenic drift are capable of greater human infection rates than existing virus, there is no marked difference in the mortality or morbidity rates within a population during an epidemic. In contrast, because of its segmented genome, shuffling of a complete gene segment of influenza A can occur, thereby introducing avian virus genes into the human influenza virus. Such genetic reassortment, or antigenic shift, can lead to a major antigenic change and result in a completely new influenza virus. The general population would not have been exposed to this new strain and hence would have no immunity to it. Consequently, mortality rates are very high during an epidemic; mortality rates of young, healthy adults may be as high as or higher than those among individuals at the two extremes of age [6, 9].

All known HA and NA subtypes of influenza A virus have been identified from and are well-established in free-flying birds, which are the major reservoir of influenza viruses in general [7]. Certain subtypes are also associated with pigs (H1, H3, N1, N2) and horses (H7, N7, N8), which seem to be intermediate hosts. Only 3 HA subtypes (H1, H2, H3) and 2 NA subtypes (N1, N2) have circulated in humans and led to pandemics in the past century. Therefore, the emergence of new human H5N1 subtypes would be entirely new to the human immune system and is likely to be associated with very high mortality rates.

Historical Background and Current Epidemiology of H5N1

The past century was marked by three major influenza pandemics that took a total of 50 to 100 million human lives. The first influenza pandemic, known as "Spanish flu", occurred in 1918 and was caused by the H1N1 strain of influenza A. It was an exceptionally devastating event in human history, and its estimated death toll was more than 40 million in less than a year [10, 11]. Most deaths were seen among young and healthy persons in the age range of 15 to 35 years. During the pandemic, an estimated 25% to 30% of the world's population fell ill, and life expectancy dropped by more than 10 years. The second influenza pandemic, known as "Asian flu", was caused by the H2N2 strain of influenza A and started in 1957. This virus came from the already circulating H1N1 strain, which had acquired the H2, N2, and PB1 genes from avian species [7]. However, the H2N2 strain was milder than the strain of the 1918 pandemic. Although by then the medical standards and technology had improved the pandemic accounted for more than 2 million deaths [8, 10]. The third influenza pandemic, "Hong Kong flu", occurred in 1968 and was caused by the H3N2 strain of influenza A, which is considered even milder than the 1957 strain. The1968 virus had genetically reassorted with duck H3 and PB1 to yield an H3N2 subtype, again possibly originating from the circulating H2N2 virus. Global mortality exceeded more than 1 million.

The 1957 and 1968 pandemics were due to a reassortment of avian and human genes, probably as a result of simultaneous coinfection of a host by human viruses and avian viruses. In contrast, the origin of the lethal 1918 virus appeared to result not from reassortment, but from the mutation of the genes of a pure avian virus that was then transmitted to humans [12].

Asian H5N1 viruses were first detected in domestic geese in southern China in 1996 [13]. In March 1997, an outbreak of H5N1 in chickens was reported in Hong Kong. Soon after in the same year, the first case of direct transmission of H5N1 virus from poultry to humans was documented [14]: a 3-year-old boy in Hong Kong was admitted to hospital with a fever and died 3 days later. The child had no known underlying diseases before admission and died of influenza pneumonia complicated by acute respiratory distress syndrome, Reye's syndrome, multiorgan failure, and disseminated intravascular coagulation. Further analysis revealed the culprit to be influenza A H5N1, a subtype previously not detected in human beings. Later, it was found that all gene segments of the A/Hong Kong/156/97 virus were purely of avian origin, with no evidence of genetic reassortment with human influenza A virus genes [14]. Hence, this was the first reported case of direct transmission of avian influenza virus from birds to humans without pigs as a "mixing vessel". More cases followed, resulting in 6 deaths among 18 infected people [15, 16]. All these Hong Kong cases involved avian virus-like gene segments that were believed to be reassortants with an HA gene from A/goose/Guangdong/1/96(H5N1) virus, an NA gene from A/teal/Hong Kong/W312/97(H6N1)-like virus, and internal genes from A/quail/Hong Kong/G1/97 (H9N2 and W312)-like viruses [14-18].

Although H5N1 was thought to be eliminated by the mass culling of all poultry in Hong Kong in 1997, it continued to circulate in domestic poultry in Hong Kong and southern China in 1999 and 2000 as diverse genotypes [13, 19, 20]. By 2000, the virus host range extended to domestic ducks, which played a key role in later outbreaks. In particular, an A/goose/Guangdong/1/96 (H5N1)-like virus was isolated during routine virological surveillance of geese and ducks imported into Hong Kong from Guangdong Province in February 1999 and February 2000 [13]. Furthermore, during this period, isolated viruses had undergone reassortment with other avian viruses to generate multiple genotypes (designated A to E) of H5N1 viruses [20]. Another mass culling of poultry was thus conducted in Hong Kong in May 2001. H5N1 was also isolated from healthy geese in live bird markets in Hanoi, Vietnam, in October 2001, which shows that H5N1 was circulating in Vietnam well before its major outbreak among poultry there in early 2004 [21].

In December 2002, new H5N1 outbreaks were reported from two Hong Kong parks and together caused deaths of many resident avian species, including waterfowl [22]. These were the first reported incidents since 1961 of mortality among aquatic birds due to influenza viruses, and were contrary to the general belief that only asymptomatic influenza infections present in wild bird species. Subsequent studies revealed novel genotypes of H5N1 (designated X, Y, and Z) [22-24]. In February 2003, H5N1 infection reemerged in humans, as a respiratory illness in a father and son; the strain was similar to that isolated from the wild water birds a few months earlier. The father subsequently died, while the son recovered fully [25]. The first documented case of natural infection of H5N1 among pigs was identified in 2003, in farms in southern China. It was an alarming finding because pigs had up to then been thought to be an intermediate host or "mixing vessel" in which virus strain acquires the ability of human-to-human transmission.

Since 2003, highly pathogenic H5N1 has become endemic in poultry in Southeast Asia. By December 2003, recurrent outbreaks of highly pathogenic H5N1 in poultry had been reported from nine Asian countries: China, South Korea, Japan, Thailand, Vietnam, Indonesia, Malaysia, Cambodia, and Laos. Human cases were recognized in Vietnam and Thailand [5, 26, 27]. Interestingly, the virulence of H5N1 strains varied by country. South Korea's report of an H5N1 outbreak among chickens and ducks in December 2003 was its first official report of this disease; however, no humans were infected [18]. Although South Korean H5N1 poultry isolates were of avian origin and contained the HA and NA genes of the A/goose/Guangdong/1/96 lineage, the topology of the phylogenetic tree clearly differentiated the Korean avian isolates from the Vietnamese and Thai human isolates [18]. A representative Korean isolate was inoculated into mice without mortality or detection of virus in the brain, although high titers of virus were found in the lungs. The same isolate, however, caused systemic infection in chickens and quail, and it killed all of the birds within 2 and 4 days of intranasal inoculation, respectively.

At about the same time, there were some anecdotal reports of H5N1 infection among cats. Later experiments demonstrated that cats could be infected after feeding on infected poultry or wild birds and could then transmit the disease to another cat [28]. This finding raised the issue of cats' role in providing an opportunity for H5N1 virus to adapt to mammalian hosts. During an outbreak in Thailand in 2003, H5N1 was isolated from two tigers (*Panthera tigris*) and two leopards (*Panthera pardus*) that died at a zoo in Suphanburi [29]. These animals had been fed fresh chicken carcasses from a local slaughterhouse. There followed an increased number of sick tigers, which demonstrated the potential of tiger-to-tiger transmission [30]. Another tiger in Sriracha tiger zoo was reportedly infected with H5N1 in October 2004 during the second outbreak of H5N1 avian influenza in Thailand.

From 2004, a single genotype (the Z genotype) of H5N1 became dominant [7, 31]. In an outbreak in Vietnam in 2004, H5N1 was found to be transmitted to pigs, which again suggested the potential role of pigs as a "mixing vessel" in which virus could reassort into a strain competent of human-to-human transmission [32]. In May 2005, an outbreak of highly pathogenic H5N1 infection among waterfowl was found in Lake Qinghaihu, Gangcha County, Qinghai Province, in western China. Several species were infected, including the bar-headed goosc (*Anser indicus*), great black-headed gull (*Larus ichthyaetus*), and brown-headed gull (*Larus brunnicephalus*). It is noteworthy that lake Qinghaihu is a breeding center for migrant birds that congregate from southeast Asia, Siberia, Australia, and New Zealand; hence, the global spread of H5N1 is inevitable [33]. During 2005, H5N1 spread to even more countries, including Russia, Kazakhstan, Mongolia, Turkey, and Croatia. Birds infected with highly pathogenic H5N1 were identified in Germany and Britain.

From November 2003 to December 2007, a total of 340 human cases of H5N1 infection have been confirmed in more than 12 countries. Of these cases, 209 have died yielding an overall case fatality rate (CFR) of 61.4%. Astonishingly, there were 51 deaths among 77 detected cases in 2007 (CFR, 74%) [34].

Transmission of H5N1

Three routes have been suggested to account for H5N1 viral transmission from its primary host, water birds: (1) from animals to humans, (2) from the environment to humans, and (3) between humans. Because H5N1 has been circulating over some time, it is evident that it has already crossed the species barrier from birds to human [9, 27]. Virus can be transmitted to humans by direct contact with infected animals or through indirect contact with animal excreta, especially bird droppings, which can survive for some time in the environment. Hence environment contamination might be an important route of viral spread in future. Person-to-person transmission of H5N1 strains is of serious concern. Ongoing surveillance for such an event has not yet found conclusive evidence of efficient person-to-person spread. However, there were probable human-to-human cases of infection reported from Thailand and Vietnam [5, 27].

The main routes of transmission have been argued to be either through fecal-oral contact or by the respiratory route. Studies have shown that avian influenza viruses are transmitted mainly by the fecal-oral route [35]. Transmission experiments in chickens have also confirmed that the 1997 Hong Kong viruses were spread by fecal-oral contact, rather than through aerosols [36]. Nevertheless, epidemiological and animals studies have shown that airborne transmission is possible for human influenza [37].

Possible Pathogenesis of H5N1 Infection

All influenza viruses adsorb to the host cell to initiate the penetration phase of the infection cycle. Receptor-binding pockets on the surface of the virus HA attach to the host cell via a surface oligosaccharide that carries a terminal sialic acid residue [6, 38]. The HA of human influenza viruses preferentially binds to host cells containing a sialic acid linked via an α-2,6 bond to galactose, whereas HA of avian influenza viruses preferentially binds receptors containing an α-2,3 sialic acid-galactose bond [6, 7, 39]. Receptors with α-2,6 bond between sialic acid and galactose are predominantly found on the surface of cells of the human respiratory epithelium. Receptors with α-2,3 linkages are present on cells of the respiratory and alimentary epithelium of birds, but also on cells of the human conjunctiva and the ciliated portion of human respiratory pseudostratified columnar epithelium. Therefore, ciliated cells may serve as primary target cells for avian viruses to initiate infection in humans. Moreover, ciliated cells of human airways have been found to be permissive to both avian and human influenza viruses in the late phase of infection. Hence, it has been postulated that these cells could be the site of gene reassortment between human and avian influenza viruses, enabling a strain with human transmissibility to be produced [39]. As the respiratory epithelium of pigs contain both the α-2,6-linked and α-2,3-linked sialic acid receptors, pigs can be infected by both human and avian influenza viruses and act as an "mixing vessel" for gene reassortment [6, 40].

To acquire the ability to sustain human-to-human transmission, the HA of avian origin must possess human receptor-binding specificity. This required change can be brought about by the mutation of only one or two amino acids [38]. A single amino acid substitution at position 226 or 228 of the HA gene has been shown to switch the receptor-binding preference from avian-specific α-2,3-linked sialic acid to human-specific α-2,6-linked sialic acid . However, whether this difference is sufficient to acquire direct human-to-human transmission is not yet known.

Mechanism of Lethal Effects of H5N1

The factors that account for the symptoms of viral influenza are still not well understood. Cytopathic effects of the virus itself and the cytokines evoked by infection are believed to account for both local and general effects [41]. Influenza virus infection and replication in the respiratory tract can injure the nasal and tracheobronchial epithelium directly, possibly as a result of virus-induced cellular apoptosis and subsequent loss of respiratory epithelial cells. This process is one of the major reasons for symptoms such as coughing, depressed tracheobronchial clearance, and altered pulmonary function.

The early phase of influenza infection also triggers a cytokine response, which serves as the first line of defense of the body against the virus [42]. Moreover, clearance of influenza virus has been shown to closely relate to the quantity of circulating interferons and tumor necrosis factor-α (TNF-α) [43]. Influenza A H5N1 evokes a major cytokine response that includes the production IL-6, TNF-α, and IFN-γ. The kinetics and magnitude of two cytokines (IL-6 and IFN-α) are closely associated with both infection and the occurrence of symptoms [44]. Interestingly, it has been observed that H5N1 influenza viruses can escape the antiviral activity of interferons, resulting in hypercytokinemia and reactive hemophagocytic syndrome, which then lead to lethal effects [42, 45].

In birds, highly virulent H5N1 can have lethal effects in several organs other than the lungs, such as the liver, spleen, kidneys, heart, and pancreas [16]. The high virulence is due to the presence of multiple basic amino acids at the HA cleavage site of H5N1. These amino acids confer the ability of viral replication in sites other than the respiratory and gastrointestinal tracts of birds. Likewise, H5N1 replication in humans is not confined to the respiratory tract and may occur in the gastrointestinal tract [5, 45, 46]. A wide array of clinical manifestations in H5N1 infection may be attributed to the diversity of tissues affected, as well as other, as yet, unknown causes. It is noteworthy that H1N1, which killed more than 40 million people worldwide in the 1918 pandemic, did not have multiple basic amino acids to allow the virus to replicate in multiple organs, thereby giving an indication of the predicted seriousness of an H5N1 pandemic [42].

Clinical Features of H5N1 Infection

The incubation period has yet to be determined for highly pathogenic H5N1. Reported cases show that it can range from 2 to 17 days [47]. H5N1 contracted from exposure to environmental sources is thought to have a longer incubation period than infection from direct contact with animals [47].

Patients who have been hospitalized with H5N1 infection have exhibited a wide range of clinical features. This broad spectrum of clinical manifestations of H5N1 influenza poses a challenge for clinical diagnosis. The main presenting complaint in most reported cases is high and/or persistent fever that is often accompanied by lower and/or upper respiratory tract symptoms. Coughing, a sore throat, headache, rhinorrhea, vomiting, malaise, and myalgia, may also be associated with a high fever [16, 27, 48]. In addition, signs of pneumonia may be seen at presentation or may develop at a later stage of infection. Surprisingly, some cases have been devoid of any clinical or radiological signs pertaining to the respiratory system [7]. Gastrointestinal symptoms (abdominal pain, vomiting, diarrhea) are the predominant symptoms at presentation or they occur later in the course of infection; watery diarrhea without blood or mucus is also a common feature [7, 16]. Occasionally, pleuretic pain and bleeding from the nose and gums have been reported early in the course of H5N1 influenza [47], and fever accompanied by gastrointestinal features (vomiting, diarrhea) can be the only initial presentation [7].

As infection progresses, patients become drowsy, convulsive, and comatose. Respiratory complications such as acute respiratory distress syndrome, pulmonary hemorrhage, pneumonia, and pleural effusion, have been observed [7, 46, 47], Progressive respiratory distress, hypoxemia, septic shock, and cardiac compromise then result in multiorgan failure and often lead to death. The wide array of clinical presentations emphasizes that H5N1 influenza infections should be vigilantly attended to and its many guises kept in mind. Accurate diagnosis is by far the most essential step, not only to save a patient's life by prompt administration of antiviral drugs and supportive care, but also to take preventive measures to minimize the spread of the disease.

Radiological Features

Radiological features of H5N1 infection also appear rapidly along with clinical deterioration. Some patients have shown radiological features of pneumonia at the time of presentation. The radiographic abnormalities seen frequently include extensive diffuse, multifocal or patchy infiltration of the lungs, interstitial infiltrates, segmented or lobular consolidation, and air bronchograms [16, 27, 37, 47]. However, in several reported cases, no initial radiological abnormalities pertaining to the respiratory system were detected [7].

Histological Features

Histological features of H5N1 infection have been mostly described from postmortem samples. Histopathologic changes due to diffuse alveolar damage such as filling of alveolar spaces with fibrous exudates, hemorrhage, hyaline membrane formation, vascular changes, alveolar infiltration with CD68+ macrophages, interstitial infiltration of CD3+ lymphocytes, and type 2 pneumocyte hyperplasia have been observed [37, 49]. Limited data indicate that this process occurs from primary viral pneumonia, usually without bacterial suprainfection at the time of hospitalization. However, superimposed fungal infection, morphologically consistent with aspergillosis, has been seen in some patients in areas of the lung [49].

Laboratory Diagnosis

The existence of highly pathogenic H5N1 highlights the need for sensitive and rapid diagnostic tools to identify as early as possible potential cases that require prompt isolation. Conventional diagnostic tools such as cell culture and serologic tests require approximately 2 days to 2 weeks for results and thus have limited usefulness in making therapeutic and infection control decisions in H5N1 influenza infections [37].

Basic hematological diagnoses are readily feasible at the time of hospital admission and are frequently carried out during the course of infection. Common features include leucopenia (especially lymphopenia), mild to moderate thrombocytopenia, hemophagocytosis, and a pronounced inversion of the CD4:CD8 ratio [16, 25, 27, 45, 48]. Biochemical evidence of liver dysfunction has been seen in the form of increased amounts of aminotransferases.

An appropriate sample from a patient should be carefully selected for accurate diagnosis and subsequent quantification of viral load. The nature of the sample depends on clinical features of the patient. The primary site of viral infection is thought to be the respiratory epithelium; hence, in general nasopharyngeal aspiration, bronchial lavage, nasopharyngeal swabbing, or throat swabbing are considered. A stool or rectal swab can be obtained in suspected cases of infection presenting with diarrhea [7]. Serum and cerebrospinal fluid are collected in patients with encephalitis. It is emphasized that in patients with suspected H5N1 infection, sampling procedures should be carried out with strict airborne precautions. The United States Centers for Diseases Control and Prevention (CDC) recommends that laboratory conditions should be met with biosafety level BSL-3C for viral diagnosis procedures [50]. However, clinical specimens can be tested by polymerase chain reaction (PCR) assays and commercially available antigen detection tests under standard BSL-2 conditions in a class II biological safety cabinet.

For a definitive diagnosis, the gold standard remains a positive culture for H5N1 virus in the Madin-Darby canine kidney (MDCK) cell line or chick embryo allantoic sac inoculated with a properly collected clinical specimen [37, 46]. Although commercially available antigen tests are known to be rapid, they seem to be less sensitive than viral cultures and are unable to subtype viruses. Therefore, a negative test does not exclude influenza A infection and a positive test does not confirm the diagnosis of H5N1 infection. On the other hand, reverse transcriptase (RT)–PCR provides the most sensitive and rapid means of detecting H5N1 and facilitates the typing and subtyping of virus. Conventional RT-PCR and confirmation of the results by Southern blot analysis or methods based on restriction fragment length polymorphism have been used for this purpose [16, 27, 48, 51]. Single-step multiplex real-time RT-PCR probes corresponding to the M, H5, and N1 genes were developed in 2004 and upgraded in 2005 [51-53]. Multiplex real-time RT-PCR seems to be more sensitive than nested RT-PCR and even more sensitive than real-time RT-PCR with a single set of primers and probes.

Management of Patients with H5N1 Infection

The most important event in the management of influenza A H5N1 is early identification. Vigorous measures can then be taken to prevent further spread of infection and cross-contamination of health care workers. However, early identification currently seems to be the critical step of empirical management, so before accurate and fast identification of viral isolates is possible, existing clues should be vigilantly investigated to allow a presumptive diagnosis. Some epidemiological markers that have been suggested to be useful to identify potential cases include travel history to endemic areas; occupations involving poultry, laboratory, or health care work; history of contact with poultry, dead, or sick birds or H5N1 patients; and clustering of infection [37]. The CDC recommends that state and local health departments, hospitals, and clinicians should enhance their efforts to identify patients who could be infected by influenza A H5N1 virus and take infection control precautions when H5N1 is suspected [50]. Testing of hospitalized patients for H5N1 infection is indicated when there is radiographically confirmed pneumonia, acute respiratory distress syndrome, or other severe respiratory illnesses for which an alternative diagnosis has not been established, plus a history of travel within 10 days of symptom onset to a country with documented H5N1 avian influenza infections in poultry or humans.

Management of potential cases depends on the infection stage of the patient. General management includes broad-spectrum antibiotics and antiviral drugs with or without corticosteroids. Respiratory support and intensive care remain the most important aspects of clinical management during the acute stage of the pneumonic illness. In addition, attention should be paid to multiorgan failure, which has been reported in numerous cases [37].

Infection Control in Hospital Settings

In an influenza pandemic, health care workers are most at risk. Therefore, adherence to strict prevention strategies is vital, not only to prevent the spread of infection, but also to prevent health care workers from being infected. Hospital-acquired infection by H5N1 virus was evident in a retrospective cohort study comparing H5N1 seropositivity in health care workers exposed to H5N1 patients with that of unexposed controls [2, 54]. Therefore, health care workers should be candidates for prior vaccination against an identified pandemic strain [37]. Although this measure may not fully protect these personnel against avian influenza, it could theoretically reduce the possibility of further genetic reassortment between human and avian influenza viruses in the same human host.

The route of infection from avian influenza–infected patients to health care workers is uncertain, although it would be reasonable to presume that inhalation of infective respiratory secretions (including large droplets and droplet nuclei) and/or contact with virus-laden secretions could be potential sources. This assumption is in line with the most common routes of infection for human influenza viruses—namely, via droplets and contact with mucous membranes. Therefore, all hospital personnel are advised to adhere strictly to CDC-recommended standard precautions [55]. Health care workers exposed to patients with H5N1 infection have shown to be at equal risk as exposure of workers to poultry. Presumably because of this consideration, and the high case-fatality rate of the disease, precautions against airborne spread should be administered in the case of patients infected by avian influenza viruses, in addition to standard precautions against contact and droplet transmission [37].

Furthermore, chemoprophylaxis has been recommended for health care workers or other personnel who might have been exposed to the highly pathogenic avian influenza viruses. In view of the widespread resistance to amantadine, NA inhibitors are currently the drugs of choice for chemoprophylaxis. The present WHO recommendation suggests giving oseltamivir 75 mg orally once a day for at least 7 days, starting as soon as possible after exposure.

Antiviral Agents

The great advantage of antiviral drugs is that they can be stockpiled for future use, thereby providing a critical management option in the first months of a pandemic and during the first great wave while a vaccine is under development. Two classes of drugs are currently available for prophylaxis and treatment of influenza virus infection: M2 ion channel blockers (amantadine and its derivative rimantadine) and NA inhibitors (zanamivir and oseltamivir).

Amantadine (1-adamantanamine hydrochloride; Symmetrel) and its derivative rimantadine (α-methyl-1- adamantanemethylamine; Flumadine) are symmetric tricyclic amine compounds that block the ion channel activity of the M2 protein of most influenza A viruses [56, 57]. Blocking M2 protein ion channels prevents fusion of the virus and host cell membranes and thus the release of viral RNA into the cytoplasm of infected cells. The transmembrane domain of the M2 protein is highly conserved in all avian and human strains of influenza A, and both amantadine and rimantadine are effective at low doses against H1N1, H2N2, and H3N2 strains [56].

Although H5N1 seemed to be susceptible to amantadine in early cases of human infection in Hong Kong in 1997 [14, 16], subsequent misuse of amantadine and rimantadine in poultry has enabled the virus to acquire resistance [23, 58]. Data from gene sequencing of genotype Z of the H5N1 virus that was isolated from Thailand and Vietnam show an asparagine residue at position 31 of the M2 protein, which invariably confers resistance to amantadine and rimantadine [59].

A second class of antivirals is NA inhibitors, such as oseltamivir and zanamivir, which interrupt an established infection in its late stages by inhibiting the release of virions from infected cells. This results in the aggregation of virions at the cell surface and the consequent inhibition of viral penetration of mucous secretions and spread to other cells. Oseltamivir (Tamiflu) is an ethyl ester prodrug with a high oral bioavailability [56] and its usual dosage is 75 mg orally twice daily for 5 days. It has been shown to reduce the median time for resolution of the infection approximately by 30% (1.5 days) and illness severity by approximately 35% in patients receiving either 75 mg or 150 mg of drug twice daily for 5 days. A higher dose of oseltamivir has been found to be associated with a larger reduction in viral load in respiratory secretions, as well as a shorter duration of illness in human influenza infections. Animal studies have shown that more beneficial protection can be obtained in administration of prolonged and higher-dose oseltamivir regimens [59]. However, some studies have yielded contradictory results and shown that the higher dose does not have further clinical benefit [56]. Nevertheless, higher doses of oseltamivir have been recommended for patients with very severe disease, especially those with diarrhoea and who thus have an impairment of drug absorption. Immunosuppressed patients such as those at the extremities of age, who may have a high initial viral load, are mandatory candidates for higher doses and longer duration of treatment [37].

The death of several patients has been reported despite the use of oseltamivir at or after 6 days of illness. Therefore, antiviral therapy is advised as early as possible, as is the case for the treatment of common, human influenza, for which clinical efficacy is maximal if given within 48 hours of onset of illness. An oseltamivir-resistant H5N1 isolate has already been reported in Vietnam [60], which highlights the importance of monitoring the emergence of drug resistance in H5N1 isolates from patients treated with NA inhibitors.

Zanamivir is a sialic acid analog developed by rational molecular design modeled on a three-dimensional structure of NA spikes [38]. Zanamivir carboxylate blocks the release of progeny virus from infected cells, which is facilitated by NA spikes. It is given by inhalation at 10 mg twice daily for 5 days. Zanamivir has shown to be more effective in reducing viral titers than oseltamivir in animal experiments and studies of isolates from patients [60]. Hence, it has been proposed that oseltamivir and zanamivir be stockpiled in the event of an H5N1 influenza pandemic. Viramidine, a purine nucleoside analog, has also gained attention owing to its high effectiveness against influenza virus in both in-vitro and in-vivo models [61]. Several other antivirals are also under consideration [56].

Vaccines

Vaccines are the most important medical tools for preventing influenza infections and reducing health consequences during a pandemic. The influenza A H5N1 outbreak in 1997 expedited the need for the production of novel vaccines against these viruses. This goal has been approached in several ways.

Vaccines produced conventionally using the H5 subunit from A/duck/Singapore/3/97 were poorly immunogenic in humans against antigenically closely related strains, even after multiple vaccination [62]. However, the use of the adjuvant, MF59 increased the antibody titer of this H5 vaccine. An alternative approach was to use inactivated "split" vaccines derived from nonpathogenic A/duck/HK/836/80 (H3N1) virus and the modified H5 HA from A/HK/156/97 (H5N1) virus. Such a vaccine induced barely detectable titers of neutralizing antibodies in mice. Taken together, although H5N1 vaccines have been well tolerated, they appear to be poorly immunogenic. Therefore, the WHO has recommended vaccine studies using new reassortant A/PR/8/34 virus with HA from A Vietnam/1203/04 (H5N1) generated by reverse genetics [62].

The main benefits of using reverse-genetics techniques are the feasibility of producing well-matched nonpathogenic H5N1 vaccine viruses at a rapid rate. Therefore, recent developments in the production of H5N1 vaccines have been based on use of plasmid-based reverse-genetic systems to construct influenza virions and vaccines [63]. Because viable viruses can be generated in this method from individually cloned cDNA copies of each of the eight viral RNA segments, reassortment can be prospectively defined and directed. Most vaccines produced to date contain the HA and NA genes of naturally circulating strains with high egg-growth capacity [64] A strain-specific vaccine could thus be created by cloning the appropriate HA and NA genes from the target virus, after removing the multiple basic amino acids at the cleavage site of the H5 HA that are associated with high virulence. Inactivated vaccine generated by plasmid-based reverse genetics from H5N1 reassortant HA and NA genes from GSGD/96 virus and 6 internal genes from the high-growth A/Puerto Rico/8/34 virus, have proved to be effective in protecting ducks and geese against highly pathogenic H5N1 [63]. However, such vaccines have to undergo extensive clinical trials to address crucial issues such as number and quantity of doses and the role of adjuvant.

siRNA

The use of RNA interference is a novel approach to antiviral therapy that specifically inhibits gene expression [65, 66]. This technique involves the use of short (21-26 nucleotide), double-stranded RNA duplexes known as small interfering RNA (siRNA) molecules that mediate the degradation of viral mRNA by cellular enzymes. Many studies have shown that siRNA can significantly suppress gene expression when delivered into mammalian cells in vitro. RNA interference has so far been studied for a number for influenza viruses with good success [67, 68]. Therefore, the use of siRNA may serve as a potential approach to develop a preventive strategy against H5N1 influenza virus. However, optimization of target sequences and delivery systems and clinical trials of siRNA are yet to be determined.

Implications of H5N1 for the Dental Practitioners

H5N1 patients are unlikely to seek dental treatment in the early acute phase of the disease owing to the rapid course of the disease and the onset of fever as a primary symptom. Nonetheless, due to the highly infectious nature of the disease, and as the modes of transmission and infectivity are not fully understood, especially in the prodromal and convalescent stages of the disease dental health care workers maybe at risk of exposure to H5N1. This is particularly the case as in dentistry the care provider has to operate in close proximity to the patient using droplet and aerosol generating procedures. The fact that the droplet spread mainly occurs within a 3 feet radius of the infective focus emphasizes this danger further.

The Significance of Droplets and Aerosols in the Transmission of Diseases

As H5N1 is likely to be transmitted via droplets, close contact and fomites. When an individual coughs or sneezes, or when aerosol generating procedures are used particles of varying size (from 0.001 μm to up to 10000 μm) are produced. Particles or droplets with a diameter greater than 100 μm, as most are, called splatter or spatter are then propelled through the air for short distances, generally 3 feet or less and settle rapidly on either animate or inanimate surfaces. Transmission of infection via droplets thus requires close contact with an index case.

On the other hand smaller droplets (or aerosols, generally under 10 μm in size) or small-particle residue of evaporated droplets are usually airborne and are entrained in the air for a lengthy period and, may carry infectious microbes. They may be dispersed widely by air currents and the disease transmission thus become airborne. It is salutary to note that the microbe-laden aerosol may also settle in surrounding areas in the clinic/office devoid of any clinical activities and it is not clear whether environmental transmission of H5N1 occurs form such fomites.

The infective dose of the organism is another important consideration that should be borne in mind when considering airborne infection. An influenza virus particle or a few spores of the *Aspergillus* fungus may have widely differing potential for causing respiratory infection and, so is the viability of the microbes and the general health of the person inhaling them.

It is the duty of all dental professionals to maintain a safe practice environment free from infectious hazards. In the event of a H5N1 crisis, practitioners should pay heed to additional precautionary measures associated with standard precautions [69] in order to help control the spread of this highly contagious disease.

Conclusion

Highly pathogenic and potentially pandemic H5N1 avian influenza viruses have not only become endemic in Asia, but have also sailed to other parts of the world in Europe and the Americas. In a relatively short period of time, H5N1 has acquired the ability to infect more and more mammalian species and result in fatal outcomes. Infected migrating birds have been the rapid carriers of the virus across the globe. Global surveillance has traced H5N1 activity over a period of time and much preparation for a possible pandemic has been undertaken. However, more health education programs are needed to alert the general public on how they should act in a pandemic—in particular, how to take preventive measures to minimize global spread. All nations, developing and developed alike, should also be armed with effective antivirals and possible vaccines. It is necessary to keep our eyes open for the emerging genetic evolution of the virus and accordingly to keep vaccines up to date. However, it is hard to predict when, whether, or in which type of H5N1 influenza A virus will acquire efficient human-to-human transmission and trigger a pandemic. Most importantly, whether we will ever have enough and sufficiently up-to-date arsenals to combat any large-scale infectious disease is still an open-ended question.

References

[1] Bartlett JG, Hayden FG. Influenza A (H5N1): will it be the next pandemic influenza? Are we ready? *Ann. Intern. Med.* 2005 Sep 20;143(6):460-2.

[2] Bridges CB, Lim W, Hu-Primmer J, Sims L, Fukuda K, Mak KH, et al. Risk of influenza A (H5N1) infection among poultry workers, Hong Kong, 1997-1998. *J. Infect. Dis.* 2002 Apr 15;185(8):1005-10.

[3] Webster RG, Bean WJ, Gorman OT, Chambers TM, Kawaoka Y. Evolution and ecology of influenza A viruses. *Microbiol. Rev*. 1992 Mar;56(1):152-79.

[4] Webster RG, Shortridge KF, Kawaoka Y. Influenza: interspecies transmission and emergence of new pandemics. *FEMS Immunol. Med. Microbiol*. 1997 Aug;18(4):275-9.

[5] Ungchusak K, Auewarakul P, Dowell SF, Kitphati R, Auwanit W, Puthavathana P, et al. Probable person-to-person transmission of avian influenza A (H5N1). *N. Engl. J. Med.* 2005 Jan 27;352(4):333-40.

[6] De Jong JC, Rimmelzwaan GF, Fouchier RA, Osterhaus AD. Influenza virus: a master of metamorphosis. *J. Infect.* 2000 May;40(3):218-28.

[7] de Jong MD, Bach VC, Phan TQ, Vo MH, Tran TT, Nguyen BH, et al. Fatal avian influenza A (H5N1) in a child presenting with diarrhea followed by coma. *N. Engl. J. Med.* 2005 Feb 17;352(7):686-91.

[8] de la Barrera CA, Reyes-Teran G. Influenza: forecast for a pandemic. *Arch. Med. Res.* 2005 Nov-Dec;36(6):628-36.

[9] Peiris JS, de Jong MD, Guan Y. Avian influenza virus (H5N1): a threat to human health. *Clin. Microbiol. Rev*. 2007 Apr;20(2):243-67.

[10] Hsieh YC, Wu TZ, Liu DP, Shao PL, Chang LY, Lu CY, et al. Influenza pandemics: past, present and future. *J. Formos Med. Assoc*. 2006 Jan;105(1):1-6.

[11] Tumpey TM, Garcia-Sastre A, Taubenberger JK, Palese P, Swayne DE, Basler CF. Pathogenicity and immunogenicity of influenza viruses with genes from the 1918 pandemic virus. *Proc. Natl. Acad. Sci. USA*. 2004 Mar 2;101(9):3166-71.

[12] Reid AH, Fanning TG, Janczewski TA, Lourens RM, Taubenberger JK. Novel origin of the 1918 pandemic influenza virus nucleoprotein gene. *J. Virol*. 2004 Nov;78(22):12462-70.

[13] Webster RG, Guan Y, Peiris M, Walker D, Krauss S, Zhou NN, et al. Characterization of H5N1 influenza viruses that continue to circulate in geese in southeastern China. *J. Virol.* 2002 Jan;76(1):118-26.

[14] Subbarao K, Klimov A, Katz J, Regnery H, Lim W, Hall H, et al. Characterization of an avian influenza A (H5N1) virus isolated from a child with a fatal respiratory illness. *Science*. 1998 Jan 16;279(5349):393-6.

[15] Claas EC, Osterhaus AD, van Beek R, De Jong JC, Rimmelzwaan GF, Senne DA, et al. Human influenza A H5N1 virus related to a highly pathogenic avian influenza virus. *Lancet*. 1998 Feb 14;351(9101):472-7.

[16] Yuen KY, Chan PK, Peiris M, Tsang DN, Que TL, Shortridge KF, et al. Clinical features and rapid viral diagnosis of human disease associated with avian influenza A H5N1 virus. *Lancet*. 1998 Feb 14;351(9101):467-71.

[17] Hoffmann E, Stech J, Leneva I, Krauss S, Scholtissek C, Chin PS, et al. Characterization of the influenza A virus gene pool in avian species in southern China: was H6N1 a derivative or a precursor of H5N1? *J. Virol*. 2000 Jul;74(14):6309-15.

[18] Lee CW, Suarez DL, Tumpey TM, Sung HW, Kwon YK, Lee YJ, et al. Characterization of highly pathogenic H5N1 avian influenza A viruses isolated from South Korea. *J. Virol*. 2005 Mar;79(6):3692-702.

[19] Cauthen AN, Swayne DE, Schultz-Cherry S, Perdue ML, Suarez DL. Continued circulation in China of highly pathogenic avian influenza viruses encoding the hemagglutinin gene associated with the 1997 H5N1 outbreak in poultry and humans. *J. Virol*. 2000 Jul;74(14):6592-9.

[20] Guan Y, Peiris JS, Lipatov AS, Ellis TM, Dyrting KC, Krauss S, et al. Emergence of multiple genotypes of H5N1 avian influenza viruses in Hong Kong SAR. *Proc. Natl. Acad. Sci. USA.* 2002 Jun 25;99(13):8950-5.

[21] Nguyen DC, Uyeki TM, Jadhao S, Maines T, Shaw M, Matsuoka Y, et al. Isolation and characterization of avian influenza viruses, including highly pathogenic H5N1, from poultry in live bird markets in Hanoi, Vietnam, in 2001. *J. Virol.* 2005 Apr;79(7):4201-12.

[22] Sturm-Ramirez KM, Ellis T, Bousfield B, Bissett L, Dyrting K, Rehg JE, et al. Reemerging H5N1 influenza viruses in Hong Kong in 2002 are highly pathogenic to ducks. *J. Virol.* 2004 May;78(9):4892-901.

[23] Guan Y, Poon LL, Cheung CY, Ellis TM, Lim W, Lipatov AS, et al. H5N1 influenza: a protean pandemic threat. *Proc. Natl. Acad. Sci. USA.* 2004 May 25;101(21):8156-61.

[24] Chen H, Smith GJ, Li KS, Wang J, Fan XH, Rayner JM, et al. Establishment of multiple sublineages of H5N1 influenza virus in Asia: implications for pandemic control. *Proc. Natl. Acad. Sci. USA.* 2006 Feb 21;103(8):2845-50.

[25] Peiris JS, Yu WC, Leung CW, Cheung CY, Ng WF, Nicholls JM, et al. Re-emergence of fatal human influenza A subtype H5N1 disease. *Lancet.* 2004 Feb 21;363(9409):617-9.

[26] Grose C, Chokephaibulkit K. Avian influenza virus infection of children in Vietnam and Thailand. *Pediatr. Infect. Dis. J.* 2004 Aug;23(8):793-4.

[27] Tran TH, Nguyen TL, Nguyen TD, Luong TS, Pham PM, Nguyen VC, et al. Avian influenza A (H5N1) in 10 patients in Vietnam. *N. Engl. J. Med.* 2004 Mar 18;350(12):1179-88.

[28] Kuiken T, Rimmelzwaan G, van Riel D, van Amerongen G, Baars M, Fouchier R, et al. Avian H5N1 influenza in cats. *Science.* 2004 Oct 8;306(5694):241.

[29] Keawcharoen J, Oraveerakul K, Kuiken T, Fouchier RA, Amonsin A, Payungporn S, et al. Avian influenza H5N1 in tigers and leopards. *Emerg. Infect. Dis.* 2004 Dec;10(12):2189-91.

[30] Thanawongnuwech R, Amonsin A, Tantilertcharoen R, Damrongwatanapokin S, Theamboonlers A, Payungporn S, et al. Probable tiger-to-tiger transmission of avian influenza H5N1. *Emerg. Infect. Dis.* 2005 May;11(5):699-701.

[31] Li KS, Guan Y, Wang J, Smith GJ, Xu KM, Duan L, et al. Genesis of a highly pathogenic and potentially pandemic H5N1 influenza virus in eastern Asia. *Nature.* 2004 Jul 8;430(6996):209-13.

[32] Choi YK, Nguyen TD, Ozaki H, Webby RJ, Puthavathana P, Buranathal C, et al. Studies of H5N1 influenza virus infection of pigs by using viruses isolated in Vietnam and Thailand in 2004. *J. Virol.* 2005 Aug;79(16):10821-5.

[33] Liu J, Xiao H, Lei F, Zhu Q, Qin K, Zhang XW, et al. Highly pathogenic H5N1 influenza virus infection in migratory birds. *Science.* 2005 Aug 19;309(5738):1206.

[34] World Health Organization. Officially confirmed Human Influenza A (H5N1) cases. Available at http://www.wpro.who.int/sites/csr/data/data_Tables.htm Accessed January 01, 2008.

[35] Sturm-Ramirez KM, Hulse-Post DJ, Govorkova EA, Humberd J, Seiler P, Puthavathana P, et al. Are ducks contributing to the endemicity of highly pathogenic H5N1 influenza virus in Asia? *J. Virol.* 2005 Sep;79(17):11269-79.

[36] Shortridge KF, Zhou NN, Guan Y, Gao P, Ito T, Kawaoka Y, et al. Characterization of avian H5N1 influenza viruses from poultry in Hong Kong. *Virology.* 1998 Dec 20;252(2):331-42.

[37] Yuen KY, Wong SS. Human infection by avian influenza A H5N1. *Hong Kong Med. J.* 2005 Jun;11(3):189-99.

[38] Suzuki Y. Sialobiology of influenza: molecular mechanism of host range variation of influenza viruses. *Biol. Pharm. Bull.* 2005 Mar;28(3):399-408.

[39] Matrosovich MN, Matrosovich TY, Gray T, Roberts NA, Klenk HD. Human and avian influenza viruses target different cell types in cultures of human airway epithelium. *Proc. Natl. Acad. Sci. USA*. 2004 Mar 30;101(13):4620-4.

[40] Ito T, Couceiro JN, Kelm S, Baum LG, Krauss S, Castrucci MR, et al. Molecular basis for the generation in pigs of influenza A viruses with pandemic potential. *J. Virol.* 1998 Sep;72(9):7367-73.

[41] Hayden FG, Fritz R, Lobo MC, Alvord W, Strober W, Straus SE. Local and systemic cytokine responses during experimental human influenza A virus infection. Relation to symptom formation and host defense. *J. Clin. Invest*. 1998 Feb 1;101(3):643-9.

[42] Seo SH, Hoffmann E, Webster RG. Lethal H5N1 influenza viruses escape host anti-viral cytokine responses. *Nat. Med*. 2002 Sep;8(9):950-4.

[43] Fritz RS, Hayden FG, Calfee DP, Cass LM, Peng AW, Alvord WG, et al. Nasal cytokine and chemokine responses in experimental influenza A virus infection: results of a placebo-controlled trial of intravenous zanamivir treatment. *J. Infect. Dis.* 1999 Sep;180(3):586-93.

[44] de Jong MD, Simmons CP, Thanh TT, Hien VM, Smith GJ, Chau TN, et al. Fatal outcome of human influenza A (H5N1) is associated with high viral load and hypercytokinemia. *Nat. Med.* 2006 Oct;12(10):1203-7.

[45] To KF, Chan PK, Chan KF, Lee WK, Lam WY, Wong KF, et al. Pathology of fatal human infection associated with avian influenza A H5N1 virus. *J. Med. Virol.* 2001 Mar;63(3):242-6.

[46] de Jong MD, Hien TT. Avian influenza A (H5N1). J Clin Virol. 2006 Jan;35(1):2-13.

[47] Beigel JH, Farrar J, Han AM, Hayden FG, Hyer R, de Jong MD, et al. Avian influenza A (H5N1) infection in humans. *N. Engl. J. Med.* 2005 Sep 29;353(13):1374-85.

[48] Chotpitayasunondh T, Ungchusak K, Hanshaoworakul W, Chunsuthiwat S, Sawanpanyalert P, Kijphati R, et al. Human disease from influenza A (H5N1), Thailand, 2004. *Emerg. Infect. Dis.* 2005 Feb;11(2):201-9.

[49] Uiprasertkul M, Puthavathana P, Sangsiriwut K, Pooruk P, Srisook K, Peiris M, et al. Influenza A H5N1 replication sites in humans. *Emerg. Infect. Dis*. 2005 Jul;11(7):1036-41.

[50] Hammel JM, Chiang WK. Update on emerging infections: news from the Centers for Disease Control and Prevention. Outbreaks of avian influenza A (H5N1) in Asia and interim recommendations for evaluation and reporting of suspected cases--United States, 2004. *Ann. Emerg. Med.* 2005 Jan;45(1):88-92.

[51] Ng EK, Cheng PK, Ng AY, Hoang TL, Lim WW. Influenza A H5N1 detection. *Emerg. Infect. Dis*. 2005 Aug;11(8):1303-5.

[52] Payungporn S, Chutinimitkul S, Chaisingh A, Damrongwantanapokin S, Buranathai C, Amonsin A, et al. Single step multiplex real-time RT-PCR for H5N1 influenza A virus detection. *J. Virol. Methods*. 2006 Feb;131(2):143-7.

[53] Payungporn S, Phakdeewirot P, Chutinimitkul S, Theamboonlers A, Keawcharoen J, Oraveerakul K, et al. Single-step multiplex reverse transcription-polymerase chain reaction (RT-PCR) for influenza A virus subtype H5N1 detection. *Viral Immunol.* 2004;17(4):588-93.

[54] Katz JM, Lim W, Bridges CB, Rowe T, Hu-Primmer J, Lu X, et al. Antibody response in individuals infected with avian influenza A (H5N1) viruses and detection of anti-H5 antibody among household and social contacts. *J. Infect. Dis.* 1999 Dec;180(6):1763-70.

[55] Samaranayake LP, Peiris M. Severe acute respiratory syndrome and dentistry: a retrospective view. *J. Am. Dent. Assoc.* 2004 Sep;135(9):1292-302.

[56] Brooks MJ, Sasadeusz JJ, Tannock GA. Antiviral chemotherapeutic agents against respiratory viruses: where are we now and what's in the pipeline? *Curr. Opin. Pulm. Med.* 2004 May;10(3):197-203.

[57] Bright RA, Medina MJ, Xu X, Perez-Oronoz G, Wallis TR, Davis XM, et al. Incidence of adamantane resistance among influenza A (H3N2) viruses isolated worldwide from 1994 to 2005: a cause for concern. *Lancet.* 2005 Oct 1;366(9492):1175-81.

[58] Cheung CL, Rayner JM, Smith GJ, Wang P, Naipospos TS, Zhang J, et al. Distribution of amantadine-resistant H5N1 avian influenza variants in Asia. *J. Infect. Dis.* 2006 Jun 15;193(12):1626-9.

[59] Yen HL, Monto AS, Webster RG, Govorkova EA. Virulence may determine the necessary duration and dosage of oseltamivir treatment for highly pathogenic A/Vietnam/1203/04 influenza virus in mice. *J. Infect. Dis.* 2005 Aug 15;192(4):665-72.

[60] Le QM, Kiso M, Someya K, Sakai YT, Nguyen TH, Nguyen KH, et al. Avian flu: isolation of drug-resistant H5N1 virus. *Nature.* 2005 Oct 20;437(7062):1108.

[61] Sidwell RW, Bailey KW, Wong MH, Barnard DL, Smee DF. In vitro and in vivo influenza virus-inhibitory effects of viramidine. *Antiviral Res.* 2005 Oct;68(1):10-7.

[62] Hoffmann E, Lipatov AS, Webby RJ, Govorkova EA, Webster RG. Role of specific hemagglutinin amino acids in the immunogenicity and protection of H5N1 influenza virus vaccines. *Proc. Natl. Acad. Sci. USA.* 2005 Sep 6;102(36):12915-20.

[63] Tian G, Zhang S, Li Y, Bu Z, Liu P, Zhou J, et al. Protective efficacy in chickens, geese and ducks of an H5N1-inactivated vaccine developed by reverse genetics. *Virology.* 2005 Oct 10;341(1):153-62.

[64] Lipatov AS, Webby RJ, Govorkova EA, Krauss S, Webster RG. Efficacy of H5 influenza vaccines produced by reverse genetics in a lethal mouse model. *J. Infect Dis.* 2005 Apr 15;191(8):1216-20.

[65] Tompkins SM, Zhao ZS, Lo CY, Misplon JA, Liu T, Ye Z, et al. Matrix protein 2 vaccination and protection against influenza viruses, including subtype H5N1. *Emerg. Infect. Dis.* 2007 Mar;13(3):426-35.

[66] Dave RS, Pomerantz RJ. RNA interference: on the road to an alternate therapeutic strategy! *Rev. Med. Virol.* 2003 Nov-Dec;13(6):373-85.

[67] Tompkins SM, Lo CY, Tumpey TM, Epstein SL. Protection against lethal influenza virus challenge by RNA interference in vivo. *Proc. Natl. Acad. Sci. USA.* 2004 Jun 8;101(23):8682-6.

[68] Zhou H, Jin M, Yu Z, Xu X, Peng Y, Wu H, et al. Effective small interfering RNAs targeting matrix and nucleocapsid protein gene inhibit influenza A virus replication in cells and mice. *Antiviral Res.* 2007 Nov;76(2):186-93.

[69] Centers for Disease Control and Prevention. Interim Recommendations for Infection Control in Health-Care Facilities Caring for Patients with Known or Suspected Avian Influenza. Available at: http://www.cdc.gov/flu/avian/professional/infect-control.htm Accessed January 01, 2008.

In: Clinical Dentistry
Editor: Scardina Giuseppe Alessandro

ISBN: 978-1-61122-354-5
© 2011 Nova Science Publishers, Inc.

Chapter 3

CLINICAL EVALUATIONS OF TWO SELF-ETCH AND ONE-TOTAL ETCH ADHESIVES IN CARIOUS CERVICAL LESION: TWO-YEAR RESULTS[§]

***Ali I. Abdalla**[*1]**, Emad Khattab**[1] **and Nabawy El Robeigy**[2]*

[1]Department of Restorative Dentistry Faculty of Dentistry,
University of Tanta, Tanta, Egypt
[2]Department of Dental Materials, Faculty of Dentistry,
University of Tanta, Tanta, Egypt

ABSTRACT

Purpose: To evaluate the clinical performance of two self-etching adhesives and one total-etch adhesive in Class V carious lesions.

Methods: Two self-etching primers, 'Clearfil SE bond' and 'Hybrid Bond' and one total etch adhesive, 'Admira bond', were placed in 244 Class V carious lesions. Restorations were evaluated at base line, one and two year using USPHS criteria.

Results: No loss of restorations was recorded after one and two year for all materials. There was no significant difference between the base line and two-year results for Admira bond and Clearfil SE bond restorations. In contrast, restorations of Hybrid bond showed significant deterioration in marginal adaptation and cavosurface marginal discoloration after two years. No significant differences were found between Admira bond and Clearfil SE bond at each recall period.

Clinical Significance: Total-etch adhesive (Admira bond) and two-step self-etch adhesive (Clearfil SE Bond) when placed in Class V carious lesions showed excellent clinical performance after two years. In contrast, one step self-etch adhesive (Hybrid

---

[§] A version of this book was also published as a chapter in *International Journal of Clinical Dentistry, Volume 1, Issue1*, published by Nova Science Publishers, Inc. It was submitted for appropriate modifications in an effort to encourage wider dissemination of research.

[*] Correspondence: Dr. Ali I. Abdalla, Department of Restorative Dentistry, Faculty of Dentistry, University of Tanta, Tanta 3111, Egypt. Tel: +2-040 3336654, +2-040 3405241, Fax: +2-040- 3331800, E-mail: ali_abdalla79@yahoo.com

Bond) showed significant deterioration with regard to the marginal adaptation and marginal discoloration.

INTRODUCTION

Today's adhesives are applied following either total-etch or self-etch technique. Several clinical studies have shown that reliable and long lasting adhesive restorations can be obtained following total-etch technique [1-6]. In contrast scarce literature is available on the clinical performance of self-etch adhesives [7-9]. When using total-etch techniques, the quality of resin-dentin adhesion can be greatly influenced by the duration of acid etching process and the amount of surface wetness left prior to adhesive application.3,10 By using this strategy, some problems could occur, such as the collapse of the collagen networks following the application of etching agent, the necessity of rinsing or the correct interpretation of the wet or dry bonding [8].

Self-etching primers use non-rinsed acidic monomers that simultaneously dissolve the smear layer, deminerlize the dentin surface beyond the smear layer and prime dentin as well as the enamel [11]. The adhesive in two-step self-etching adhesives agent is often a solvent-free component. Newer self-etching systems combine the etchant, primer and adhesive in one container [12]. As they etch, they also infiltrate the exposed collagen with hydrophilic monomers, where after they copolymerize with the placed adhesive resin to the same depth in dentin. The result is the formation of a hybridized complex; a hybridized smear layer and hybrid layer which thickness is related to the aggressiveness of the self-etching agent [13]. With these systems the smear layer is a bonding substrate. Moreover, these systems are used under dry bonding conditions.

Laboratory studies evaluating self-etch materials showed diverging findings. Some studies have reported that self-etch adhesives bond less effectively to enamel than total etch systems [14-17]. Other, however, have reported that both self-etch and total-etch adhesive systems perform equally well on ground enamel [18-20].

Self-etch adhesives have also been reported to less effectively interact with dentin compared to total etch ones [21-23]. In particular with regard to bond durability, a bond produced by self-etch adhesives appears more vulnerable to degradation due to areas of increased permeability present at the hybridized adhesive dentin interface [24]. Water was suggested to be incompletely removed and resulted in regions of incomplete polymerization making the interface permeable and more degradation sensitive.

Though new *in vitro* testing methodology tends to better predict clinical performance, clinical trials remain needed to ultimately evaluate the clinical efficacy of such self-etch adhesives.

The objective of this study was to evaluate the clinical effectiveness of two self-etch and one total-etch adhesive for the restoration of Class V carious lesions during two years of function.

MATERIALS AND METHODS

Sixty-nine patients with age ranging between 18-52 years participated in this study. A total of 244 Class V carious were restored. Only carious lesions were selected in maxillary and mandibular premolars and maxillary anterior (incisors and cuspid) teeth (Table 1). Patients were selected so that each one must had at least three class V carious lesions. Patients having only one or two lesions were not included. So the three tested adhesives were placed under the same condition.

Patients with a compromised medical history, severe or chronic periodontitis, high caries risk, heavy smoking and abnormal occlusion were excluded from the study. All procedures were explained to the patients and their written consents were obtained.

Table 1. Composition of the adhesive systems used in the study

Adhesive system	Component	Composition	Manufacturer
Admira Bond	Acid Bond	36% Phosphoric acid Acetone, bonding ormocer, Dimethacrylate, functionizing methacrylates, initiators, stabilizer	Voco, Germany
Clearfil SE bond	Primer Adhesive	HEMA, Hydrophilic Dimethacrylate, 10-MDP Toluidine, Camphorquinone, Water 10-MDP, BIS-GMA, HEMA, hydrophilic dimethacrylate, microfillre.	Kuraray, Japan
Hybrid Bond	Brush Adhesive	Sodium p-toluenesulfinate, Sodium N-phenylglycine (NPG-Na) Methylmethacrylate (MMA), 4-methacryloxyethyltrimetillic acid anhydride tri (2-hydroxyethyl)-isocyanurat-triacrylate (THIT), HEMA, Acetone, Water.	Sun Medical, Japan

Restorative Procedures

Operative procedures were carried out by the first author. Local anaesthesia was applied with 2% Lidocaine solution (Mepacaine). All restorative procedures were done under rubber dam isolation using gingival retraction clamps. The teeth to be restored were first cleaned with a non-fluoridated prophylaxis paste on a rubber cup and subsequently rinsed with water. A Class V cavity was prepared on the buccal surface of each tooth using a # 56 bur at high speed with water coolant. If the carious lesion permits an attempt was made to prepare cavities of comparable size; 3-4 mm occlusogingivally, 2-3 mm mesiodistally and 1 mm deep in dentin. Cavities that exceeded these dimension or those that were difficult to be isolated properly were excluded from the study. Deep caries, if found, was removed with # 4 round bur at low speed and a thin layer of calcium hydroxide 'Dycal'[a] was placed on the deep portion of the cavity.

The materials (Table 2) were applied according to manufacturer's instructions as follows:

Admira Bond[b]

The entire cavity was etched for 15s with 36% phosphoric acid[b], rinsed with water spray. Excess water was removed with air blast for 3s leaving the dentin moist. Admira bond[b] was applied with disposable brush, thinned with mild air for 2-3s and light cured for 20s using a visible light curing device (Heliolux DLX)[c]. The output of the light curing unit was regularly checked with a curing radiometer (Demetron Research Corp., Danbury, CT, USA) to be at least 600 mW/mm^2.

Table 2. Distribution of materials and tooth location

Adhesive system	Maxillary anterior	Maxillary premolars	Mandibular premolars	total
Admira	30	26	28	84
Clearfil SE bond	35	20	30	85
Hybrid Bond	27	23	25	75
total	92	69	83	244

Clearfil SE Bond[d]

The SE primer[d] was applied to the cavity for 20s using a disposable brush and air thinned. SE bond[d] was then applied, thinned with gentle stream of air and light cured for 20s.

Hybrid Bond[e]

Hybrid bond[e] was dispensed into the mixing well. A hybrid bond brush[e] was dipped into the solution, stirred shortly and then applied to the cavity for 20s. The adhesive was thinned with gentle blast of air for 5s and light cured for 20s. All cavities were restored with resin composite Clearfil APX[d] using an incremental condensation technique. Each increment was (thickness < 2mm) light cured for 40s. Finishing was accomplished using contouring diamond at high speed and polishing was done with flexible discs and finishing strips at low speed hand piece with water cooling (Sof-Lex Pop-on set, 3M Espe, AG, Seefeld, Germany.

[a] Dentsply Caulk, Milford, DE, USA
[b] Voco, Cuxhaven, Germany.
[c] Vivadent, Schaan, Liechtenstein.

Evaluation Procedures

Each restoration was clinically evaluated after finishing and polishing (base line), after one and two year in accordance with the US Public Health Service (USPHS) criteria [25]. Two independent evaluators who have used the same criteria in a similar investigations were chosen for evaluation. Evaluation was done in a blind base so both evaluators were not aware of the tested adhesive. When disagreement occurred during evaluation, consensus evaluations were obtained between evaluators. An initial agreement of at least 85% between evaluators was considered statistically significant.

The obtained data were tabulated and statistically analysed with McNemar test at a significance level of 5 % ($P < 0.05$).

RESULTS

The data for colour match, anatomic form, marginal adaptation and cavosurface marginal discoloration for the tested materials are presented in Table 3.

After one year, 227 restorations were available for evaluation (recall rate 93 %). No loss of restoration was recorded (retention rate 100%).

Table 3. Clinical evaluation of the tested materials after one and two year

Adhesive system	Colour match A B C	Anatomic form A B C	Marginal adaptation A B C	Marginal discoloration A B C	Retention rate (%)
Admira					
Base line (84)	84 0 0	84 0 0	84 0 0	84 0 0	100%
One year (78)	78 0 0	78 0 0	78 0 0	78 0 0	100%
Two year (70)	67 3 0	70 0 0	69 1 0	67 3 0	100%
Clearfil SE Bond					
Base line (85)	85 0 0	85 0 0	85 0 0	85 0 0	100%
One year (80)	80 0 0	80 0 0	77 3 0	76 4 0	100%
Two year (77)	77 0 0	77 0 0	73 4 0	70 7 0	100%
Hybrid Bond					
Base line (75)	75 0 0	75 0 0	75 0 0	75 0 0	100%
One year (69)	69 0 0	69 0 0	64 4 1	60 7 2	100%
Two year (62)	60 2 0	57 5 0	48 10 4	42 12 8	100%

( ) indicate the number of restorations evaluated.

Restorations of Admira bond showed Alfa ratings for all the inspected criteria. For SE bond, all restorations showed Alfa rating regarding colour match and marginal adaptation.

Three restorations (3.7 %) and four restorations (5%) showed Bravo rating for marginal quality and marginal discoloration respectively. Hybrid bond restorations showed 100% Alfa rating for colour match and anatomic form. For marginal adaptation four restorations (5.8%) showed Bravo score and one restoration showed Charlie score. For cavosurface marginal discoloration seven restorations (10%) were rated Bravo and two restorations were rated Charlie. Statistical analysis revealed no significant differences (P>0.05) between the one-year and base-line evaluation for Admira and SE bond. Also there were no significant differences between the three tested materials after one year. For Hybrid Bond a significant difference (P=0.05) between the base-line and one-year results was observed. Also these values were a significantly higher than that of the other materials (p=0.04).

After two year, 209 restorations were available (recall rate 85.6%). No loss of restorations was recorded for any of the tested materials. All restorations of Admira bond showed Alfa ratings for anatomic form. For colour match, three restorations showed Bravo score. For marginal adaptation, one restoration showed Brave rating. For cavosurface marginal discoloration, three restorations showed Brave score.

All restorations of SE bond showed Alfa ratings for colour match and anatomic form. For marginal adaptation, four (5.2%) restorations showed Brave rating. For cavosurface marginal discoloration, seven (9%) restorations showed Brave score. These marginal discrepancies and discoloration were mainly located at the enamel margins.

For Hybrid Bond, two restorations were rated Bravo for colour match and four restorations showed Bravo rating for anatomic form. For marginal adaptation, ten restorations (16.6%) showed Bravo rating and two showed Charlie rating. For cavosurface marginal discoloration, twelve restorations (19.3%) showed Brave and six restorations (6.9%) received Charlie scores. In contrast to SE bond restorations, these defects were located at the enamel and dentinal margins.

Statistical analysis revealed no significant differences (P>0.05) between the two-year and base-line evaluation results for Admira bond and SE bond. In contrast, the data for Hybrid Bond was significantly different (P=0.02) from the base-line ones. Also these values was a significantly higher than that of the other materials (p = 0.002).

No caries recurrence was recorded at any recall period. Also no tooth became non vital, due to the cervical restoration.

Discussion

In the present study two self-etch and one total-etch adhesives were evaluated regarding their effectiveness to restore Class V carious lesions after one and two years.

This clinical trial revealed that both total-etch adhesive, Admira bond and two-step self-etch adhesive, SE bond were effective in restoring Class V carious lesion after two years. In contrast, restorations of Hybrid bond showed significant deterioration during the evaluation period. This difference in clinical performance between the tested adhesive systems may be attributed the nature of adhesive-tooth bond with regard to durability under *in-vivo* condition.

The favourable clinical effectiveness of Admira bond may have been resulted from the strong and reliable bond obtained when the material applied to etched tooth tissues. The bonding mechanism of Admira to dentin is diffusion-based and depends on hybridization or infiltration of resin within the exposed collagen mesh as well as into dentinal tubules [26]. After *in situ* polymerization, the hybrid layer created with this adhesive system provides a reliable micromechanical retention. Another contributing factor to such favorable performance of Admira is the presence of ormocer (organic modified ceramic) in the bonding resin. Ormocer was reported to have a calcium complexing function which enhances the bond strength to tooth structure [27]. In addition; it reduces the rate of release of residual monomers in comparison with conventional composites which, if not polymerized thoroughly, may be washed out in time leading to bond degradation. Admira bond also contains acetone as a solvent which is capable of displacing water carrying resin monomers to the interfibiller spaces formed by etching [22].

All restorations of SE bond rated Alfa as regarding all the criteria after one year. After two year, four restorations showed localised area of marginal discrepancies at the enamel margin. Also seven restorations showed small area of stain at the enamel margin. This marginal enamel discrepancies and stains may raise the concern about the etching capability of self-etch adhesives. The enamel etching pattern resulting from self-etch adhesive is less defined when compared to that resulting from phosphoric acid etching [28]. Clearfil SE bond is a two-step mild self-etching primer-adhesive system. The primer of SE bond contains 10-MDP as functional monomer dissolved in water and ethanol to result in a pH around 2. On dentin, Clearfil SE does not remove the smear layer but hybridizes it to the underlying dentin. It impregnates smear plugs fixing it at the internal tubular walls. The bonding mechanism of SE bond was suggested to result from the simultaneous demineralization and infiltration of enamel and dentin to form a continuum in the substrate incorporating the smear plug in the resin tag [29]. This leads to a shallow but uniform resin-infiltrated interface. Besides simplifying bonding technique, the elimination of both rinsing and drying steps reduces the possibility of over-wetting or over-drying as they have a negative effect on adhesion [30]. Also, the presence of the highly hydrophilic 10-MDP monomer is believed to improve the wetting to moist tooth surface [31]. In addition, 10-MDP has two hydroxyl groups that may chelate the calcium ions of dentin. Moreover, the residual hydroxyapatite around the exposed collagen fibrils remain available for additional chemical interaction with the functional monomers [32].

Another factor that may have contributed to the favourable performance of SE bond is the fact that SE bond is filled adhesive that contain 10 wt% silica nanofiller, resulting in a thicker adhesive layer and thus more flexible interface that thought to relieve interfacial tensile stress between the shrinking composite and the rigid dentin interface [33].

The results of Hybrid Bond showed significant marginal discrepancies and marginal discoloration at the enamel and dentinal margins of several restorations after one year. Such deterioration continues for the second year. Hybrid Bond contains 4-META as an active monomer component. In an aqueous environment this monomer is converted to the dicarboxylic acid 4-MET, the etching component of Hybrid bond with pH around 1.34 This high acidity resulted in rather aggressive demineralization, collagen was exposed and nearly all hydroxyapatite crystallites were dissolved. Consequently, the underlying mechanism of bonding of Hybrid Bond is primarily diffusion-based, like that of the total-etch approach. In spite of such bonding mechanism which may be comparable to that of total etch, poor clinical performance was observed in our study. Frankenberger and Tay [34] reported inferior performance of one step self- etching adhesives compared to two-step self- etch after thermal and mechanical load cycling. This was attributed to the absence of coupling hydrophobic bonding agent in the all in one adhesives, which made these materials to behave as permeable membranes after polymerization. In the absence of more hydrophobic coating in the simplified adhesive system, rapid water sorption can occur via the hydrophilic and permeable adhesive layer [22]. In addition, water sorption and dissolution of the incompletely polymerized resin containing amphiphilic monomers may result in deterioration of the hybrid bond *in-vivo* [35] Moreover, the higher acidity and hydrophilicity of the acidic monomers increase the risk of hydrolytic degeneration [36].

Although a single-step adhesive is desirable in the clinical situation, the combination of water, acids, hydrophilic and hydrophobic monomers into single solution has been reported to compromise bonding. Recent reports on their bond strengths indicate that such all-in-one adhesive systems do not perform well [37-39].

References

[1] Browning WD, Brackett WW, Gilpatrick RO. Two-year clinical comparison of a microfilled and a hybrid resin-based composite in non-carious Class V lesions. *Oper. Dent.* 2000; 25: 46-50.

[2] van Dijken JW. Clinical evaluation of three adhesive systems in class V non-carious lesions. *Dent. Mater.* 2000; 16: 285-291.

[3] Van Meerbeek B, De Munck J, Yoshida Y, Inoue S, Vargas M, Vijay P, Van Landuyt K, Lambrechts P, Vanherle G. Buonocore memorial lecture. Adhesion to enamel and dentin: current status and future challenges. *Oper. Dent.* 2003; 28: 215-235.

[4] Van Meerbeek B, Perdigao J, Lambrechts P, Vanherle G. The clinical performance of adhesives. *J. Dent.* 1998; 26: 1-20.

[5] Van Meerbeek B, Peumans M, Gladys S, Braem M, Lambrechts P, Vanherle G. Three-year clinical effectiveness of four total-etch dentinal adhesive systems in cervical lesions. *Quintessence Int.* 1996; 27: 775-784.

[6] Van Meerbeek B, Peumans M, Verschueren M, Gladys S, Braem M, Lambrechts P, Vanherle G. Clinical status of ten dentin adhesive systems. *J. Dent Res.* 1994; 73: 1690-1702.

[7] Brackett WW, Covey DA, St Germain HA, Jr. One-year clinical performance of a self-etching adhesive in class V resin composites cured by two methods. *Oper. Dent.* 2002; 27: 218-222.

[8] Swift EJ, Jr. Dentin/enamel adhesives: review of the literature. *Pediatr. Dent.* 2002; 24: 456-461.

[9] Turkun SL. Clinical evaluation of a self-etching and a one-bottle adhesive system at two years. *J. Dent.* 2003; 31: 527-534.

[10] Tay FR, Gwinnett AJ, Wei SH. The overwet phenomenon: a transmission electron microscopic study of surface moisture in the acid-conditioned, resin-dentin interface. *Am. J. Dent* 1996; 9: 161-166.

[11] De Munck J, Van Meerbeek B, Yoshida Y, Inoue S, Vargas M, Suzuki K, Lambrechts P, Vanherle G. Four-year water degradation of total-etch adhesives bonded to dentin. *J. Dent. Res.* 2003; 82: 136-140.

[12] Tay FR, Pashley DH. Dental adhesives of the future. *J. Adhes. Dent.* 2002; 4: 91-103.

[13] Perdigao J. Dentin bonding as a function of dentin structure. *Dent. Clin. North Am.* 2002; 46: 277-301, vi.

[14] Hara AT, Amaral CM, Pimenta LA, Sinhoreti MA. Shear bond strength of hydrophilic adhesive systems to enamel. *Am. J. Dent.* 1999; 12: 181-184.

[15] Kanemura N, Sano H, Tagami J. Tensile bond strength to and SEM evaluation of ground and intact enamel surfaces. *J. Dent.* 1999; 27: 523-530.

[16] Tay FR, Pashley DH, Suh BI, Carvalho RM, Itthagarun A. Single-step adhesives are permeable membranes. *J. Dent.* 2002; 30: 371-382.

[17] Torii Y, Itou K, Nishitani Y, Yoshiyama M, Ishikawa K, Suzuki K. Effect of self-etching primer containing N-acryloyl aspartic acid on enamel adhesion. *Dent. Mater.* 2003; 19: 253-258.

[18] Hannig M, Reinhardt KJ, Bott B. Self-etching primer vs phosphoric acid: an alternative concept for composite-to-enamel bonding. *Oper. Dent.* 1999; 24: 172-180.

[19] Ibarra G, Vargas MA, Armstrong SR, Cobbb DS. Microtensile bond strength of self-etching adhesives to ground and unground enamel. *J. Adhes. Dent.* 2002; 4: 115-124.

[20] Pashley DH, Tay FR. Aggressiveness of contemporary self-etching adhesives. Part II: etching effects on unground enamel. *Dent. Mater.* 2001; 17: 430-444.

[21] Inoue H, Inoue S, Uno S, Takahashi A, Koase K, Sano H. Microtensile bond strength of two single-step adhesive systems to bur-prepared dentin. *J. Adhes. Dent.* 2001; 3: 129-136.

[22] Oliveira SS, Pugach MK, Hilton JF, Watanabe LG, Marshall SJ, Marshall GW, Jr. The influence of the dentin smear layer on adhesion: a self-etching primer vs. a total-etch system. *Dent. Mater.* 2003; 19: 758-767.

[23] Tay FR, Pashley DH. Aggressiveness of contemporary self-etching systems. I: Depth of penetration beyond dentin smear layers. *Dent. Mater.* 2001; 17: 296-308.

[24] Tay FR, King NM, Chan KM, Pashley DH. How can nanoleakage occur in self-etching adhesive systems that demineralize and infiltrate simultaneously? *J. Adhes. Dent.* 2002; 4: 255-269.

[25] Cvar JF, Ryge G. Reprint of criteria for the clinical evaluation of dental restorative materials. 1971. *Clin. Oral Investig.* 2005; 9: 215-232.

[26] Abdalla AI, Davidson CL. Bonding efficiency and interfacial morphology of one-bottle adhesives to contaminated dentin surfaces. *Am. J. Dent.* 1998; 11: 281-285.

[27] Tagtekin DA, Yanikoglu FC, Bozkurt FO, Kologlu B, Sur H. Selected characteristics of an Ormocer and a conventional hybrid resin composite. *Dent. Mater*. 2004; 20:487-97.

[28] Perdigao J, Geraldeli S. Bonding characteristics of self-etching adhesives to intact versus prepared enamel. *J. Esthet. Restor. Dent.* 2003; 15: 32-41; discussion 42.

[29] Perdigao J, May KN, Jr., Wilder AD, Jr., Lopes M. The effect of depth of dentin demineralization on bond strengths and morphology of the hybrid layer. *Oper Dent.* 2000; 25: 186-194.

[30] Van Meerbeek B, Yoshida Y, De Munck J, Inoue S, Vargas M, Lambrechts P, Vanherle G. Correlative morphologic and clinical characterization of tooth biomaterial interaction In: Self-etching primer: current status and its evolution. Proceedings of the international symposium ' 01, Tokyo 2001; P. 41-55

[31] Yoshida Y, Nagakane K, Fukuda R, Nakayama Y, Okazaki M, Shintani H, Inoue S, Tagawa Y, Suzuki K, De Munck J, Van Meerbeek B. Comparative study on adhesive performance of functional monomers. *J. Dent. Res.* 2004; 83: 454-458.

[32] Misra DN. Adsorption from solutions on synthetic hydroxyapatite: nonaqueous vs. aqueous solvents. *J. Biomed. Mater. Res.* 1999; 48: 848-855.

[33] Kemp-Scholte CM, Davidson CL. Marginal integrity related to bond strength and strain capacity of composite resin restorative systems. *J. Prosthet. Dent.* 1990; 64: 658-664.

[34] Frankenberger R, Tay FR. Self-etch vs etch-and-rinse adhesives: effect of thermo-mechanical fatigue loading on marginal quality of bonded resin composite restorations. *Dent. Mater.* 2005; 21: 397-412.

[35] Blunck U, Roulet JF. Effect of one year water storage on the effectiveness of dentin adhesive in class V composite resin restorations. *J. Dent. Res.* 2002;81:A-39 (Abstr 946).

[36] van Dijken JW. Durability of three simplified adhesive systems in Class V non-carious cervical dentin lesions. *Am. J. Dent.* 2004; 17: 27-32.

[37] German Cecilia C, Garcia Ballesta C, Cortes Lillo O, Perez Lajarin L. Shear bond strength of a self-etching adhesive in primary and permanent dentition. *Am. J. Dent.* 2005; 18: 331-334.

[38] Moll K, Park HJ, Haller B. Effect of simulated pulpal pressure on dentin bond strength of self-etching bonding systems. *Am. J. Dent.* 2005; 18: 335-339.

[39] O'Keefe KL, Pinzon LM, Rivera B, Powers JM. Bond strength of composite to astringent-contaminated dentin using self-etching adhesives. *Am. J. Dent.* 2005; 18: 168-172.

In: Clinical Dentistry
Editor: Scardina Giuseppe Alessandro

ISBN: 978-1-61122-354-5
© 2011 Nova Science Publishers, Inc.

Chapter 4

THE SITE-SPECIFIC NATURE OF THE VOLUMETRIC FEATURES AND ENZYMATIC PROFILE OF GINGIVAL CREVICULAR FLUID (GCF): ANALYSIS OF MYELOPEROXIDASE (MPO) ACTIVITY AT DISTINCT SAMPLING SITES[#]

Hasan Hatipoğlu[1], Nermin Yamalik[2], Asuman Kılınç[3], Kamer Kılınç[3], Atilla Berberoğlu[*2], Erdem Karabulut[4] and Kenan Eratalay[2]

[1]Dumlupinar University, Research and Training Hospital,
Dental Clinic/Periodontology, Kütahya / Turkey
[2]Department of Periodontology, Faculty of Dentistry,
University of Hacettepe, Ankara, Turkey
[3]Department of Biochemistry, Faculty of Medicine,
University of Hacettepe, Ankara-Turkey
[4]Department of Biostatistics, Faculty of Medicine,
University of Hacettepe, Ankara-Turkey

ABSTRACT

The site-specific nature of the volumetric features and enzymatic profile of gingival crevicular fluid (GCF): Analysis of myeloperoxidase (MPO) activity at distinct sampling sites.

[#] This study is presented in International Association for Dental Research/CEDandID divisional meeting held in Thessalonica, Greece, 26-29 September 2007.

[*] Corresponding author: Dr. Atilla Berberoğlu, Professor, Department of Periodontology, Faculty of Dentistry, University of Hacettepe, 06100 Ankara – Turkey, Phone: + 90 312 305 22 17, + 90 312 305 24 05, Fax: + 90 312 442 15 98, E-mail: aberbero@hacettepe.edu.tr

Purpose: Further clarification of the biodynamics and the site-specific nature of gingival crevicular fluid (GCF), in terms of volume and content, may serve both for a better understanding of periodontal pathogenesis and developing reliable diagnostic tools. Thus, the aim of the present study was to analyze, on a site-specific basis, the potential variances in GCF volume and its myeloperoxidase (MPO) content and the relationship of these two measures with the clinical periodontal status.

Methods: At a total of 719 sites, representing either clinical periodontal health (n=175), or gingivitis (n=308), or periodontitis (n=236), clinical parameters were recorded, GCF samples were obtained and MPO activity was spectrophotometrically determined. Statistical analyses considered the comparison of the three periodontal conditions, multi-rooted or single-rooted teeth, and mesio-buccal (MB) and disto-buccal (DB) sites, and the correlations among the clinical parameters, GCF volume and MPO activity.

Results: There were clear differences between all site-analysis and analysis of distinct sites. For all sites clinical parameters, GCF volume, and GCF MPO activity generally presented with a disease-related spectrum; healthy<gingivitis<periodontitis ($p<0.05$). However, differences in GCF volume and MPO profile between multi-rooted and single-rooted sites and between MB and DB sites were observed ($p<0.05$). Site–specific differences were also observed regarding the presence/absence of GCF and MPO and correlations.

Clinical Significance: The site-specific nature of periodontal diseases and the apparent variances in both the GCF volume and its enzymatic profile at the individual sites needs to be taken into account for a precise GCF-methodology and also for the correct interpretation of the GCF-related data.

Keywords: Gingival crevicular fluid (GCF), myeloperoxidase (MPO), inflammation, pathogenesis, periodontal diseases.

INTRODUCTION

Although clinical periodontal status is among the major determinants of the volumetric features of gingival crevicular fluid (GCF) [1-11], it seems that it is not the only factor. The great fluctuations in the GCF resting volume among individual sites with similar clinical periodontal conditions and the clear volumetric overlaps between different categories of periodontal diseases (e.g. gingivitis and periodontitis) address the presence of other determinants that affect the volumetric features of this biological fluid [6-15]. The GCF sampling strategy [4, 9, 10, 13, 16], the process of volume determination and the related environmental conditions [17], and the GCF sampling site [6-10, 12, 15, 18, 19] are among such determinants.

When the difficulties of sampling of the entire dentition and the extent of the site-specific variations in GCF volume are concerned, identification of the appropriate subset of GCF sampling sites becomes a key factor [6-10, 12, 18]. However, a universal standardization of the sampling site does not seem to exist as most studies rely on different criteria for the identification/preference of the sampling site (e.g. probing depths (PD), clinical periodontal status, the susceptibility/resistance to periodontal destruction, anatomical relation of sites, or distinct teeth groups) [4, 5, 7-10, 19, 20-22]. In recent years, the need for developing of an ideal GCF sampling strategy, including the selection of the sampling area, is frequently mentioned. Such attempts may serve for the improvement of the reliability of GCF-related studies and thus the diagnostic potential of this biological fluid, including its volumetric features [2-5, 7, 18, 19, 23, 24].

Myeloperoxidase (MPO) is a leukocyte-derived enzyme located within the primary granules of these cells [25, 26] and it can even serve as an indicator of PMN infiltration [25]. MPO particularly catalyzes the formation of a number of reactive oxidant species [25, 26], and it generates H_2O_2 and halides from reactive species, thus it is considered as an antibacterial enzyme [27-29]. Its antibacterial activity is shown to be non-specific and effective against both Gram (+) and Gram (-) bacteria [18, 30, 31], including Actinobacillus actinomycetemcomitans [28, 29] and Escherichia coli [32]. This microbicidal activity places MPO among the important protective enzymes and makes it an integral component of the immune response [18, 27-29, 30, 31]. However, there is also the risk for the MPO-derived oxidants to contribute to tissue damage during inflammation [26, 33]. Evidence suggests for a link between MPO and the generation of reactive oxygen metabolites, as nitric oxide (NO) is shown to influence MPO and the capability of MPO to convert nitrite and peroxides to a nitrating agent for proteins and lipids [26, 34]. Medical literature also provides some evidence about the interaction of NO metabolism and MPO in inflammation [26, 34].

MPO is a well-described component of GCF and the periodontal tissues, and the increased amount of MPO activity is suggested to play a significant role in destructive periodontal diseases [25, 35, 36, 37, 38]. Its significant contribution to connective tissue breakdown is suggested to be via providing appropriate conditions for the destructive activity of most proteases by changing the protease/antiprotease balance through activating latent proteases [39, 40]. MPO is suggested to be a good indicator of periodontal disease [37], and also a good indicator of neutrophil activity at failed peri-implant sites [41, 42].

All of these studies reveal that, we have considerable amount of evidence regarding the involvement of MPO in the pathogenesis of periodontal diseases [25, 35-37, 43], and regarding the general features of GCF [2-5, 7, 19, 14, 15, 17, 18, 23, 24, 35]. However, for a more reliable interpretation of GCF-related data, a better understanding of the biodynamic and site-specific nature of the volumetric features and the enzymatic profile of GCF are likely to be needed. Such attempts seem to be particularly important when the site-specific nature of periodontal diseases is concerned. Thus, the aim of the present study is to analyze the potential site-specific variations in GCF volume and its MPO content based on the location of the sampling area, and the relationship of these two measures with the clinical periodontal status.

Materials and Methods

Criteria for selection of the participants: Special care was taken to ensure that the individuals (23 female, 28 male; mean age: 32.06 yrs) who voluntarily participated to this study had no history of any systemic disorder, no antibiotics/antiinflammatory/antidepressant drugs and/or no periodontal therapy within the past 3 months. This was considered to be important for the study design as all of these factors have been proven to have the potential to affect GCF volume. All of these participants had available maxillary multi-rooted or single-rooted teeth sites that are designated as either clinical periodontal health, or gingivitis or periodontitis. No age limits were set, however the equal distribution of the gender of the participants was a particular concern. The participants were provided with the necessary information regarding the purpose of the study and the experimental design, and their informed consent was obtained according to the study protocol which was approved by The Ethical Council of Hacettepe University (HEK 02/18-9).

Determination of the clinical periodontal status and classification of the individual sampling sites: For the entire dentition (except 3rd molars) PDs were measured and plaque index (PI), gingival index (GI) [44] and gingival bleeding time index (GBTI) [45] scores were recorded. These recordings served both for a basis for the clinical periodontal diagnosis and for the subsequent selection of the appropriate subset of GCF sampling sites. To eliminate the risk of interfering with the actual GCF volume, clinical measures and GCF sampling was not performed on the same day. All clinical measurements were recorded by the same periodontist. By a thorough clinical and radiographic examination, the sites were categorized as three experimental groups (clinical periodontal health, gingivitis, and periodontitis) based on the clinical periodontal status of a particular sampling area. Sites with clinical periodontal health presented with no signs of inflammation, bleeding on probing, and attachment and/or bone loss. Radiographic examination revealed no apparent periodontal pathology. Gingivitis sites only exhibited clinical signs of gingival inflammation and with no apparent clinical and radiographic periodontal destruction of deep periodontal tissues. There were no signs of any attachment and/or bone loss, and pathological deepening of the gingival sulci. Sites with periodontitis presented with PD > 4 mm, gingival inflammation, and attachment and alveolar bone loss. No further attempt was to identify different periodontitis forms or determine the severity of the periodontal destruction. In order to minimize the potential inter-individual volumetric variances, in each participant, a minimum of six (or more sites if available) were sampled. To be able to analyze the impact of distinct tooth types, the sites from three disease categories were further divided into two subgroups as multi-rooted (MR) and single-rooted (SR). For the evaluation of the distinct location of the sampling site, MB and DB sites were separately analyzed.

Sampling of GCF and electronic volume quantification: GCF was sampled according to the method defined by Rüdin et al. [46] at the selected subset of sampling sites. In brief, to minimize the risk of contamination with saliva the sampling area was isolated with cotton rolls, and supragingival plaque was removed to eliminate the risk of plaque contamination. After gentle air drying, GCF was collected by use of standardized Periopaper® (#593525, OraFlow Inc., Amityville, NY, USA) strips that were inserted 1mm into the sulcus/pocket and left there for 30 seconds. Samples with evidence of gingival bleeding were excluded. In spite of the potential affect of gravity on GCF volume and flow, sampling was limited with the maxillary sites. To assure accessibility and isolation, GCF samples were obtained only from the buccal sites, and for the same purpose maxillary 3rd molars were excluded. To achieve a distinct standardization of the sampling site, GCF sampling was performed only in buccal-interproximal sites and buccal-median sites were not included. Two GCF samples were simultaneously harvested in each of the selected teeth, as mesio-buccal (MB) or disto-buccal (DB) samples. Likewise the recording of the clinical parameters, clinical GCF sampling and electronic volume determination was performed by the same periodontist. For precise volume determination, prior to the first reading, Periotron 8000® (OraFlow Inc.) was switched on and was allowed to warm up before zero adjustment [47]. Standardized Periopaper® strips and a standardized syringe (Hamilton 0-1.0μl micro syringe - Hamilton 80100, Hamilton Company, Reno, Nevada, USA) graduated with 10nl markings was used to generate the calibration curve in triplicate readings with the test fluid (distilled water) [47]. To immediately transfer the paper strips to Periotron 8000® for electronic volume quantification (within 0-2 seconds) and to eliminate the potential risk or evaporation, the device was placed in a chair side manner. The paper strip containing GCF was placed to a standard distance between the electrodes of the device as recommended by Ciantar and Caruana [48]. Digital readout (Periotron unit–PU) was obtained within 16 seconds and was converted to micro liter by MLCONVERT.EXE software version 2.52 (Ora Flow, Inc., New York, USA). After each measurement, the electrodes of the device were dried by use of sterile cotton tissue, to eliminate the risk of any contamination between multiple readings. The calibration curve was periodically checked and was generated again based on a 5 PU change in any particular volume [49]. These attempts were considered to be necessary for precise electronic volume quantification.

Determination of MPO content of GCF: MPO activity of PISF/GCF was measured using the spectrophotometric MPO assay that is a modification of the method reported by Suzuki and colleagues [50]. Briefly, the assay mixture consisted of 50 mM phosphate buffer (pH 5.4), 1.6 mM synthetic substrate tetramethyl benzidine (TMB), 0.5% hexadecyltrimethyl ammonium bromide, 1mM H_2O_2, and 50 µl GCF extract. The reaction was initiated by the addition of H_2O_2, and the rate of TMB oxidation was followed at 655 nm using a recording spectrophotometer. Considering the initial and linear phase of the reaction, the absorbance change per minute was determined. One unit of MPO activity was expressed as the amount of enzyme producing one absorbance change under assay conditions. MPO activity in PISF/GCF samples was calculated and expressed both as enzyme concentration and the total enzyme activity.

Statistical analysis: Kolmogorov-Smirnov test was used to analyze the normality of data [51]. Because, distributions of variables were not normal, the differences among all sites regarding the clinical parameters, GCF volume and MPO levels were analyzed by using Kruskal-Wallis Variance Analysis [51] and the subsequent pair wise comparisons were made by Mann-Whitney U-test with Bonferroni correction [51]. Multi-rooted and single-rooted sampling sites and MB and DB sites were compared by using Mann-Whitney U-test. Correlations between the clinical parameters of a distinct sampling site and the corresponding Vr values and MPO levels were analyzed by Spearman's rank order correlation coefficient [51].

RESULTS

In fact the total number of sites was 735. However, due to technical problems (n=12) and spectrophotometric errors (n=4) MPO analysis could not be performed at 16 of the sites. A total of 719 sites in a total of 51 participants (age range: 17-60; mean age 32.06 ± 9.26) were analyzed. The age range of the three periodontal categories were quite homogenous (healthy: 32.89 ± 8.66, gingivitis: 32.38 ± 9.48, periodontitis: 33.17 ± 9.48). Of the 719 sites, 175 were designed as clinically healthy, 308 as gingivitis, and 236 as periodontitis. Number of multi-rooted and single-rooted sites and MB and DB sites are provided in the related tables. Approximately 7% (n=48) of the sites lacked detectable levels of MPO; clinical periodontal health (13.7%), gingivitis (5.8%), and periodontitis (2.5%).

All sites: Table 1 shows descriptive statistical data from all sites regarding the clinical parameters, GCF volume and GCF MPO levels. In general, all of the clinical parameters (except PI) were higher at diseased sites than non-diseased sites, being higher for sites with periodontitis than with gingivitis ($p<0.05$). GCF volume and GCF total MPO activity a disease-related pattern; healthy < gingivitis < periodontitis ($p<0.05$). A discrepancy existed between total MPO activity and MPO concentration, as the lowest MPO concentration was observed at healthy sites ($p<0.05$) and there was not any significant difference between the sites with periodontitis and gingivitis ($p>0.05$). Correlations between the clinical parameters and GCF volume and MPO activity and the actual p values are provided in Table 2. At healthy sites GCF volume presented significant correlations with PI ($r=0.173$, $p=0.022$) and PD ($r=0.299$, $p=0.0001$), GCF MPO levels were significantly correlated with PI ($r=0.185$, $p=0.014$) and GCF volume ($r=0.464$, $p=0.0001$). More significant correlations were observed for sites with gingivitis ($p<0.05$), as at gingivitis sites GCF volume and MPO were correlated with all of the clinical parameters ($p<0.05$). GCF MPO generally presented positive and significant correlations with the clinical parameters reflecting the inflammatory status (GI, GBTI, GCF volume) in both of the diseased groups ($p<0.05$).

Single-rooted and multi-rooted sites: Statistical data regarding single-rooted and multi-rooted sites are shown in Table 3. Except the PD at healthy sites, PI at sites with gingivitis, and GI and GBTI at periodontitis sites, clinical parameters between single-rooted and multi-rooted sites were similar ($p>0.05$). GCF volume at multi-rooted sites were higher than single-rooted sites in all of clinical conditions, being significant at both of the diseased sites ($p<0.05$). At healthy and gingivitis sites MPO activity was similar between single-rooted and multi-rooted sites ($p>0.05$), while at periodontitis sites higher MPO activity was observed at single-rooted sites ($p=0.001$). At single-rooted sites, the clinical parameters, GCF volume and MPO activity increased at diseased sites. The difference in MPO levels among the three periodontal conditions were significant ($p<0.05$). At multi-rooted sites, the clinical parameters, GCF volume and MPO activity increased at diseased sites. MPO activity was increased at both of the diseased groups, however the difference between gingivitis and periodontitis was not significant ($p>0.05$). Correlations regarding the clinical parameters, GCF volume and GCF MPO levels are provided in Table 2. Similar to all sites, significant correlations were mostly observed at diseased sites, and particularly at sites with gingivitis. However, when SR and MR sites were comparatively analyzed, it was observed that not all correlations were absolutely matching and there were some differences in the correlations between SR and MR sites (e.g. between GCF-PI, GCF-PD, MPO-PI, MPO-PD).

MB and DB sites: Table 4 shows descriptive statistical data from MB and DB sites regarding the clinical parameters, GCF volume and GCF MPO levels. For all of the clinical parameters higher scores were observed in the diseased groups than the healthy group and the differences among the three groups were significant at MB and DB sites ($p<0.05$). However there were differences between MB and DB sites regarding GCF volume and MPO activity ($p<0.05$). GCF volume and MPO activity generally was higher at diseased sites than healthy sites ($p<0.05$). At MB sites periodontitis sites had higher GCF volume and MPO activity than gingivitis sites ($p<0.05$), however at DB sites GCF volume and MPO activity presented no significant difference between gingivitis and periodontitis ($p>0.05$). When the MB and DB sites were compared, there were no significant differences in any of the clinical parameters ($p>0.05$).

Table 1. Descriptive statistical data regarding clinical parameters, and GCF volume, and MPO levels for all sampling sites

Categories (n)		PI	PD (mm)	GI	GBTI	GCF(μl)	T-MPO (U/site)	MPO-C (U/μl)
Healthy (175)		0,23 ± 0,43	1,91 ± 0,65	0 ± 0	0 ± 0	0,11 ± ,09	0,216 ± 0,32	2,136 ± 3,010
		(0-2)	(1-3)	(0-0)	(0-0)	(0-0,47)	(0-2,094)	(0-15,197)
Gingivitis (308)		1,33 ± 1,02	2,56 ± 0,55	2,03 ± 0,66	1,94 ± 1,18	0,18 ± 0,13	0,414 ± 0,44	2,559 ± 2,565
		(0-3)	(1-3)	(1-3)	(0-3)	(0,01-0,65)	(0-2,499)	(0-14,404)
Periodontitis (236)		1,78 ± 1,03	4,80 ± 1,29	2,43 ±0,66	2,44 ± 0,93	0,23 ± 0,13	0,548 ± 0,59	2,483 ± 2,448
		(0-3)	(2-11)	(1-3)	(0-3)	(0,01-0,68)	(0-3,298)	(0-19,078)
	X^2	234,228*	500,871*	454,689*	363,987*	127,41*	75,296*	23,739*
Healthy-Gingivitis	z	-12,281*	-10,040*	-19,210*	-15,974*	-7,601*	-6,752*	-4,297*
Healthy-Periodontitis	z	-14,465*	-17,234*	-18,124*	-17,957*	-11,040*	-8,321*	-4,457*
Gingivitis-Periodontitis	z	-5,002*	-19,312*	-7,244*	-5,376*	-4,999*	-2,587**	-0,009

Arithmetic mean ± S.D.(minimum-maximum).

* Significant p<0.001.

** Significant p< 0.05.

Kruskal-Wallis variance analysis was used for differences among groups and Mann-Whitney U-test was used for pairwise comparisons.

Table 2. Correlations between clinical parameters, and GCF volume and MPO levels for all sites and for distinct sampling sites

	sites (n)	measure		PI	PD (mm)	GI	GBTI	GCF (μl)	T-MPO (U/site)
Healthy (n=175)	All sites (175)	GCF-Vr (μl)	r	0.173	0.299	0.014	N/A	1.000	0.464
			p	0.022**	0.0001*	0.851	N/A		0.0001*
		T-MPO (U/site)	r	0.185	0.147	0.120	N/A	0.464	1.000
			p	0.014**	0.051	0.113	N/A	0.0001*	
	Single-rooted (104)	GCF-Vr (μl)	r	0.199	0.359	N/A	N/A	1.000	0.506
			p	0.043**	0.0001*	N/A	N/A		0.0001*
		T-MPO (U/site)	r	0.085	0.184	N/A	N/A	0.506	1.000
			p	0.389	0.062	N/A	N/A	0.0001*	
	Multi-rooted (71)	GCF-Vr (μl)	r	0.171	0.160	-0.009	N/A	1.000	0.386
			p	0.154	0.182	0.942	N/A		0.001**
		T-MPO (U/site)	r	0.384	0.077	0.175	N/A	0.386	1.000
			p	0.001**	0.524	0.144	N/A	0.001**	
	MB (84)	GCF-Vr (μl)	r	0.216	0.269	N/A	N/A	1.000	0.416
			p	0.049**	0.013**	N/A	N/A		0.0001*
		T-MPO (U/site)	r	0.317	0.167	N/A	N/A	0.416	1.000
			p	0.003**	0.129	N/A	N/A	0.0001*	
	DB (91)	GCF-Vr (μl)	r	0.127	0.325	0.016	N/A	1.000	0.496
			p	0.232	0.002**	0.880	N/A		0.0001*
		T-MPO (U/site)	r	0.072	0.109	0.177	N/A	0.496	1.000
			p	0.499	0.304	0.093	N/A	0.0001*	

Table 2. (Continued)

	sites (n)	measure		PI	PD (mm)	GI	GBTI	GCF (µl)	T-MPO (U/site)
Gingivitis (n=308)	All sites (308)	GCF-Vr (µl)	r	0.420	0.214	0.316	0.318	1.000	0.484
			p	0.0001*	0.0001*	0.0001*	0.0001*		0.0001*
		T-MPO (U/site)	r	0.178	0.154	0.336	0.358	0.484	1.000
			p	0.002**	0.0001*	0.0001*	0.0001*	0.0001*	
	Single-rooted (197)	GCF-Vr (µl)	r	0.339	0.184	0.354	0.390	1.000	0.581
			p	0.0001*	0.0001*	0.0001*	0.0001*		0.0001*
		T-MPO (U/site)	r	0.217	0.169	0.360	0.305	0.581	1.000
			p	0.02**	0.018**	0.0001*	0.0001*	0.0001*	
	Multi-rooted (138)	GCF-Vr (µl)	r	0.501	0.281	0.307	0.225	1.000	0.333
			p	0.0001*	0.003**	0.001**	0.018**		0.0001*
		T-MPO (U/site)	r	0.148	0.127	0.289	0.447	0.333	1.000
			p	0.122	0.185	0.002**	0.0001*	0.0001*	
	MB (170)	GCF-Vr (µl)	r	0.380	0.227	0.308	0.300	1.000	0.525
			p	0.0001*	0.0001*	0.0001*	0.0001*		0.0001*
		T-MPO (U/site)	r	0.136	0.216	0.315	0.345	0.525	1.000
			p	0.077	0.005**	0.0001*	0.0001*	0.0001*	
	DB (138)	GCF-Vr (µl)	r	0.457	0.215	0.325	0.339	1.000	0.434
			p	0.0001*	0.011**	0.0001*	0.0001*		0.0001*
		T-MPO (U/site)	r	0.221	0.076	0.354	0.364	0.434	1.000
			p	0.009**	0.377	0.0001*	0.0001*	0.0001*	

Table 2. (Continued)

	sites (n)	measure		PI	PD (mm)	GI	GBTI	GCF (µl)	T-MPO (U/site)
	All sites (236)	GCF-Vr (µl)	r	0.204	0.036	0.148	0.057	1.000	0.442
			p	0.002**	0.582	0.023**	0.386		0.0001*
		T-MPO (U/site)	r	-0.014	0.152	0.205	0.344	0.442	1.000
			p	0.828	0.019**	0.002**	0.0001*	0.0001*	
	Single-rooted (119)	GCF-Vr (µl)	r	0.169	-0,006	0.24	0.089	1.000	0.556
			p	0.042	0.939	0.004	0.288		0.0001*
		T-MPO (U/site)	r	-0.014	0.152	0.292	0.324	0.556	1.000
			p	0.867	0.069	0.0001*	0.0001*	0.0001*	
Periodontitis (n=236)	Multi-rooted (117)	GCF-Vr (µl)	r	0.291	0.131	0.083	0.107	1000	0.412
			p	0.005**	0.217	0.436	0.313		0.0001*
		T-MPO (U/site)	r	-0.062	0.105	-0.005**	0.261	0.412	1000
			p	0.559	0.322	0.964	0.012	0.0001*	
	MB (119)	GCF-Vr (µl)	r	0.187	-0.027	0.151	0.042	1.000	0.435
			p	0.042**	0.771	0.101	0.649		0.0001*
		T-MPO (U/site)	r	0.025	0.148	0.185	0.340	0.435	1.000
			p	0.789	0.148	0.185	0.340	0.435	
	DB (117)	GCF-Vr (µl)	r	0.219	0.089	0.143	0.068	1.000	0.453
			p	0.018**	0.339	0.124	0.467		0.0001*
		T-MPO (U/site)	r	-0.063	0.156	0.220	0.340	0.453	1.000
			p	0.501	0.093	0.017**	0.0001*	0.0001*	

N/A= not available. Spearman's rank order correlation coefficient was used for all correlations.

* Significant $p<0.001$.

** Significant $p< 0.05$.

Table 3. Descriptive statistical data regarding clinical parameters and GCF volume at single-rooted and multi-rooted sites

	Categories (n)		PI	PD (mm)	GI	GBTI	GCF (µl)	T-MPO (U/site)
Single-rooted	Healthy (104)		0.27 ± 0.467	1.83 ± 0.630	0 ± 0	0 ± 0	0.10 ± 0.09	0.192 ± 0.262
			(0-2)	(1-3)	(0-0)	0 ± 0	(0-0.41)	(0-1.520)
	Gingivitis (197)		1.20 ± 1.008	2.53 ± 0.576	2.06 ± 0.675	1.97 ± 1.182	0.17 ± 0.13	0.416 ± 0.454
			(0-3)	(1-3)	(1-3)	(0-3)	(0.01-0.64)	(0-2.499)
	Periodontitis (145)		1.81 ± 0.986	4.88 ± 1.195	2.50 ± 0.614	2.62 ± 0.791	0.21 ± 0.12	0.642 ± 0.649
			(0-3)	(2-9)	(1-3)	(0-3)	(0.01-0.67)	(0-3.298)
		X^2	141.768*	322.753*	279.671*	234.671*	75.337*	62.139*
Multi-rooted	Healthy (71)		0.17 ± 0.377	2.03 ± 0.654	0 ± 0	0 ± 0	0.12 ± 0.09	0.251 ± 0.380
			(0-1)	(1-3)	(0-0)	0 ± 0	(0-0.47)	(0-2.094)
	Gingivitis (111)		1.56 ± 1.009	2.60 ± 0.510	1.97 ± 0.625	1.87 ± 1.192	0.21 ± 0.12	0.411 ± 0 .419
			(0-3)	(2-3)	(1-3)	(0-3)	(0.02-0.65)	(0-1.798)
	Periodontitis (91)		1.74 ± 1.094	4.68 ± 1.429	2.31 ± 0.710	2.15 ± 1.064	0.25 ± 0.13	0.399 ± 0.443
			(0-3)	(2-11)	(1-3)	(0-3)	(0.03-0.68)	(0-2.169)
		X^2	98.819*	177.755*	175.726*	133.183*	56.717*	19.857*
Single-rooted	Healthy-Gingivitis	z	-8.451*	-8.367*	-14.981*	-12.416*	-5.422*	-5.444*
	Healthy-Periodontitis	z	-11.369*	-13.540*	-14.177*	-14.323*	-8.598*	-7.599*
	Gingivitis-Periodontitis	z	-5.511*	-15.654*	-6.146*	-5.653*	-4.293*	-3.596*
Multi-rooted	Healthy-Gingivitis	z	-9.028*	-5.713*	-11.985*	-10.019*	-5.746*	-4.042*
	Healthy-Periodontitis	z	-8.921*	-10.565*	-11.276*	-10.905*	-7.038*	-3.860*
	Gingivitis-Periodontitis	z	-1.166	-11.282*	-3.971*	-1.744	-2.701**	-0.382
Single-rooted vs. multi-rooted	Healthy	z	-1.434	-2.008**	-1.210	0.0001	-1.654	-0.783
	Gingivitis	z	-3.176**	-0.884	-1.077	-0.630	-3.169**	-0.061
	Periodontitis	z	-0.467	-1.491	-2.169**	-3.640*	-2.413**	-3.361**

Arithmetic mean ± S.D.(minimum-maximum). Kruskal-Wallis variance analysis was used for differences among groups and Mann-Whitney *U*-test was used for pairwise comparisons.

* Significant $p<0.001$.

** Significant $p< 0.05$.

Table 4. Descriptive statistical data regarding clinical parameters and GCF volume at mesio-buccal and disto-buccal sites

	Categories (n)		PI	PD (mm)	GI	GBTI	GCF (µl)	T-MPO (U/site)
MB	Healthy (84)		0,23 ± 0,421	1,90 ± 0,652	0 ± 0	0 ± 0	0,10 ±0,08	0,236 ± 0,383
			(0-1)	(1-3)	(0-0)	(0-0)	(0-0,47)	(0-2,094)
	Gingivitis (170)		1,28 ± 1,012	2,56 ± 0,565	2,01 ± 0,648	1,91 ± 1,196	0,17 ± 0,11	0,393 ±0,427
			(0-3)	(1-3)	(1-3)	(0-3)	(0,01-0,64)	(0-2,101)
	Periodontitis (119)		1,80 ± 1,046	4,82 ± 1,228	2,48 ± 0,609	2,50 ± 0,901	0,23 ±0,12	0,578 ± 0,,601
			(0-3)	(2-10)	(1-3)	(0-3)	(0,04-0,67)	(0-3,129)
		X^2	113,807*	257,225*	233,893*	183,177*	78,242*	41,361*
DB	Healthy (91)		0,23 ± 0,449	1,91 ± 0,644	0 ±0	0 ± 0	0,11 ± 0,09	0,197 ±0,238
			(0-2)	(1-3)	(0-0)	(0-0)	(0-0,41)	(0-1,177)
	Gingivitis (138)		1,39 ± 1,035	2,55 ± 0,541	2,06 ± 0,670	1,96 ± 1,174	0,20 ±0,14	0,441 ± 0,458
			(0-3)	(1-3)	(1-3)	(0-3)	(0,01-0,65)	(0-2,499)
	Periodontitis (117)		1,77 ± 1,012	4,79 ± 1,357	2,38 ± 0,704	2,38 ±0,962	0,22 ±0,13	0,518 ± 0,578
			(0-3)	(2-11)	(1-3)	(0-3)	(0,01-0,68)	(0-3,298)
		X^2	120,854*	242,818*	220,464*	180,964*	53,612*	35,682*
MB	Healthy-Gingivitis	z	-8,429*	-7,167*	-13,669*	-11,144*	-5,432*	-4,566*
	Healthy-Periodontitis	z	-10,051*	-12,066*	-12,810*	-12,722*	-8,409*	-6,247*
	Gingivitis-Periodontitis	z	-4,079*	-14,037*	-6,075*	-4,601*	-5,048*	2,756**
DB	Healthy-Gingivitis	z	-8,943*	-6,986*	-13,429*	-11,414*	-5,519*	-5,073*
	Healthy-Periodontitis	z	-10,377*	-12,271*	-12,787*	-12,654*	-7,172*	-5,488*
	Gingivitis-Periodontitis	z	-2,907**	-13,219*	4,106*	-2,973**	-1,828	-0,826
MB vs. DB	Healthy	z	-0,062	-0,081	-0,961	0,0001	-0,71	-0,326
	Gingivitis	z	-0,926	-0,287	-0,773	-0,36	-2,0267**	-1,121
	Periodontitis	z	-0,244	-0,565	-0,992	-1,239	-0,581	-0,810

Arithmetic mean ± S.D.(minimum-maximum); Kruskal-Wallis variance analysis was used for differences among groups and Mann-Whitney *U*-test was used for pairwise comparisons; * Significant $p<0.001$; ** Significant $p< 0.05$.

Table 5. Statistical data regarding the distinct sampling sites as single-rooted and multi-rooted plus mesio-buccal and disto-buccal

		Categories (n)	PI	PD (mm)	GI	GBTI	GCF (µl)	T-MPO (U/site)
Healthy	MB	Single-rooted (48)	0.27 ± 0.449 (0-1)	1.87 ± 0.672 (1-3)	0.00 ± 0.000 (0-0)	0.00 ± 0.000 (0-0)	0.09 ± 0.065 (0-0.27)	0.181 ± 0.283 (0-1.52)
		Multi-rooted (36)	0.17 ± 0.378 (0-1)	1.94 ± 0630 (1-3)	0.00 ± 0.000 (0-0)	0.00 ± 0.000 (0-0)	0.12 ± 0.099 (02-0.47)	0.31 ± 0.480 (0-21)
	DB	Single-rooted (56)	0.27 ± 0.486 (0-2)	1.79 ± 0.594 (1-3)	0.00 ± 0.000 (0-0)	0.00 ± 0.000 (0-0)	0.011 ± 0.098 (0-0.41)	0.20 0.245 (0-1.18)
		Multi-rooted (35)	0.17 ± 0.382 (0-1)	2.11 ± 0.676 (1-3)	0.03 ± 0169 (0-1)	0.00 ± 0.000 (0-0)	0.11 ± 0.089 (0-0.37)	0.20 ± 0.231 (0-0.90)
Gingivitis	MB	Single-rooted (107)	1.20 ± 995 (0-3)	2.51 ± 0.589 (1-3)	2.01 ± 0.680 (1-3)	1.92 ± 1.214 (0-3)	0.15 ± 0.119 (0.1-0.64)	0.38 ± 0.409 (0-2.10)
		Multi-rooted (62)	1.42 ± 1.033 (0-3)	2.63 ± 0.517 (2-4)	2.00 ± 0.596 (1-3)	1.90 ± 1.174 (0-3)	0.19 ± 0.132 (0.3-0.57)	0.48 ± 0.457 (0-1.80)
	DB	Single-rooted (90)	1.20 ± 1.030 (0-3)	2.54 ± 0.564 (1-4)	2.12 ± 0.668 (1-3)	2.03 ± 1.146 (0-3)	0.18 ± 0.132 (0.1-0.56)	0.46 ± 0.501 (0-2.499)
		Multi-rooted (48)	1.75 ± 0.957 (0-3)	2.56 ± 0.501 (2-3)	1.94 ± 0.665 (0-3)	1.83 ± 1.226 (0-3)	0.24 ± 0.144 (0.2-0.65)	0.40 ± 0.367 (0-1.681)
Periodontitis	MB	Single-rooted (70)	1.83 ± 1.1021 (0-3)	5.03 ± 1.154 (3-8)	2.56 ± 0.555 (1-3)	2.70 ± 0.729 (0-3)	0.21 ± 0.116 (0.6-0.67)	0.69 ± 0.674 (0-3.129)
		Multi-rooted (49)	1.76 ± 1.090 (0-3)	4.51 ± 1.277 (2-10)	2.37 ± 0.668 (0-3)	2.22 ± 1.046 (0-3)	0.26 ± 1.130 (0.4-0.61)	0.41 ± 0.435 (0.26-1.677)
	DB	Single-rooted (75)	1.80 ± 0.959 (0-3)	4.73 ± 1.223 (2-9)	2.45 ± 0.664 (0-3)	2.55 ± 0.843 (0-3)	0.21 ± 1.122 (0.1-0.58)	0.59 ± 0.625 (0-3.298)
		Multi-rooted (42)	1.71 ± 1.111 (0-3)	4.88 ± 1.580 (2-11)	2.45 ± 0.759 (0-3)	2.07 ± 1.091 (0-3)	0.24 ± 0.136 (0.3-0.68)	0.38 ± 04457 (0-2.169)

Table 5. (Continued)

		Categories (n)	PI	PD (mm)	GI	GBTI	GCF (µl)	T-MPO (U/site)
Healthy	MB	Single-rooted Multi-rooted	-1.123	-0.508	0.0001	-1.830	-1.830	-1.027
	DB	Single-rooted Multi-rooted	-0.909	-2.325**	-1.265	0.0001	-0.552	-0.004
Gingivitis	MB	Single-rooted Multi-rooted	-1.464	-1.067	-0.095	-0.088	-2.400**	-0.053
	DB	Single-rooted Multi-rooted	-3.136**	-0.116	-1.464	-0.834	-2.147**	-0.013
Periodontitis	MB	Single-rooted Multi-rooted	-0.334	-2.365**	-1.548	-2.772**	-2.280**	-2,675**
	DB	Single-rooted Multi-rooted	-0.346	-0.204	-1.602	-2.494**	-1.066	-2.083**
Healthy	Single-rooted	MB DB	-0.184	-0.642	0.0001	0.0001	-1.055	-0.689
	Multi-rooted	MB DB	-0.053	-1.101	-1.014	0.0001	-0.219	-0.311
Gingivitis	Single-rooted	MB DB	-0.067	-0.167	-1.165	-0.589	-1.609	-0.961
	Multi-rooted	MB DB	-1.641	-0.688	-0.401	-0.260	-1.963**	-0.610
Periodontitis	Single-rooted	MB DB	-0.215	-1.649	-0.825	-1.341	-0.091	-0.995
	Multi-rooted	MB DB	-0.170	-0.968	-0.766	-0.742	-0.988	-0.239

Arithmetic mean ± S.D.(minimum-maximum); Mann-Whitney *U*-test was used for pairwise comparisons.
* Significant $p<0.001$; ** Significant $p< 0.05$.

No difference in healthy and periodontitis groups were observed regarding GCF volume and MPO activity (p>0.05). However, GCF volume at DB (0.20 μl) sites with gingivitis was higher than MB (0,17 μl) sites (p=0.039). Correlations regarding the clinical parameters, GCF volume and GCF MPO levels are provided in Table 2. Again, significant correlations were mostly observed at diseased sites, particularly at sites with gingivitis. However, when MB and DB sites were comparatively analyzed, it was observed that not all correlations were absolutely matching and there were some differences between DB and MB sites in the significant correlations (e.g. between MPO-PI, MPO-PD, GCF-PI).

MB and DB sites of single-rooted and multi-rooted teeth: When the 719 sites were further grouped as single-rooted and multi-rooted plus MB and DB sites, analysis confirmed the site-specific nature of both GCF and MPO activity and revealed that differences could be observed in GCF volume and local MPO production at these distinct sites (Table 5).

Discussion

In the present study, GCF volume presented with a disease-related spectrum; healthy < gingivitis < periodontitis). GCF volume also exhibited significant correlations with the clinical parameters, especially the parameters reflecting the clinical inflammatory status of the site (GI, GBTI). This was particularly observed at the diseased sites. These findings are in line with the previous studies which underlined the impact of the gingival inflammation [1-10, 12, 46], and periodontitis and pathological pockets [6-8, 11, 18, 21, 24] on the volumetric features of GCF.

Although the mean GCF volume had a disease-related spectrum and clearly discriminated the three clinical categories from each other (healthy: 0.11μl, gingivitis: 0.18 μl, and periodontitis 0.23 μl) , at the individual sites GCF volume presented with a wide range of distribution and clear overlaps among the three categories: healthy (0.0-0.47 μl), gingivitis (0.01-0.65 μl), periodontitis (0.01-0.68 μl). Previous studies are available highlighting the great variations in the volumetric features of GCF at sites with a similar clinical appearance [6, 7, 9, 12-15, 19]. It has been shown that under similar conditions, more GCF is available at interproximal than buccal [6], posterior than anterior [7, 9, 14], mandibular than maxillary [12], upper molar teeth than lower canine [19], interproximal posterior sites than anterior labial sites [8] , and interproximal sites of multi-rooted teeth than single-rooted teeth [15]. Even some volumetric differences were found between interproximal MB and DB sites [15], and the limited validity of GCF volume in the discrimination between gingivitis and periodontitis sites was suggested [15]. As similar differences between single-rooted and multi-rooted, and MB and DB sites were observed, the present study generally support the evidence for great fluctuations in GCF volume at distinct sampling sites [6, 7, 9, 12, 13, 15, 19]. Such significant volumetric variances may highlight the impact of standardization of the distinct location of the sampling-site on improvement of reliability [7, 9, 12]. These site-specific fluctuations also remind for caution when interpreting the clinical meaning of the GCF volume at an individual site [14, 15, 24].

Based on the findings of most studies suggesting the preference of total activity mode of data presentation, in the present study only the total MPO activity was considered when interpreting the GCF MPO profile. The generally increased GCF MPO activity at diseased sites observed in the present study is not a new finding as the role of MPO in periodontal diseases was highlighted in many of the previous studies, where GCF MPO levels were generally shown to increase with the severity of periodontal diseases [25, 35, 37-38, 43], and decrease following periodontal treatment [36, 38]. The increased MPO activity was attributed to the increased number of neutrophils and to their degranulation as a result of the increased antigenic stimulus in periodontal diseases [43].

In the present study, GCF MPO content also exhibited a disease-related spectrum; healthy < gingivitis < periodontitis. However, this pattern could be detected via the statistical analysis where all sites were included and these sites were broadly categorized as healthy, gingivitis and periodontitis. On the other hand, when the distinct teeth groups and distinct sampling sites (single-rooted vs. multi-rooted sites, or MB vs. DB sites) were concerned, differences were observed in GCF MPO activity and its pattern. Further, in the present study approximately 7% of the sites lacked detectable amount of MPO. On the contrary to the lack of GCF only at healthy sites, sites lacking detectable levels of MPO were not solely healthy sites (13.7%), but also involved sites with gingivitis (5.8%) and periodontitis (2.5%). There also were clear overlaps between the healthy (0-2.094 U/site), gingivitis (0-2.449 U/site) and periodontitis (0-3.298 U/site) sites. All of these findings address the apparent variations in GCF MPO activity among the individual sites and the need for further interest and concern regarding the site-specific nature of the enzymatic profile of this biologic fluid.

While limited correlations were observed at healthy sites, at diseased sites GCF MPO generally presented positive and significant correlations with the clinical parameters, in particular with the clinical parameters reflecting the inflammatory response (GI, GBTI, GCF volume). There is likely to be some discrepancies among the previous studies regarding the correlations between the clinical parameters, GCF volume and GCF MPO activity. Positive and strong [46], moderate [55] correlations between gingival inflammation and GCF flow, weak correlations between GCF volume and the clinical parameters [36], and lack of constant correlations between the clinical measures and GCF volume [14] are all reported. On the other hand, studies that reveal a positive correlation between MPO and some clinical [25, 35, 37, 38, 43] and microbiological parameters [38], weak correlations with the clinical parameters and GCF volume [36], a significant correlation between GI scores and GCF MPO activity [37] and no association [36] are all available. The lack of correlations between GCF volume and the clinical parameters was attributed to the fact that GCF volume and clinical parameters could act as two different measures [14] , and volumetric features of GCF are suggested as early and reliable measures of gingival inflammation than most clinical parameters [14, 24]. When MPO profile of GCF was concerned, the weak correlations of MPO activity, GCF volume and the clinical parameters were suggested to be related to the possibility that the magnitude of neutrophil migration and GCF volume could vary at sites with gingivitis and periodontitis [36].

Despite the general positive correlations at all sites between GCF volume, the clinical parameters reflecting inflammatory status, and the GCF MPO activity, discrepancies regarding the presence/absence of GCF and MPO existed at individual sites. At sites lacking MPO, detectable amounts of GCF was available. While all of the sites that lacked detectable amount of GCF (PU=0) was the non-inflamed sites, there were periodontally-diseased sites that lacked detectable MPO activity. This finding indicates that despite the overall positive correlation at all sites, an absolute correlation between GCF volume and its MPO content may not be expected at all sites and at all periodontal circumstances. An explanation for this discrepancy may be the flow of GCF (e.g. an osmotically-mediated process in response to any kind of bacterial or mechanical irritation) and the migration of neutrophils (e.g. in response to chemotactic factors) to be two distinct phenomenon under the control of different regulatory mechanisms [1]. The discrepancy also may be associated with the variances in the severity of sub-clinical inflammation [14] and the presence/availability of bacteria within the sulci at the individual sites. Based on the fact that only clinically-healthy sites lacked detectable amount of GCF, while there were diseased sites that lacked MPO activity, it may be speculated that lack of GCF could be more related than MPO with site-specific periodontal health [15].

Further, this may be interpreted as a limitation of the diagnostic value of GCF MPO as a site-specific measure. Despite the generally higher GCF MPO levels at the diseased sites, GCF MPO levels did not seem to serve for a clear-cut discrimination among periodontal disease forms (e.g. chronic periodontitis and aggressive periodontitis) [35]. In the present study, when distinct sampling sites, such as single-rooted and multi-rooted, and MB and DB, and the MB and DB sites of single-rooted and multi-rooted teeth were concerned, correlations between GCF and clinical parameters and between MPO activity and clinical parameters also presented variances among these distinct sampling sites. These findings also support the site-specific nature of GCF volume, GCF MPO profile, and may also suggest the possibility that the relationship of these measures with the clinical periodontal status may also be site-specific.

It seems that study designs using broad categories are likely to provide limited information regarding the individual sites and the site-specific GCF MPO profile or even may underestimate the great fluctuations in GCF volume and its enzymatic content among individuals and sites. There is no doubt that both the GCF volume and its MPO content are related to pathogenesis of periodontal diseases [1, 4-10, 11, 25, 35-37, 38]. However, the clear fluctuations in GCF volume and MPO production among the sites, and the discrepancy of these two measures on a site-specific basis needs to be taken into account for more correct interpretation of the GCF-related data. Sampling of as many sites as possible and attempts for the standardization of the distinct sampling area may serve for more reliability and for a better understanding of the dynamics of this biologic fluid. On the other hand, besides its MPO profile, the possibility of other GCF components to also present with such similar site-specific variances also needs to be considered. It is clear that, a better clarification of the distinct site-specific nature of GCF (volume and content) is likely to be an advantage when dealing with site-specific pathologies, likewise periodontal diseases.

ACKNOWLEDGMENT

This study is supported by the grant 05 T0 9102002 from The Research Foundation of Hacettepe University.

References

[1] Kowashi Y, Jaccard F and Cimasoni G. Sulcular polymorphonuclear leukocytes and gingival exudate during experimental gingivitis in man. *J. Periodontal. Res.* 1980; 15:151-158.

[2] Tsuchida K, Hara K. Clinical significance of gingival fluid measurements by Periotron. *J. Periodontol.* 1981; 52: 697-700.

[3] Cimasoni G. *Crevicular fluid updated.* 2 nd ed Basel Newyork: Krager; 1983; 29-45.

[4] Lamster, IB, Oshrain RL, Gordon JM. Enzyme activity in human gingival crevicular fluid: considerations in data reporting based on analysis of individual crevicular sites. *J. Clin. Periodontol.* 1986; 13:799-804.

[5] Lamster, IB, Oshrain, RL, Florello, et al. A comparison of four methods of data presentation for lysosomal enzyme activity in gingival crevicular fluid. *J. Clin. Periodonto*l. 1988; 15, 347-352.

[6] Lamster IB, Oshrain RL, Ceelenti R, et al. Correlation analysis for clinical and gingival crevicular fluid parameters at anatomically related sites. *J. Clin. Periodontol.* 1991; 18: 272-277.

[7] Smith QT, Au GS, Freese PL, et al. Five parameters of gingival crevicular fluid from eight surfaces in periodontal health and disease. *J. Periodontal. Res.* 1992; 27:466-475.

[8] Booth V, Young S, Cruchley A, et al. Vascular endothelial growth factor in human periodontal disease. J. *Periodontal. Res.* 1998; 33:491-499.

[9] Özkavaf A, Aras H, Huri CB, Yamalık N, et al. Relationship between quantity of gingival crevicular fluid and clinical periodontal status. *J. Oral Sci.* 2000; 42:231-238.

[10] Özkavaf A, Aras H, Huri CB, Yamalık N, et al. Analysis of factors that may affect the enzymatic profile of gingival crevicular fluid: sampling technique, sequential sampling and mode of data presentation. *J. Oral Sci.* 2001; 43:41-48.

[11] Jin L, Yu C, Corbet ET. Granulocyte elastase activity in static and flow gingival crevicular fluid. *J. Periodontal. Res.* 2003; 38:303-310.

[12] Smith QT, Geegan SJ. Repeated measurements of crevicular fluid parameters at different sites. *J. Clin. Periodontol.* 1991; 18: 171-176.

[13] Page RC. Host response tests for diagnosing periodontal disease. *J. Periodontol.* 1992; 63:356-366.

[14] Griffiths GS. Formation, collection and significance of gingival crevicular fluid. *Periodontology 2000* 2003; 31: 32-42.

[15] Hatipoglu H, Yamalik N, Berberoğlu A, et al. Impact of the distinct sampling area on volumetric features of gingival crevicular fluid. *J. Periodontol.* 2007; 78:705-715.

[16] Persson GR, Page RC. Effect of sampling time and repetition on gingival crevicular fluid and aspartate aminotransferase. *J. Periodontal. Res.* 1990; 25:236-242.

[17] Tozum TF, Hatipoglu H, Yamalik N, et al. Critical steps in electronic volume quantification of gingival crevicular fluid: the potential impact of evaporation, fluid retention, local conditions and repeated measurements. *J. Periodontal. Res.* 2004; 39: 344-357.

[18] Uitto VJ, Overall CM, McCulloch C. Proteolytic host cell enzymes in gingival crevicular fluid. *Periodontology* 2000 2003; 31: 77-104.

[19] Griffiths GS, Sterne JAC, Wilton JMA, et al. Association between volume and flow rate of GCF and clinical assessments of gingival inflammation in a population of British male adolescents. *J. Clin. Periodontol.* 1992; 19:464-470.
[20] Matthias B, Cimasoni G. The pH of human crevicular fluid measured by a new microanalytical technique. *J. Periodontal. Res.* 1985; 20: 35-40.
[21] Villela B, Cogen RB, Batolucci AA, et al. Crevicular fluid collagenase activity in healthy, gingivitis, chronic adult periodontitis and localized juvenile periodontitis patients. *J. Periodontal. Res.* 1987; 22: 209-211.
[22] Curtis MA, Griffiths GS, Price SJ, et al. The total protein concentration of gingival crevicular fluid. Variation with sampling time and gingival inflammation. *J. Clin. Periodontol.* 1988; 15:628-632.
[23] Champagne CM, Buchanan W, Reddy MS, et al. Potential for gingival crevice fluid measures as predictors of risk for periodontal diseases. *J. Periodontol.* 2000 2003; 31: 167-180.
[24] Goodson JM. Gingival crevicular fluid flow. *Periodontology* 2000 2003; 31: 43-54.
[25] Cao CF, Smith QT. Crevicular fluid myeloperoxidase at healthy, gingivitis and periodontitis sites. *J. Clin. Periodontol.* 1989;16:17-20.
[26] Eiserich JP, Hristova M, Cross CE, et al. Formation of nitric oxide-derived inflammatory oxidants by myeloperoxidase in neutrophils. *Nature* 1998; 391:393-397.
[27] Klebanoff SJ. Myeloperoxidase-halide-hydrogen peroxide antibacterial system. *J. Bacteriol.* 1968; 95:2131-2138.
[28] Miyasaki KT, Wilson ME, Brunetti AJ, et al. Oxidative and nonoxidative killing of Actinobacillus actinomycetemcomitans by the human neutrophils. *Infect. Immun.* 1986; 53:154-160.
[29] Miyasaki KT, Wilson ME, Genco RJ. Killing of Actinobacillus actinomycetemcomitans by the human neutrophil myeloperoxidase-hydrogen peroxide-chloride system. *Infect. Immun.* 1986; 53: 161-165.
[30] Delima AJ, Van Dyke TE. Origin and function of the cellular components in gingival crevicular fluid. *Periodontol.* 2000 2003; 31:55-76.
[31] McRipley RJ, Sbarra AJ. Role of phagocyte in host-parasite interactions XII. Hydrogen peroxide-myeloperoxidase bactericidal system in the phagocyte. *J. Bacteriol.* 1967; 94:1425-1430.
[32] Thomas EL. Myeloperoxidase, hydrogen peroxide, chloride antimicrobial system: Nitrogen-chlorine derivatives of bacterial components in bactericidal action against Escheria coli. *Infect Immun.* 1979; 23:522-531.
[33] Nicholls SJ, Hazen SL. Myeloperoxidase and cardiovascular disease. *Arterioscler. Thromb. Vasc. Biol.* 2005; 25:1102-1111.
[34] Dedon PC, Tannenbaum SR. Reactive nitrogen species in the chemical biology of inflammation. *Arch. Biochem. Biophys.* 2004;423:12-22.
[35] Yamalik N, Çağlayan F, Kilinc K, et al. The importance of data presentation regarding gingival crevicular fluid myeloperoxidase and elastase-like activity in periodontal disease and health status. *J. Periodontol.* 2000; 71:460-467.
[36] Smith QT, Hinrichs JE, Melynk RS. Gingival crevicular fluid myeloperoxidase at periodontitis sites. *J. Periodontol. Res.* 1986; 21:45-56.
[37] Kowolik MJ, Grant M. Myeloperoxidase activity in human gingival crevicular neutrophils. *Arch. Oral Biol.* 1983; 28:293-295.

[38] Wolff LE, Smith QT, Synder WK, et al. Relationship between lactate dehydrogenase and myeloperoxidase levels in human gingival crevicular fluid and clinical and microbiological measurements. *J. Clin. Periodontol.* 1988; 15:110-115.
[39] Weiss SJ. Tissue breakdown by neutrophils. *N. Engl. J. Med.* 1989; 320: 365-376.
[40] Clark RA, Stone PJ, Hag AE, et al. Myeloperoxidase-catalyzed inactivation of alpha-1 protease inhibitor by human neutrophils. *J. Biol. Chem.* 256:3348-3353, 1981.
[41] Boutros SM, Michalowicz BS, Smith QT, et al. Crevicular fluid enzymes from endosseous dental implants and natural teeth. *Int. J. Oral. Maxillofac Implants* 1996; 11:322-330.
[42] Liskmann S, Zilmer M, Vihalemm T, et al. Correlation of peri-implant health and myeloperoxidase levels: a cross-sectional clinical study. *Clin. Oral Implants Res.* 2004; 15:546-552.
[43] Över C, Yamalik N, Yavuzyılmaz E, et al. Myeloperoxidase activity in peripheral blood neutrophil, crevicular fluid and whole saliva of patients with periodontal disease. *J. Nihon Univ. Sch. Dent.* 1993; 35:235-240.
[44] Löe H. The gingival index, the plaque index and the retention index systems. *J. Periodontol.* 1967; 38:610-616.
[45] Nowicki D, Vogel RI, Melcer S, et al. The gingival bleeding time index. *J. Periodontol.* 1981; 52:260-262.
[46] Rüdin HJ, Overdiek, HF, Rateitschack, KH. Correlations between sulcus fluid rate and clinical and histological inflammation of the marginal gingiva. *Helv. Odonto Acta* 1970; 14, 21-26.
[47] Chapple IL, Landini G, Griffiths GS, et al. Calibration of Periotron 8000 and 6000 by polynomial regression. *J. Periodontal. Res.* 1999; 34: 79-86.
[48] Ciantar M, Caruana DJ. Periotron 8000: Calibration characteristics and reliability. *J. Periodontal. Res.* 1998; 33: 259-264.
[49] Deinzer R, Mossanen BS, Herforth A. Methodological considerations in the assessment of gingival crevicular fluid volume. *J. Clin. Periodontol.* 2000; 27:481-488.
[50] Suzuki K, Ota H, Sasagawa S, et al. Assay method for myeloperoxidase in human polymorphonuclear leukocytes. *Anal. Biochem.* 1983; 132: 345-352.
[51] Siegel S, Castelan NJ. *Nonparametric statistic for the behavioral sciences*. 2nd ed, New York: McGraw-Hill Inc; 1988; 144-244.

In: Clinical Dentistry
Editor: Scardina Giuseppe Alessandro

ISBN: 978-1-61122-354-5
© 2011 Nova Science Publishers, Inc.

Chapter 5

EPIDEMIOLOGY OF MAXILLOFACIAL TRAUMA AND ASSOCIATED FACTORS IN PATIENTS AGED 1-18 YEARS[#]

***Alessandro Leite Cavalcanti*[*1], *Priscilla Kelly, Medeiros Bezerra*[2] *and David Moraes de Oliveira*[3]**

[1]DDS, MSc, PhD, Professor, Department of Pediatric Dentistry, School of Dentistry, State University of Paraíba, Campina Grande, Brazil
[2]Undergraduate student, Department of Pediatric Dentistry, School of Dentistry, State University of Paraíba, Campina Grande, Brazil
[3]Post-graduate student, Bucomaxillofacial Surgery and Traumatology Program, School of Dentistry, University of Pernambuco, Camaragibe, Brazil

ABSTRACT

Aim: A retrospective study was undertaken to assess causes of maxillofacial trauma in Recife, Pernambuco, Brazil.

Method: A review of 126 patients with maxillofacial injuries aged 1 and 18 years old seen and treated at the Hospital da Restauração between January and December 2006 was conducted and were analyzed according to age, sex, etiology, site of fracture, dentoalveolar trauma and alcohol abuse. Analysis was made in Epi Info using the Chi-square and Fisher's Exact Tests.

Results: It was found that maxillofacial injuries were most frequent in males (69%) and in the 11-18 year age group (50.8%). Falls (34.1%) and pedestrian accidents (19%) were the most common aetiological factor. The most common facial fracture was

---

[#] A version of this book was also published as a chapter in *International Journal of Clinical Dentistry, Volume 1, Issue 1*, published by Nova Science Publishers, Inc. It was submitted for appropriate modifications in an effort to encourage wider dissemination of research.

* Address Correspondence and Reprint Requests to: Prof. Dr. Alessandro Leite Cavalcanti, Avenida Manoel Moraes, 471/802 – Manaíra, 58038-230 João Pessoa, PB, Brasil. Phone: +55 83 3315-3326. E-mail: dralessandro@ibest.com.br

mandible (40%), followed by the zygomatic-orbital complex (23.1%). A positive association between the presence of facial fracture and age (P=0.000) and alcohol consumption was strongly associated with facial fracture (P = .008). Dentoalveolar injuries were present in 14.3% of patients.

Conclusion: The incidence of facial fractures in children is higher than previously reported elsewhere. There were most common in male patients, mainly due to falls and pedestrian accidents. Therefore, strategies to prevent pedestrian related accidents need to be identified, evaluated, and implemented.

Keywords: Epidemiology. Pediatric dentistry. Surgery, Oral. Jaw fractures.

Introduction

Injuries to the craniomaxillofacial area affect a significant number of trauma patients, and consequences of trauma to this region can include any combination of dental, bone, or soft tissue injury [1].

The aetiology and incidence of facial fractures are influenced by social, cultural and environmental factors and hence vary from one country to another [2]. The incidence of facial fractures is higher in boys than in girls [3, 4]. Road traffic accidents, sporting injuries, falls and assaults have been reported to be the most common causes of maxillofacial fractures [1, 5, 6].

The location of a facial fracture depends on the cause and force of the injury as well as the child's stage of development [2]. Anatomically, the most frequently encountered pediatric facial fracture is the mandible, followed by the midface and the upper face [3, 7].

Although few studies on paediatric maxillofacial fractures from Brazil are found in medical literature [8, 9].

The aim of the present study was to analyze the etiology and pattern of craniomaxillofacial injuries in children aged 1 and 18 years in the Recife City, Pernambuco, Brazil.

Methods

The protocol was approved by the State University of Paraiba ethics review committee. The records of all children with facial injuries between the ages of 1 and 18 years who were treated at the Hospital da Restauração, Recife, Brazil, between the beginning of January 2006 and the end of December 2006 were retrospectively examined.

Patients were stratified into two ages classes for analysis. The first stratum encompasses patients from 1 to 10 years (Group A) and the second from 11 to 18 years of age (Group B). Data were analyzed according to age, sex, etiology of the injury, anatomic location of facial fractures, dentoalveolar injury and alcohol abuse.

The etiology was classified as: traffic accidents (cars, motorcycles and pedestrian), physical violence, accidental falls, sports accidents, weapon injuries (knife and fire gun), bicycle accidents and other causes. Mandibular fractures were grouped into condylar, coronoid, ramus, angle, body, parasymphyseal, symphyseal, and dentoalveolar. Dentoalveolar injuries included: avulsion, tooth fracture, luxation and concussion.

Data analysis included descriptive statistics such as frequency distribution and cross tabulation. Comparisons of data were evaluated statistically using the Chi-square and Fisher's Exact Tests at a significance level of 5% ($p<0.05$). Odds ratio (OR) with confidence intervals to 95% were calculated (IC95%). They were calculated using the Epi Info Software (Centers for Disease Control and Prevention, CDC, Atlanta, USA).

RESULTS

Age and Sex Distribution

The average age was 9.7 (SD 5.3 years). There were 87 boys (69%) and 39 girls (31%), a ratio of 2.2:1. Sixty-two children (49.2%) were aged 10 years or younger, and 64 (50.8%) were between 11 and 18 years (Table 1). The ratio of males to females varied considerably with each age and the overall distribution showed that the ratio of males to females in Group A was 1.9:1, but the ratio of males to females in Group B was 2.5:1.

Table 1. Distribution of patients by sex and age

Sex	Age				Total	
	Group A		Group B			
	n	%	n	%	n	%
Male	41	47.1	46	52.9	87	69.0
Female	21	53.8	18	46.2	39	31.0
TOTAL	62	49.2	64	50.8	126	100.0

Etiology

On closer examination, obvious differences between the ages in the causes of fracture are readily apparent (Table 2).

Table 2. Patterns of cause varied by age

Cause	Age				Total	
	Group A		Group B			
	n	%	n	%	n	%
Falls	30	69.8	13	30.2	43	34.1
Bicycle accidents	6	50.0	6	50.0	12	9.5
Physical violence	-	-	3	100.0	3	2.4
Traffic accidents/car	3	60.0	2	40.0	5	4.0
Traffic accidents/motorcycle	-	-	5	100.0	5	4.0
Traffic accidents/pedestrian	11	45.8	13	54.2	24	19.0
Fire gun	1	6.2	15	93.8	16	12.7

Table 2. (Continued)

Cause	Age				Total	
	Group A		Group B			
	n	%	n	%	n	%
Knife	4	80.0	1	20.0	5	4.0
Sports accidents	-	-	2	100.0	2	1.6
Animal attacks	1	50.0	1	50.0	2	1.6
Other	6	66,7	3	33,3	9	7.1
Total	62	49.2	64	50.8	126	100.0

The most frequent cause was a fall, with 43 cases (34.1%), followed by pedestrian accidents with 24 cases (19%). The third most common cause was fire gun (16 cases; 12.7%). Accidental falls were the most causes of facial injuries in children of 10 years or less (Group A). However, in Group B, the causes of the trauma were more diverse. All violence-associated trauma and motorcycle and 93.7% of the fire gun-related injuries occurred in children older than 10 years. There were two accidents related to animal attacks.

Type and Location of Fractures

A total of 65 facial fractures were diagnosed in the 44 patients (34.9%). This sample consisted of 30 boys (68.2%) and 14 girls (31.8%) and no statistically significant difference between sex and facial fracture was found (P = .961). Thirty-two patients (72.7%) sustained single fractures, whereas twelve patients (27.3%) had multiple (two or more) fractures. The only case of five facial fractures in a patient was recorded in a 17-year-old boy.

The most common facial fracture was mandible (40%), followed by the zygomatic-orbital complex (23.1%), maxilla (13.8%), frontal (10.8%), nasal (6.1%) and naso-orbital-ethmoid (6.1%). The most common mandibular fracture site were the angle (21.4%), the condyle (21.4%), the symphyseal and parasymphyseal regions (21.4%), the body (17.8%), the ramus (7.2%), the mandibular dentoalveolar (7.2%), and the coronoid (3.6%).

The table 3 shows a positive association between the presence of facial fracture and age (P=0.000). According to these data, children between 11 and 18 years (Group B) have 5.89 times more chance of have facial fracture. Alcohol consumption was strongly associated with facial fracture (P = .008) (Table 4). According to these data, patients who reported drinking alcohol have 16.04 times more chance of have facial fracture.

Table 3. Distribution of the children according to the age and the presence of facial fracture

Age	Facial Fracture				P value[1]	Odds Ratio (IC=95%)
	Yes		No			
	n	%	n	%		
Group A	10	16.1	52	83.9		1
Group B	34	53.1	30	46.9	P=0.000*	5.89 (2.55-13.59)
Total	44	34.9	82	65.1		

(*) Statistically significant association at 1% significance level; ([1]) Yates' chi-square test.

Dentoalveolar trauma was present in 14.3% and there were no statistically significant relationships between the age of the patients (P = .855), sex distribution (P = .968), and presence of dentoalveolar trauma. The most common injury was avulsion with 10 cases (50%), followed by teeth fractures (25%), subluxation (15%) and concussion (10%).

A positive association between dentoalveolar trauma and facial fracture is shown in Table 5 (P = .024). According to these data, children with facial fractures have 3.57 times more chance of have dentoalveolar trauma.

Table 4. Distribution of the children according to the facial fracture and alcohol involvement

Facial Fracture	Alcohol involvement[a]				P value[1]	Odds Ratio (IC=95%)
	Yes		No			
	n	%	n	%		
Yes	10	29.4	24	70.6		1
No	2	2.5	77	97.5	P=0.000*	16.04 (3.28-78.33)

[a]Data on alcohol involvement were unavailable for 13 of the 126 patients in the study. (*) Statistically significant association at 1% significance level; ([1]) Yates' chi-square test.

Table 5. Distribution of the children according to the facial fracture and dentoalveolar trauma

Facial Fracture	Dentoalveolar Trauma				P value[1]	Odds Ratio (IC=95%)
	Present		Absent			
	n	%	n	%		
Yes	11	25	33	75		1
No	7	8.5	75	91.5	P=0.024*	3.57 (1.27-10.02)

(*) Statistically significant association at 5% significance level; (1) Yates' chi-square test.

DISCUSSION

The incidence of facial fractures increasing with age in our study. We found that maxillofacial fractures are most common in the age to 11 to 18 years (Group B), consistent with much of the international literature [10, 11]. Children below the age of 5 years live in a protected environment, which is thought to be the main reason for the extremely low rate of facial fractures in this group. After the age of 5 years, children's social environment changes and they have more contact with the outside world. They go to school and start to participate in sports. Their height, weight, strength, and aggressiveness also increase[12]. In addition, children older than 12 years tend to become more independent and involved in more social activities with less parental protection [13].

This study supports earlier studies [1, 7, 11, 12] that reported higher incidence of paediatric facial injuries in boys than in girls of all age groups. A male preponderance was found in this study with a ration of 2.3:1. This ratio was similar that reported in Japan [6, 14], but lower than found in Malaysia [7]. This male-to-female ratio is attributed to the fact that men are more involved in outdoor activities and more frequently exposed to violent interactions [1].

The main causes of maxillofacial injuries were falls and pedestrian accidents. Therefore, strategies to prevent pedestrian related accidents need to be identified, evaluated, and implemented. The numerous causes of facial injuries reported in the literature include traffic accidents [7, 12], falls [6], sports injuries [3], bicycles accidents and attacks by animals [1]. Physical violence and fire gun are rare causes of facial injuries in children, and when they occur, are commonly seen in older age groups as confirmed in our study.

Similar to previous studies [6, 12, 13], the distribution of causes and ages revealed that the incidence of the fall-related injuries decreased in patients older than 10 years. However, motorcycle accidents and fire gun became a common cause in patients older than 10 years [7, 11].

Children are distinctive individuals and in relation to injury, they demonstrate different pattern of clinical features depending on the stage of their bone maturation [7].

Anatomically, the most frequently encountered pediatric facial fracture is the mandible [1,7 , 11, 13], followed by the midface and the upper face [12]. Naso-orbital-ethmoidal injuries were present in 6.1% of the sample.

In this study, the most common mandibular fracture site were the angle, the condyle and the symphyseal and parasymphyseal regions. According to previous reports the condyle [3] and parasymphyseal regions [11] are the most frequently injured region of the mandible. This type of injury, especially in the pediatric age group, is amenable to less aggressive therapy.

In the study reported here, alcohol was associated with about 29.4% of facial fractures, a proportion significantly higher. This result may be explained by the illegal sale and consumption of alcohol by adolescents. Some studies have shown a high correlation between alcohol consumption and maxillofacial injuries [15-17]. Our finds showed that alcohol consumption was strongly associated with the occurrence of facial fractures. Clearly there is evidence of increased morbidity in patients who abuse alcohol and present with facial fractures.

Dentoalveolar injury showed a lower incidence in the pediatric population. Avulsions and teeth fractures were the more prevalent types of dental trauma. A positive association between dentoalveolar trauma and facial fracture was observed.

Conclusion

The results of this study have shown that the incidence of facial fractures in children is higher than previously reported elsewhere. The proper knowledge and treatment of these injuries leads to an often expected good recovery from injury with the reestablishment of pretrauma form and function.

References

[1] Al-Khateeb T, Abdullah FM. Craniomaxillofacial injuries in the United Arab Emirates: A retrospective study. *J. Oral Maxillofac. Surg.* 2007; 65:1094-1101.

[2] Zimmermann CE, Troulis MJ, Kaban LB. Pediatric facial fractures: recent advances in prevention, diagnosis and management. *Int. J. Oral Maxillofac. Surg.* 2005: 34:823-833.

[3] Haug RH, Foss J. Maxillofacial injuries in the pediatric patient. *Oral Surg. Oral Med. Oral Pathol. Oral Radiol. Endod.* 2000; 90:126-134.

[4] Zerfowski M, Bremerich A. Facial trauma in children and adolescents. *Clin. Oral Investig.* 1998; 2:120-124.

[5] Bataineh AB. Etiology and incidence of maxillofacial fractures in the north of Jordan. *Oral Surg Oral Med. Oral Pathol. Oral Radiol. Endod.* 1998; 86:31-35.

[6] Iida S, Matsuya T. Paediatric maxillofacial fractures: their aetiological characters and fracture patterns. *J. Craniomaxillofac. Surg.* 2002; 30:237-241.

[7] Rahman RA, Ramli R, Rahman NA, Hussaini HM, Idrus SM, Hamid AL. Maxillofacial trauma of pediatric patients in Malaysia: a retrospective study from 1999 to 2001 in three hospitals. *Int. J. Pediatr. Otorhinolaryngol.* 2007; 71:929-936.

[8] Brasileiro BF, Passeri LA. Epidemiological analysis of maxillofacial fractures in Brazil: a 5-year prospective study. *Oral Surg. Oral Med. Oral Pathol. Oral Radiol. Endod.* 2006; 102:28-34.

[9] Rezende FM, Gaujac C, Rocha AC, Peres MP. A prospective study of dentoalveolar trauma at the Hospital das Clínicas, São Paulo University Medical School. *Clinics* 2007; 62:133-138

[10] Fasola AO, Denloye OO, Obiechina AE, Arotiba JT. Facial bone fractures in Nigerian children. *Afr. J. Med. Med. Sci.* 2001; 30:67-70.

[11] Ogunlewe MO, James O, Ladeinde AL, Adeyemo WL. Pattern of paediatric maxillofacial fractures in Lagos, Nigeria. *Int. J. Paediatr. Dent.* 2006; 16:358-362.

[12] Iizuka T, Thorén H, Annino DJ Jr, Hallikainen D, Lindqvist C. Midfacial fractures in pediatric patients. Frequency, characteristics, and causes. *Arch. Otolaryngol. Head Neck. Surg.* 1995;121:1366-71.

[13] Shaikh ZS, Worrall SF. Epidemiology of facial trauma in a sample of patients aged 1-18 years. *Injury* 2002;33:669-71.

[14] Tanaka N, Uchide N, Suzuki K, Tashiro T, Tomitsuka K, Kimijima Y, Amagasa T. Maxillofacial fractures in children. *J. Craniomaxillofac. Surg.* 1993; 21:289-93.

[15] Lee KH, Snape L, Steenberg LJ, Worthington J. Comparison between interpersonal violence and motor vehicle accidents in the aetiology of maxillofacial fractures. *ANZ J. Surg.* 2007;77:695-8.

[16] Eggensperger N, Smolka K, Scheidegger B, Zimmermann H, Iizuka T. A 3-year survey of assault-related maxillofacial fractures in central Switzerland. *J. Craniomaxillofac. Surg.* 2007;35:161-7.

[17] Goodisson D, MacFarlane M, Snape L, Darwish B. Head injury and associated maxillofacial injuries. *NZ Med. J.* 2004;117(1201):U1045.

In: Clinical Dentistry
Editor: Scardina Giuseppe Alessandro

ISBN: 978-1-61122-354-5
© 2011 Nova Science Publishers, Inc.

Chapter 6

INDIRECT COMPOSITE RESTORATIONS IN THE POSTERIOR REGION - CASE REPORTS[§]

Giuseppe Lo Giudice*, Frank Lipari*, Angelo Lizio*, Gabriele Cervino* and Marco Cicciù*

[*]Dept. of Odontostomatology - University of Messina

[**]Private practice

ABSTRACT

Objectives: Techniques relying on the use of II generation laboratory composites to carry out indirect restorations ensure long-lasting and predictable results also in posterior teeth. The evolution of restorative materials and adhesive systems improved chemical-physical characteristics of resins (resistance to stress and to wear, hardness) and allowed to perform bonded restorations that respect the biologic and aesthetic principles.

Methods: We have clinically evaluated different types of indirect composite restorations (inlay, onlay and overlay) performed to treat carious lesions in posterior teeth.

After analyzing occlusion and structural factors, the treatment plan included the cavity preparation and, if necessary, a preliminary build-up with a nano-hybrid composite (Filtek Supreme, 3M ESPE). After cavity preparation, indirect composite restorations were fabricated using post-polymerized laboratory composite (Sinfony, 3M ESPE). The following cementation procedure was carried out with the same adhesive system and composite resin used in the preliminary build-up step.

Results: According to our clinical evaluation, the operative protocols applied have proved to be efficient, versatile and simple to perform, providing effective solutions for all the analyzed cases. The technique we have standardized allowed to obtain satisfactory results both for functional and aesthetic aspects.

[§] A version of this book was also published as a chapter in *International Journal of Clinical Dentistry, Volume 1, Issue 1*, published by Nova Science Publishers, Inc. It was submitted for appropriate modifications in an effort to encourage wider dissemination of research.

[*] Address: Dept. of Odontostomatology, AOU Policlinico "G. Martino", Via C. Valeria Messina, Tel: +390902216922, Fax: +390902216910.

Conclusion: indirect composite restorations allow maximum preservation of sound dental structure, better plaque control, good marginal seal and high resistance of the tooth-restoration complex, because of the homogeneous biomechanical properties of the different parts of the restoration.

Clinical Significance

The analysis of the case reports demonstrates the wide application field of indirect composite restorations. This technique allows overcoming some of the limits related with direct restorations and is particularly indicated in posterior teeth.

Introduction

The advancements in adhesive dentistry have brought significant changes in the treatment of caries. Direct composite restorations are preferred over indirect composite restorations when treating caries in posterior teeth because they require minimal intervention and cavity preparation. However, indirect composite restorations are usually recommended when teeth require large restorations. As indirect restorations rely on cements to remain in place, the final outcome depends on the successful selection of the cement. The recent improvement of the chemical-physical properties and biocompatibility of adhesive systems and aesthetic materials has considerably changed restorative techniques of the latero-posterior dentition (Mangani F.M. et al.).

These developments allow to carry out an adhesive restoration that has aesthetic features and is capable of reinforcing the remaining dental structure, besides being as conservative as possible (Ferrari P., Patroni S.).

The materials that mostly fulfil these aesthetic and functional requirements are composites and adhesive resins that can now guarantee stability and predictable outcomes (Veneziani M. ; Skeeters T.M.).

However the posterior region is characterized by some limitations due to the chemical-physical properties of these materials and due to the cavity's shape and site (Mangani F.M. et al.).

In fact, an incomplete degree of conversion achieved during the polymerization reaction, negatively influences the surface properties of the restorations that, in this region, are exposed to remarkable occlusal loading (Ho C.T. et al.; Campanella V.).

An unfavourable C-factor, composite's high viscosity and polymerization shrinkage are further negative factors that may cause poor marginal adaptation of composite restoration in posterior teeth (Manhart J. et al.; Brenna F. et al.).

A cervical margin located in the radicular cement, a dental structure where adhesive's effectiveness is reduced, represents a further risk factor in carrying out direct posterior restorations (Fichera G.).

These limits may be overcome by techniques that make use of II generation laboratory composite restorations (Dietschi D., Spreafico R.).

These kind of restorations, according to Dietschi's classification, can be placed among the indirect techniques (Dietschi D., Holz J.; Fichera G.).

Considering that there is no clinical or statistic evidence in favour of ceramic restorations compared to II generation laboratory composites, there are various factors that lead to choose composite resins (Mangani F.M. et al.; Fichera G.; Goracci G., Andreasi Bassi M.).

In fact, second generation composites show good compressive strength, wear resistance and adequate stiffness. Furthermore, compared to the previous generation, they show less risk of pigmentation and also less fractures and marginal gap formation. The improved mechanical properties are due to the resin's and the filler's composition and, to some extent, also to the post-polymerization process that allows to achieve a higher degree of conversion (Ho C.T. et al.; Ferracane J.L., Condon J.; Watts DC.).

The process makes use of heat, light and vacuum variously combined depending on the different market product's properties and devices used to complete the polymerization reaction. The final effect of this procedure is an improvement of some physical properties evaluated by means of parameters such as: solubility, fragility, Young modulus and thermal expansion coefficient.

The restoration's extra-oral fabrication allows a better marginal adaptation in the most difficult areas (cervical and occlusal margins) resulting in a polymerization-shrinkage stress reduction due to the need of a thin layer of luting agent required during the cementation procedure (Sanches Borges A.F. et al.; Yilmaz D.,Gemalmaz D.; Dietschi D. et al.).

The technique so far described can be associated to procedures, performed before the indirect restoration is fabricated, that require resin composites and fiber posts to carry out the build-up (Fichera G.).

In this case direct and indirect restorative techniques are combined and the goal is to use composite resins with similar physical-chemical properties during different restoring steps in order to achieve a functional monoblock. Consequently, the indirect composite restoration technique allows to solve, effectively and in a simple way, many critical problems concerning the restoration of posterior teeth.

Table 1 shows the advantages and the disadvantages of this technique.

The decision to choose an indirect composite restoration, after an accurate clinical evaluation, must respect some operative parameters that characterize the technique's field of application (Table 2) (Dietschi D.; Mangani F.M. et al)

Table 1. The indirect composite restoration technique: advantages and disadvantages

ADVANTAGES
1. Lower absolute polymerization-shrinkage values
2. Extra-oral fabrication
3. Better marginal adaptation especially in cement
4. Ideal interproximal contacts
5. Structural homogeneity with the build-up (if present)
6. Better surface properties
7. Occlusal stability
8. Low wear of counterpart teeth
9. Possibility to be repaired
10. Good aesthetics
11. Not very expensive

Table 1. (Continued)

DISADVANTAGES
1. Need to work under isolation
2. More operative steps
3. The restoration must be fabricated by a technician
4. Need to perform an adhesive luting procedure

Table 2. Indirect technique choosing parameters from Dietschi and Mangani – modified

1. Size and number of restorations
2. Location of the margins
3. Location of the tooth inside the dental arch
4. Tooth anatomy and resistance
5. Isolation of the operative field
6. High standard of oral hygiene
7. Low susceptibility to decay
8. Absence of parafunctions

Mangani and other authors have analyzed in detail these parameters dividing them in general and local parameters.

These authors emphasize how this technique is particularly suitable for patients who require the performance of multiple restorations.

As a matter of fact, the extra-oral occlusal modelling allows to achieve ideal interarch contacts (Mangani F.M. et al.).

The cavity preparation technique allows to preserve thin cavity walls and gingival margins at less than 1 mm. from the cemento-enamel junction allowing a very conservative approach to the carious lesion (Fichera et al.).

Furthermore, this kind of restoration improves the resistance of the residual tooth structure also in teeth that are exposed to remarkable occlusal load in relation to their position within the dental arch.

As for all the adhesive procedures, in order to make the best composite's potentiality, it is necessary to guarantee a complete isolation of the operative field with rubber dam.

Depending on the aesthetic requirements, functional needs and cavity's configuration it's possible to carry out all the different types of laboratory composite indirect restorations (inlay, onlay and overlay).

The authors have evaluated the aesthetic and functional outcomes, the technique's versatility and the stability of various indirect restorations.

Materials and Methods

The indirect composite technique's clinical evaluation has been carried out on four patients with carious lesion of different sizes located in the latero-posterior area.

The restorative treatment plan, which in some cases included endodontic therapy, was finalized by an indirect composite restoration (inlay, onlay or overlay).

For the teeth with no need for endodontic treatment, the first step is represented by the rubber dam placement, followed by the complete removal of carious dentine with the aid of a caries detector dye and the elimination of the damaged enamel.

A build-up was performed in all the teeth in order to achieve dentinal and enamel seal, reinforment of the remaining tooth structure, and also to block out the undercuts and optimize the cavity configuration.

The build-up was performed by etching with 37% phosphoric acid (dentin for 15" and enamel for 30"), applying the adhesive system (Scotchbond 1, 3M Espe™,St. Paul, MN, USA®), applying a thin layer of flowable composite (Filtek Flow, 3M Espe™,St. Paul, MN, USA®) and then a microhybrid composite with nanofillers and nanoclusters (Filtek Supreme, 3M Espe™,St. Paul, MN, USA®).

The composite was photo-polymerized by a L.E.D. curing device (T-LED dna Anthos™,Imola, Bo, Italy®) with a increasing power program (10" at 100 mW/cm^2 ; 10" ramp mode; 20" at 500 mW/cm^2). Subsequently, after the analysis of the central and peripheral structural factors and of the occlusion according to the principles proposed by Fichera, the cavity preparation was completed (Fichera G.).

The principles followed during the preparation are summarized in Table 3.

Table 3. Cavity preparation's principles

- Divergent cavity walls
- Round internal angles
- Occlusal isthmus width must be at least 2 mm
- 1,5 - 2.0 mm of occlusal reduction
- Smooth preparation walls
- No undercuts
- Supragingival margins
- Smooth enamel margins
- Cervical margin with a butt joint

Therefore, we consider in detail the clinical cases we performed.

Case n. 1 – INLAY

Patient: A.C., 31 years old, female

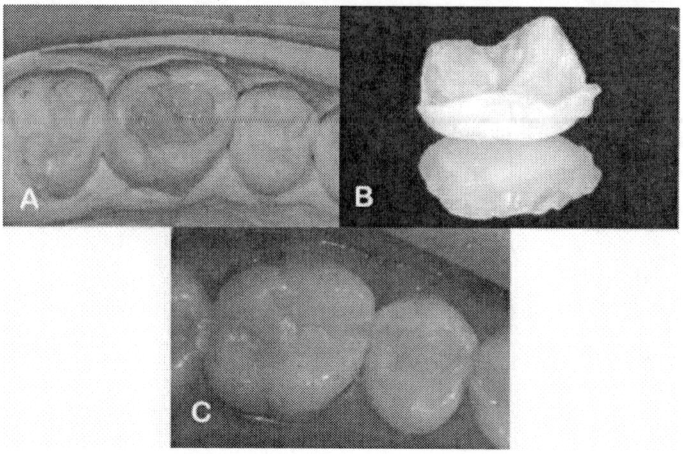

Figure 1. Case 1 - 1.6 Inlay; A. Occlusal view of the inlay on the working model; B. Laboratory-processed composite inlay; C. Final result after cementation.

Objective exam: The patient presents a class I carious lesion of tooth 1.6. No sign of pulpal pathology.

Therapeutic choice: an indirect composite inlay that allows an ideal aesthetic integration of the restoration (Figure 1).

Case n. 2 – ONLAY

Patient: S.B., 27 years old, female

Objective exam: The mesial side of tooth 1.6 presents a wide coronal destruction. The pulp vitality tests were positive.

Therapeutic choice: An indirect composite onlay, preserving the distal marginal ridge and contact point. The occlusal restoration includes mesial cusps replacement providing an adequate functional and aesthetic integration. (Figure 2).

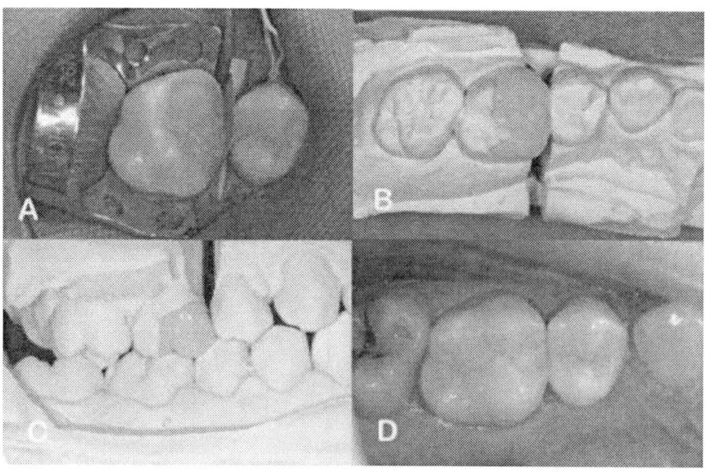

Figure 2. Case 2 1.6 Onlay; A. Wide coronal destruction of 1.6; B. Model showing the occlusal view of the onlay; C. Buccal view of the onlay on the model; D. Final view of the bonded onlay.

Case n. 3 – ONLAY

Patient: F.M., 40 years old, male

Objective exam: The patient presents a defective composite restoration with marginal infiltration and the absence of the mesial marginal ridge on tooth 3.6 that has been already endodontically treated.

Therapeutic choice: A partial cusp coverage indirect composite onlay preserving the vestibular sound tooth structure. The preparation design requires the removal of the lingual and mesial walls and part of the distal wall preserving the contact point. (Figure 3).

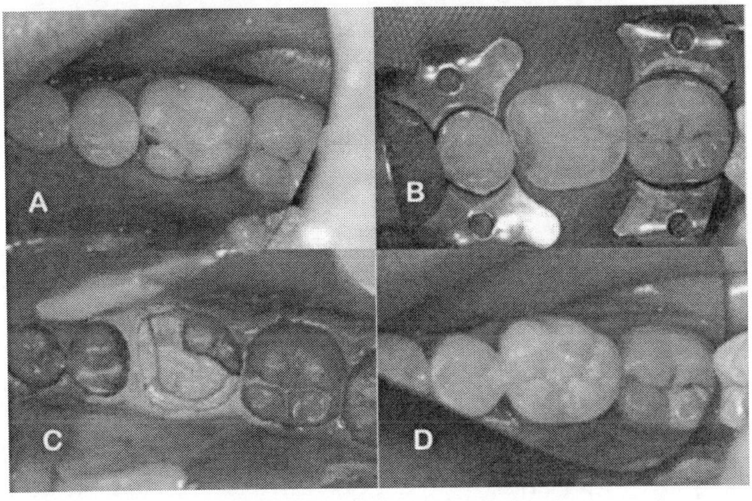

Figure 3. Case 3 - 3.6 Onlay; A. Composite restoration with marginal infiltration of 3.6; B. The preparation design; C. Impressions made using a polyether material and a one-step/two-viscosity techinique; D. View after cementation procedure.

Case n. 4 – OVERLAY

Patient: A.P., 28 years old, female

Objective exam: A large coronal destruction is present on tooth 1.6 . Chronic pulpal pathology is present.

Therapeutic choice: After endodontic treatment the build-up was carried-out using a fiber post. A MOD and a full-coverage cavity preparation was executed in order to perform an indirect composite overlay. (Figure 4)

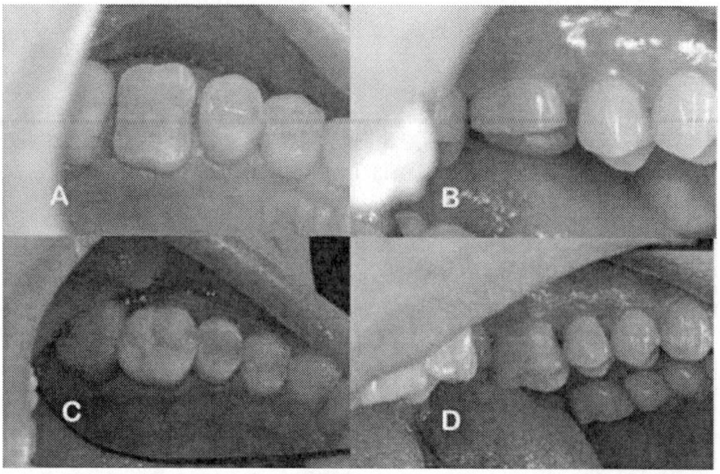

Figure 4. Case 4 – 1.6 Overlay; A. Occlusal view of the build-up carried out using a fiber post of 1.6.; B. Buccal view of cavity design; C. Occlusal view showing the overlay luted; D. Buccal view showing the final result.

Results

Our evaluation, based on clinical evidence, shows the versatility of this restorative technique that allows to face and effectively solve various clinical situations involving coronal lesions in the posterior region.

The results, achieved with an easy and not expensive technique, turned out to be positive both under a functional and an aesthetic point of view.

Analyzing in detail the clinical results it is evident that one important advantage is represented by a relevant preservation of dental structure that this technique permits.

The possibility to locate most margins in areas far away from the periodontal tissues consents better plaque control procedures consequently minimizing the risk of secondary decays and periodontal lesions.

Extra-oral modelling of the interproximal boxes' margins and the cementation procedures that we used, and that allows to optimize the marginal seal and the excess' removal, contribute to this positive outcome.

A further positive factor is represented by the homogeneity between the composite inlay, the build-up, the fiber posts and the luting agents that causes positive biomechanical behaviour of the various components.

The extra-oral modelling permits to obtain correct occlusal relations. This condition is stable over time since the second generation laboratory composites show a better wear resistance than the composites conventionally used in direct restorations.

This technique allows to achieve a good aesthetic restoration that can be used in place of ceramic inlays.

At last, this technique seems to be inexpensive and easy to carry out. At the same time it reduces the operative time, and the tooth-restoration complex may represent a pre-treatment in the case a conventional fixed prosthodontic treatment is needed.

CONCLUSIONS

Since it's not possible to have a restorative material with ideal properties, the use of composite indirect restorations can minimize some peculiar limits of the composite resins.

Actually, the convergence of more than one restorative technique allows the use of composites also in the posterior region taking maximum advantage of this material's versatility and of the potentiality offered by dentin-enamel adhesive systems.

Microleakage in the proximal walls of direct and indirect posterior resin slot restorations was analyzed by Fruits et al. (Fruits TJ. et al.) In this study, the author's purpose was to compare the degree of microleakage in the proximal walls of direct and indirect resin slot restorations in relation to the types of dentin bonding systems and the location of gingival margins. Significant differences were found in the degree of microleakage observed in the various restorative groups. Generally, the group restored with indirect resin showed less microleakage than the direct resin groups. Factors, such as type of dentin bonding system and location of gingival margins, exert a substantial influence on the degree of microleakage that occurred along the walls of proximal resin restorations.

Marginal gap formation, residual internal stress and the possible enamel margin fractures due to the unavoidable polymerization-shrinkage can be relevantly minimized using this restorative technique.

This outcome is possible thanks to the use of thin layers of composite, particularly during cementation and to the extra-oral polymerization of the most part of the restorative material.

The influence of cavity preparation design on fracture strength and mode of fracture of laboratory-processed composite resin restorations was evaluated by Fonseca et al. (Fonseca RB. et al.) After an in vitro study the authors concluded that the different cavity preparation designs evaluated had no effect on the fracture strength of teeth restored with a laboratory-processed composite resin, but intact teeth were always more resistant to fracture than teeth prepared, irrespective of the type of restoration.

According to Magne et al. composite resins demonstrate a resilient component that favors stress transfer within the tooth/restoration complex. (Magne P. et al.) In spite of that, high elastic modulus materials tend to develop high tensile stresses directly below their interface with the resin cement at the loaded area.(Kelly JR. ; Chen HY. et al. ; Yoshinari M., Derand T.).

With new equipment and techniques for cavity preparation and new or improved restorative materials, the preservation of tooth structure has become an important trend in modern dentistry. However, as Hood reported, "the natural consequence of dental treatment is continued replacement of restorations.". (Hood J.A.) Removing defective Class II restorations typically leads to an extension of the preparation, which is associated with an increase in the cusp height and the isthmus width. It is known that for Class II preparations, the depth and width of the preparation have a role in postoperative fracture resistance. (Vale W.A,, Blaser P.K. et al., Larson T.D. et al.).

Additionally, occlusal relationships and cusp structure may affect tensile and compressive stresses in the tooth structure (Mondelli J. et al.; Lin C.L. et al.;).

At last, the stability over time of the aesthetic and functional outcomes is due to the improvement of the surface properties achieved with the post-curing processes.

In order to optimize the results, it is essential to preliminarily analyze the morphologic and structural factors of the residual sound tooth tissue that guide to the cavity configuration.

A correct preliminary planning consents to solve a variety of clinical situations using all the different kinds of indirect composite restorations.

When the preparation size is of the extent that direct composite is not indicated, ceramic or processed composite inlays provide an alternative when a tooth-colored restoration is selected. (Roberson T.M. et al.) Indirect restorations have better physical properties than direct composite restorations being fabricated under relatively ideal laboratory conditions.

So it's possible to plan more conservative treatments performing partial coronal preparations, also in complex restorations, taking advantage of adhesive techniques and assembling a more homogeneous structure in it's physical properties, using similar materials.

So we can achieve a restorative monoblock which is functionally integrated with the tooth structure allowing an ideal resistance of the tooth-restoration complex.

The outcome is an effective and predictable restoration, with functional and aesthetic features, that turns out to be stable over time.

References

Blaser P.K, Lund M.R., Cochran M.A., Potter R.H. Effect of designs of class 2 preparations on resistance of teeth to fracture. *Oper. Dent.* 1983; 8:6–10.

Brenna F, Porro S, Artioli G. Clinica e laboratorio nella realizzazione di restauri estetici indiretti nei settori posteriori - *Dent. Mod.* 2002, 05:23-49.

Campanella V. Restauri indiretti in composito nei settori posteriori: nuova tecnica costruttiva e cementazione sotto pressione G. *It. Cons.* 2003; 1(1): 8-15.

Chen HY, Hickel R, Setcos JC, Kunzelmann KH. Effects of surface finish and fatigue testing on the fracture strength of CAD-CAM and pressed-ceramic crowns, *J. Prosthet. Dent* 1999; 82:468–75.

Dietschi D, Holz J. Restaurations des dentes postérieures Rev. Mens. *Suisse Odontostomatol* 1990; 100:1325-32.

Dietschi D, Olsburgh S, Krejci I, Davidson C. In vitro evaluation of marginal and internal adaptation after occlusal stressing of indirect class II composite restorations with different resinous bases. – *Eur. J. Of Oral Scien.* 2003; 111(1): 73-80.

Dietschi D, Spreafico R. Adhesive metal-free restorations: current concepts for the esthetic treatment of posterior teeth Berlin: Quintessence Publishing Co Ltd, 1997.

Ferracane JL, Condon J. Postcure heat treatment for composite. *Dental Materials* 1992; 8:290.

Ferrari P, Patroni S. Attuali orientamenti nel trattamento conservativo dei settori posteriori *Dent. Mod.* 2000, 4:85-100.

Fichera G, Dinapoli C, Re D. Restauri estetico-adesivi indiretti: modello per diagnosi di configurazione cavitaria. *Dent. Mod.* 2003; 2: 21-59.

Fichera G. Restauri indiretti in composito nei settori posteriori. Prima parte: piano di trattamento, materiali e indicazioni *Dent. Mod.* 2001; 10:105-24.

Fichera G. Restauri indiretti in composito nei settori posteriori. Seconda parte: principi di preparazione cavitaria – *Dent. Mod* 2002; 05:73-93.

Fonseca RB, Fernandes-Neto AJ, Correr-Sobrinho L, Soares CJ. The influence of cavity preparation design on fracture strength and mode of fracture of laboratory-processed composite resin restorations. *J. Prosthet. Dent.* 2007 Oct; 98(4):277-84.

Fruits TJ, Knapp JA, Khajotia SS. Microleakage in the proximal walls of direct and indirect posterior resin slot restorations. *Oper. Dent.* 2006 Nov-Dec; 31(6):719-27.

Goracci G., Andreasi Bassi M. Aesthetic inlays in the dental practice – *Dental News* 1999; 6(2):11-15.

Ho CT, Vijayaraghavan TV, Lee SY, Tsai A, Huang HM, Pan LC. Flexural behaviour of post-cured composites at oral-simulating temperatures. *J. of Oral Rehab.* 2001; 28:658-67.

Hood J.A. Biomechanics of the intact, prepared and restored tooth: some clinical implications. *Int. Dent. J.* 1991; 41: 25–32.

Kelly JR. Clinically relevant approach to failure testing of all-ceramic restorations. – *J. Prosthet. Dent.* 1999; 81:652–61.

Larson T.D., Douglas W.H., Geistfeld R.E. Effect of prepared cavities on the strength of teeth. *Oper. Dent.* 1981;6:2–5.

Lin C.L., Chang C.H., Ko C.C. Multifactorial analysis of an MOD restored human premolar using auto-mesh finite element approach. *J. Oral Rehabil.* 2001; 28:576–85.

Magne P, Perakis N, Belser UC, Krejci I. Stress distribution of inlay-anchored adhesive fixed partial dentures: a finite element analysis of the influence of restorative materials and abutment preparation design, *J. Prosthet. Dent.* 2002; 87:516–27.

Mangani FM, Sigalot C,Vanini L. Intarsi in resina composita nel restauro estetico dei settori latero-posteriori. *Dent. Mod.* 2001, 02:25-58.

Manhart J, Neuerer P, Scheibenbogen-Fuchsbrunner A, Hickel R. Three-year clinical evaluation of direct and indirect composite restorations in posterior teeth. *J. Prosthet. Dent.* 2000; 84:289-96.

Mondelli J, Steagall L., Ishikiriama A., de Lima Navarro M.F., Soares F.B. Fracture strength of human teeth with cavity preparations. *J. Prosthet. Dent.* 1980; 43:419–422

Roberson T.M., Heymann H.O., Swift E.J. Jr. In: *Sturdevant's art and science of operative dentistry* (4th ed ed.), Mosby, St. Louis 2001; 571.

Sanches Borges AF, Correr GM, Coelho Sinhoreti MA, Consani S, Correr Sobrinho L, Puppin Rontani RM. Compressive strength recovery by composite onlays inprimary teeth. Substrate treatment and luting agent effects - *Journal of dentistry* 2006; 34:478-84.

Skeeters TM. A resin composite for posterior restorations. 15 years results. *J. Dent. Res.* 1998; 77 (Special Issue B).

Vale W.A. Cavity preparation. *Irish Dent. Rev.* 1956; 2:33–41.

Veneziani M. Riabilitazione conservativa di due quadranti antagonisti. *Dent. Mod.* 2002; 11:37-41.

Watts DC. Surface hardness development in light cured composite. *Dental Materials* 1987; 3:256.

Yilmaz D, Gemalmaz D. Clinical evaluation of class II Targis inlays: preliminary results after 1 year - *Journal of Oral Rehabilitation* 2003; 30:855–60.

Yoshinari M, Derand T. Fracture strength of all-ceramic crowns. *Int. J. Prosthodont.* 1994; 7:329–338.

In: Clinical Dentistry
Editor: Scardina Giuseppe Alessandro

ISBN: 978-1-61122-354-5
© 2011 Nova Science Publishers, Inc.

Chapter 7

CLINICAL SUCCESS RATE OF FISSURE SEALINGS WITH RESIN MODIFIED GLASS-IONOMER CEMENT OR BIS-GMA AFTER THREE YEARS[#]

***Stefan Zimmer**[*1], **Nadine Bastendorf**[2], **Klaus-Dieter Bastendorf**[2], **Axel Bartsch**[3], **Hermann Lang**[1] and **Claudia R. Barthel**[1]*

[1]Heinrich-Heine-University,
Dept. of Operative and Preventive Dentistry and Endodontics,
Moorenstr. 5, D-40225 Düsseldorf, Germany
[2]Private Practice, Gairenstr. 6, 73054 Eislingen, Germany
[3]An der Schütt 12, 97922 Lauda-Königshofen, Germany

ABSTRACT

The aim of the present study was to evaluate retention and clinical success rate of a resin modified glass ionomer cement (compomer) fissure sealant in comparison to a bis-GMA sealant. Three hundred and fifty-two fissure sealings (Helioseal or Ionosit Seal) were placed in 1st and 2nd permanent molars of 95 patients using a split-mouth design. The subjects were five to 15 years old. All 352 sealed teeth could be included in the final analysis. The mean observation time was 3.16 (SD 0.5) years. Over the entire observation period, 90.4% of the bis-GMA based sealants (6.8% partial loss, 2.8% complete loss) and 5.1% of the resin modified glass ionomer sealants (18.1% partial loss, 76.8% complete loss) remained intact. Established caries was found in ten occlusal surfaces sealed with resin modified glass ionomer and in two cases when the bis-GMA sealer was used. In one case each, caries developed after partial loss, whereas in all the other cases complete loss was preceding caries. The caries frequency was not statistically significantly different between the materials (Fisher's exact test, $p=0.35$). With "established caries" as failure

---

[#] A version of this book was also published as a chapter in *International Journal of Clinical Dentistry, Volume 1, Issue 2*, published by Nova Science Publishers, Inc. It was submitted for appropriate modifications in an effort to encourage wider dissemination of research.

[*] Corresponding author: Stefan Zimmer, Heinrich-Heine-University, Dept. of Operative and Preventive Dentistry and Endodontics, Building 18.13. Moorenstr. 5, D-40225 Düsseldorf, Germany; Fone: +49-(0)211-8119880; Fax: +49-(0)211-8119244 ; Email1: zimmer@med.uni-duesseldorf.de; Email2: stefan.zimmer@t-online.de

criteria, the three-year survival rate was 96.7% for the resin modified glass ionomer sealants and 99.5% for the bis-GMA sealants (Kaplan-Meier analysis). Log-rank analysis showed a statistically significant difference between the materials (p=0.02). From a clinical point of view, however, it can be concluded that a resin modified glass ionomer sealer is as effective in caries prevention as a bis-GMA sealer after three years.

Clinical Significance

The present study shows that fissure sealings made with resin modified glass-ionomer cement are as effective as bis-GMA based sealers in preventing caries over a three-year-period. However, the resin modified glass-ionomer cement sealants were almost completely lost after three years. This can be interpreted as an advantage over bis-GMA sealers since a sealer must protect a caries susceptible fissure during the first years in the oral cavity and may be useless in the following years. A long term follow-up of the present study group is planned to answer this question.

Introduction

The sealing of fissures is proven to be an effective measure in preventing caries on occlusal surfaces of permanent molars (Simonsen 1991). Carvalho et al. demonstrated that the risk of fissure caries in permanent first molars is increased during tooth eruption. More plaque was found in erupting teeth as opposed to fully erupted teeth with antagonistic contact. The proportion of active lesions was reduced and arrested lesions were increased in the latter group. As main reason for these findings, it was discussed that functional usage of teeth in addition to improved access for toothbrushing promotes arrestment of lesions initiated during eruption. (Carvalho et al. 1989). According to Ekstrand et al., the mean duration of eruption of permanent molars varies between 15.0 (1st molar, boys) and 27.9 months (2nd molars, girls) (Ekstrand et al. 2003). Therefore, it can be argued, that fissure sealants have to protect occlusal surfaces of permanent molars during tooth eruption and that they may be no longer necessary after the teeth are fully erupted. The retention of methacrylate-based sealants usually by far exceeds this time span. For example, Lygidakis and Oulis found retention rates of 77,0 and 89.0% after four years of service (Lygidakis and Oulis 1999) and Albani et al. of 81.7% after five years (Albani et al. 2005). On the other hand, sealings made of conventional glass-ionomer cement or resin modified glass ionomer cement were completely lost by 74.2% and 89.0% after five years (Pardi et al. 2003), which seems much more appropriate under the described conditions. It was therefore the aim of the present study to evaluate retention and clinical success rate of a resin modified glass ionomer cement (compomer) fissure sealant in comparison to a bis-GMA sealant.

Materials and Methods

In a private dental practice in Eislingen/Germany, 352 fissure sealings were placed in 95 patients (49 female, 46 male). The subjects were five to 15 years old. All first and second molars being newly erupted since the last visit were designated to be sealed.

The materials used were the bis-GMA based Helioseal (Ivoclar/Vivadent, Schaan, Liechtenstein) and the resin modified glass ionomer Ionosit Seal (DMG, Hamburg, Germany). Both materials are light curing. The split-mouth experimental design was used to allocate the two materials to the teeth that were designated to be sealed. This resulted in 177 sealings in newly erupted contralateral permanent first and second molars per material. One pair of teeth was sealed in 14 subjects, two in 80 and three in one.

Clinical Procedure

All sealings were placed by one dentist (KDB) with support of a chair side dental assistant. The operator used 2x magnifying glasses (Carl Zeiss, Jadent, Aalen, Germany). Before starting the placement of the sealants, cotton rolls were placed to keep dry conditions. The occlusal surfaces were dried by air syringe and the fissures were cleaned using a powder jet cleaner (Rondoflex 2013, KaVo, Biberach, Germany). Thereafter, the fissures were etched for 60 seconds using 35% phosphoric acid (Ultra-Etch, Ultradent Products, South Jordan/Utah, USA). After rinsing for 20 seconds the fissures were air dried followed by the application of acetone. Subsequently cotton rolls were carefully changed while preventing the etched enamel surface from being contaminated by saliva. The sealer was placed and light-cured after a 20 seconds waiting period, allowing the material to penetrate the fissure system. Curing time was according to the manufacturer's recommendations. Static and dynamic occlusion was checked by the use of an 8 micron foil (Haniel-Roeko, Langenau, Germany). Finally, the sealant was polished using a conical silicone polisher (Komet 9662/9663, Lemgo, Germany) and a fluoride varnish (Duraphat, Colgate, Hamburg) was applied. According to the individual risk of the patient, a follow-up was appointed three or six months later.

Follow Ups

Within the study period, two to eleven follow-up examinations were administered, reflecting the different observation periods and risk categories of the subjects. All follow-up examinations were performed under dry conditions (cotton rolls, air syringe) using magnifying glasses, a dental mirror (Stoma Size 5, plane, Emmingen- Liptingen, Germany) and a dental probe (3A, Henry Schein, Stuttgart, Germany). All intermediate follow-up examinations were performed by one single examiner (KDB), whereas another examiner who had not placed the sealings performed the final examination (NB). All sealings were tactilely checked with the dental probe for intact sealing, complete, or partial loss. Caries was visually diagnosed according to WHO criteria (WHO 1987). Date of examination as well as condition of the sealing and tooth were recorded on a examination form. If a failure was detected at a routine check up or at the final examination, the medium day between the preceding examination without failure and the actual examination was noted as day of failure.

Statistical Analysis

All recorded data were transferred to the SPSS 12.0 (SPSS Inc. Chicago, Illinois, USA) program. For statistical analysis of categorical data chi²-test and Fisher's exact test were used. Student's t-test and Mann-Whitney U-test were used to compare mean values. Kaplan-Meier analysis with log-rank-test was used to calculate the survival rate. For all statistical analyses, SPSS 12.0 was used.

RESULTS

All 352 sealed teeth could be included in the final analysis. The median age of the subjects was 9.06 (25th percentile 7.6, 75th percentile 12.95) years. The number of follow-ups per subject was between two and eleven with a mean of six. The observation time was between 1.50 and 4.14 years with a mean value of 3.16 (SD 0.5) years. 90.4% of the bis-GMA based sealants remained intact (6.8% partial loss, 2.8% complete loss) over the entire observation period whereas this was only true for 5.1% of the resin modified glass ionomer sealants (18.1% partial loss, 76.8% complete loss). Sealant loss was statistically significant different between the two materials (chi², $p < 0.001$). For the resin modified glass ionomer sealants Kaplan-Meier-analysis showed a median longevity of 1.65 years and for the bis-GMA sealants of 3.75 years for „partial loss" as failure criteria (Figure 1). The three-year survival rate was app. 4% for the resin modified glass ionomer sealants and 91.8% for the bis-GMA sealants. Log-rank-analysis showed a statistically significant difference between the materials ($p < 0.0001$).

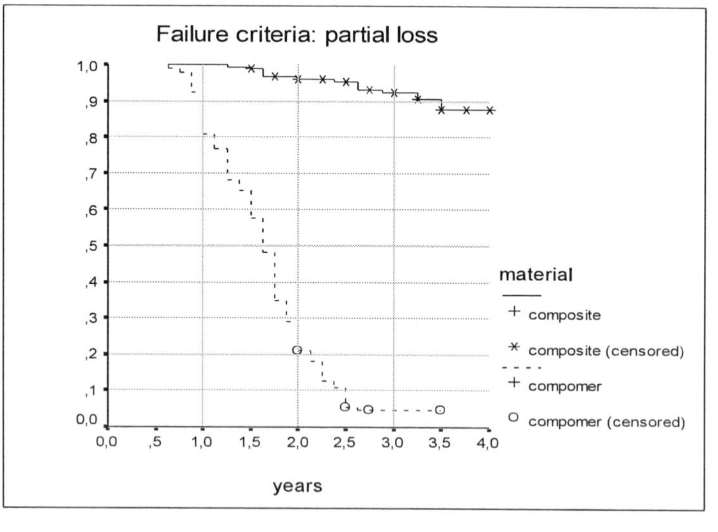

Figure 1. Kaplan-Meier survival analysis with partial loss as failure criteria. "Partial loss" includes "complete loss".

When “complete loss” was defined as failure criteria, the median longevity was 2.80 years for the resin modified glass ionomer sealants and 3.95 years for the bis-GMA sealants (Figure 2). The three-year survival rate was 30.2% for the resin modified glass ionomer sealants and 96.5% for the bis-GMA sealants. Log-rank-analysis showed a statistically significant difference between the materials ($p < 0.0001$).

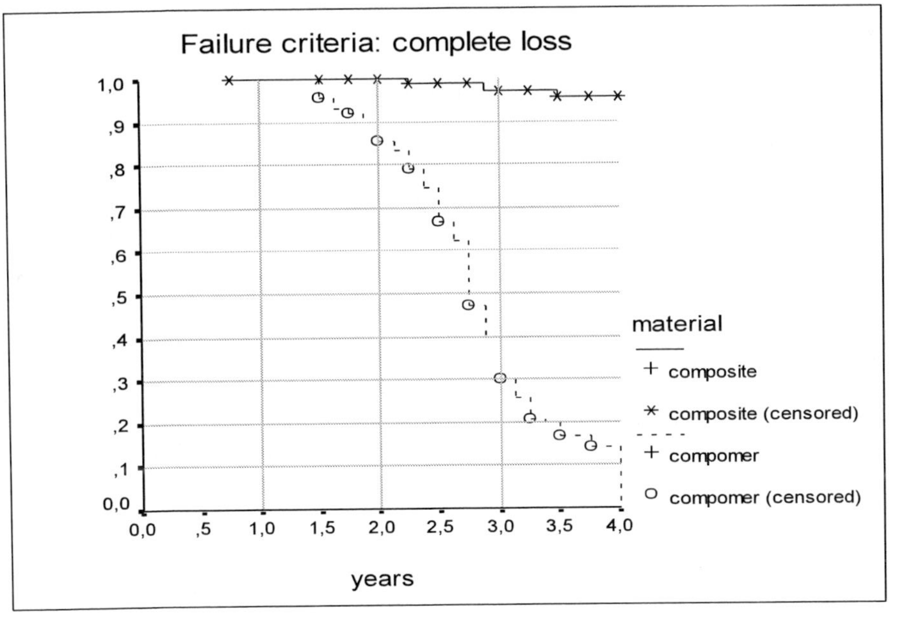

Figure 2. Kaplan-Meier survival analysis with complete loss as failure criteria.

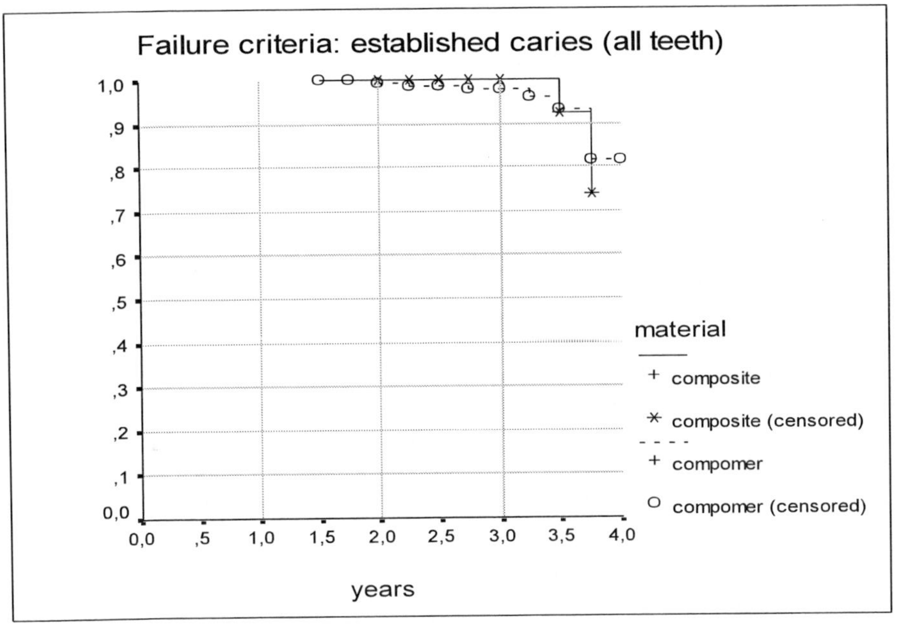

Figure 3. Kaplan-Meier survival analysis with established caries as failure criteria.

Established caries was found in ten occlusal surfaces sealed with resin modified glass ionomer and in two cases when the bis-GMA sealer was used. In one case each, caries developed after partial loss whereas in all the other cases, complete loss was preceding caries. The caries frequency was not statistically significant different between the materials (Fisher's exact test, p=0.35). With "established caries" as failure criteria, the median longevity was 3.91 years for the resin modified glass ionomer sealants and 3.98 years for the bis-GMA sealants (Figure 3). The three-year survival rate was 96.7% for the resin modified glass ionomer sealants and 99.5% for the bis-GMA sealants. Log-rank-analysis showed a statistically significant difference between the materials (p=0.02).

Discussion

In the present study, the complete retention rate of the bis-GMA based sealer was 94.4% after three years, whereas it was 5.1% for the resin modified glass ionomer sealer. Thus, the assumption, that the resin modified glass ionomer material would be lost after the tooth eruption was completed, was fulfilled. The retention rates are in accordance with the results of other clinical studies (Lygidakis and Oulis 1999; Albani et al. 2005; Pardi et al. 2003).

Since the effectiveness of resin-based sealants in preventing caries is well documented, e.g. in a in a systematic Cochrane review (Ahovuo-Saloranta et al. 2004), it is not justifiable to perform a no-treatment controlled clinical study to demonstrate the effectiveness of a resin modified glass ionomer sealant. This ethical judgement resulted in a limitation of the present study. It was only possible to compare the effectiveness of the resin modified glass ionomer to an established bis-GMA sealant. In comparison to this, an equivalent effectiveness in preventing caries was demonstrated. An explanation for the contradictory results for retention and effectiveness in caries prevention may be the fact, that even if the glass ionomer sealant is clinically lost, remnants of the material can be found on the bottom of the fissure, as shown by Mejare and Mjör (Mejare and Mjör 1990). These remnants may have some sealing function and release fluoride.

However, another recently published three-year split-mouth study failed to demonstrate an equivalent effectiveness of a chemically curing glass ionomer cement in comparison to a light-curing resin-based sealant material (Kervanto-Seppälä et al. 2008). In contrast to the present study, the population of the study of Kervanto-Seppälä et al. was 12-16 years old and only permanent 2nd molars were sealed. In the present trial, 1st (n=212) and 2nd (n=140) molars were treated. An explanation for the contradictory results may be the fact, that the eruption of 2nd molars takes about one year longer than for 1st molars (Ekstrand et al. 2003). It can be speculated that the retention of the glass ionomer cement was not long enough to protect 2nd molars.

The result of the present study is supported by data of Puppin-Rontani et al. In their clinical study, they found equal effectiveness in caries prevention for a resin-based sealer and for a compomer after 24 months. The subjects were 7-9 years old and only 1st molars were sealed. (Puppin-Rontani et al. 2006).

In their review, Bürkle and Hickel concluded, that the caries inhibition of glass ionomer cement sealants is similar to resin based sealants. However, since the retention rate of the latter ones was higher in eight from ten analyzed studies and a significantly better caries inhibition was found in two from nine studies (glass ionomer cement was never superior), the authors favour resin based sealers. (Bürkle and Hickel 2003). Based on the results of the present study, it can be concluded that a resin modified glass ionomer sealer is as effective in caries prevention as a bis-GMA sealer after three years. A follow-up of the present study group is planned to evaluate if this comparability persists on a long term basis.

REFERENCES

Ahovuo-Saloranta A, Hiiri A, Nordblad A, Worthington H, Mäkelä M. Pit and fissure sealants for preventing dental decay in the permanent teeth of children and adolescents. *Cochrane Database Syst. Rev*. 2004;(3):CD001830.

Albani F, Ballesio I, Campanella V, Marzo G. Pit and fissure sealants: results at five and ten years. *Eur. J. Paediatr. Dent*. 2005; 6: 61-65.

Bürkle V, Hickel R. Fissurenversiegelung mit Glasionomerzementen – eine Literaturübersicht. *Dtsch Zahnärztl* Z 2003; 58: 207-211.

Carvalho JC, Ekstrand KR, Thylstrup A. Dental plaque and caries on occlusal surfaces of first permanent molars in relation to stage of eruption. *J. Dent. Res*. 1989; 68: 773-779.

Ekstrand KR, Christiansen J, Christiansen ME. Time and duration of eruption of first and second permanent molars: a longitudinal investigation. *Community Dent. Oral Epidemiol*. 2003; 31: 344-350.

Kervanto-Seppälä S, Lavonius E, Pietilä I, Pitkäniemi J, Meurman JH, Kerosuo E. Comparing the caries-preventive effect of two fissure sealing modalities in public health care: a single application of glass ionomer and a routine resin-based sealant programme. A randomized split-mouth clinical trial. *Int. J. Paediatr. Dent*. 2008; 18: 56-61.

Lygidakis NA, Oulis KI. A comparison of Fluroshield with Delton fissure sealant: four year results. *Pediatr. Dent*. 1999; 21: 429-431.

Mejare I, Mjör IA. Glass ionomer and resin-based fissure sealants: a clinical study. *Scand. J. Dent. Res*. 1990; 98: 345-350.

Pardi V, Pereira AC, Mialhe FL, Meneghim Mde C, Ambrosano GM. A 5-year evaluation of two glass-ionomer cements used as fissure sealants. *Community Dent. Oral Epidemiol*. 2003; 31: 386-391.

Puppin-Rontani RM, Baglioni-Gouvea ME, deGoes MF, Garcia-Godoy F. Compomer as a pit and fissure sealant: effectiveness and retention after 24 months. *J. Dent. Child* 2006; 73: 31-36.

Simonsen RJ. Retention and effectiveness of dental sealant after 15 years. *J. Am. Dent. Assoc*. 1991; 122: 34-42.

WHO. *Oral Health Surveys. Basic Methods*. Third Edition. Geneva: WHO, 1987; 34-37.

In: Clinical Dentistry
Editor: Scardina Giuseppe Alessandro

ISBN: 978-1-61122-354-5
© 2011 Nova Science Publishers, Inc.

Chapter 8

EVALUATION OF THE FLUORESCENCE OF CLINICALLY SIMULATED ALL-CERAMIC MATERIALS[#]

Jin-Soo Ahn and Yong-Keun Lee*
Department of Dental Biomaterials Science and Dental Research Institute
School of Dentistry, Seoul National University
Seoul, Korea

ABSTRACT

Purpose: Since the ultraviolet (UV) component of a light can brighten a fluorescent material like human teeth, a color difference between tooth and a non-fluorescent esthetic material would be more apparent when viewed under the UV included light. The purpose of this study was to evaluate the fluorescence of simulatedly layered all-ceramic materials at a clinically relevant thickness with a color-measuring spectrophotometer.

Methods: Seven all-ceramic core materials of Vita A2-corresponding shade, one sintering ceramic and one alloy core as references, were prepared in clinically relevant thicknesses (0.4 to 0.8 mm). A2- and A3-corresponding shades of each recommended veneer ceramic were fabricated so that the thickness of the layered specimens was 1.5 mm. Color and spectral reflectance of layered ceramics were measured over a white background according to the CIELAB color scale. An UV filter of the spectrophotometer was inserted or removed to exclude or include the UV component of illuminant D65 to determine the fluorescence. Seven specimens were made for each group and each specimen was measured three times. Difference in color (ΔE*ab-FL) and color coordinates by the fluorescence was calculated. From the spectral reflectance values, subtraction spectrum by the inclusion and the exclusion of the UV component was

---

[#] This paper was originally presented in the International Dental Materials Congress on November 23rd, 2007 in Bangkok, Thailand.

* Direct correspondence to: Dr. Yong-Keun Lee, DDS, PhD Professor, Department of Dental Biomaterials Science, School of Dentistry, Seoul National University, 28 Yeongeon-dong, Jongro-gu, Seoul, Korea, Tel: 82-2-740-8693, Fax: 82-2-740-8694, E-mail: ykleedm@snu.ac.kr

calculated. Three-way ANOVA was performed for the differences in color and color coordinates with the fixed factors of the type of core, the type of veneer and the shade of the veneer (α=0.05).

Results: ΔE*ab-FL was 0.6 to 4.3 for the A2-veneer layered ceramics and 0.4 to 2.1 for the A3-veneer layered ceramics. Differences in color and color coordinates were significantly influenced by the three factors ($p<0.05$).

Clinical Significance

Color difference by the fluorescence induced by the UV component of the illuminant D65 of all-ceramics varied by the material and was higher than that of natural dentin. Therefore, these color discrepancies by the fluorescent emission should be considered in clinical shade matching. Shade matching of ceramics should be performed under the light most clinically relevant.

Introduction

Fluorescence by definition is the absorption of light by a substance and the spontaneous and immediate emission of light in a longer wavelength (Nassau [1]). A fluorescent object can radiate more visible light than is incident on it, making it look brighter than a non-fluorescent object (Berns 2). Therefore, color measurement of a fluorescent object should be more exacting than that for a non-fluorescent object because relative contribution of reflected and fluorescent radiations varies with the characteristics of illuminants (ASTM [3]). In the same specification (ASTM [3]), measurement protocol for the ultraviolet (UV)-activated fluorescence, which indicates the fluorescence resulting principally from absorption of the UV radiant flux; shorter than 380 nm in wavelength, is specified. In another ASTM specification (ASTM [4]), a standard practice for detecting fluorescence in an object by spectrophotometry is provided.

Natural teeth emit blue fluorescence under the action of the UV light, in which the UV light is absorbed and bluish light is emitted (Spitzer and ten Bosch [5]). The fluorescence spectrum of tooth enamel has a peak around 450 nm, which makes teeth whiter and brighter in daylight (Monsenego *et al.* [6]). When human dentin is irradiated with 365 nm light, blue fluorescence is observed with a peak at 440±10 nm (Matsumoto *et al.* [7]). For human dentine, color difference (ΔE^*_{ab}) by the blue fluorescence was 0.73 ± 0.04 and yellow-blue coordinate difference (Δb^*) was -0.10 ± 0.03 by spectrophotometry (Lee *et al.* [8]).

Esthetic restorative materials should have similar fluorescence to that of natural teeth. If it is absent, the esthetic quality of a restoration would suffer under the UV light. Since the UV light can brighten a fluorescent object such as human teeth (Spitzer and ten Bosch 5) and fluorescent esthetic materials (Monsenego *et al.* 6; Wozniak and Moore 9; Lee and Powers 10), color differences between human teeth and non-fluorescent resin composites would be apparent when viewed under the UV included light (Lee *et al.* 8; Lee *et al.* 10; ten Bosch and Coops [11]). Fluorescence also adds to the natural look of a restoration and minimizes the metameric effect (Chu *et al.* [12]). Fluorescence spectra of direct esthetic restorative materials varied by the material (Panzeri *et al.* [13]). It was also reported that many of the porcelain teeth and powders had clearly different luminescence characteristics from those of natural teeth (Wozniak and Moore [9]).

For the evaluation of color match, color difference (ΔE^*_{ab}) value is usually used. There have been arguments on the threshold levels for the perceptible or acceptable color differences (Ruyter *et al.* [14]; Seghi *et al.* [15]; Douglas and Brewer [16]). However, these thresholds were determined under optimal in vitro conditions, which may not apply to clinical settings. As a clinical perceptibility threshold, 3.7 ΔE^*_{ab} units was proposed (Johnston and Kao [17]). Recently, based on an actual clinical scenario using spectroradiometric instrumentation, it was reported that the predicted color difference at which 50% of the dentists could perceive a color difference was 2.6 ΔE^*_{ab} units and the value at which 50% of the subjects would remake the restoration due to color mismatch was 5.5 ΔE^*_{ab} units (Douglas *et al.* [18]). It was also reported that the color difference value should be differentially correlated with the clinical situation depending on the shifting direction of the hue (Douglas and Brewer [16]). In the present study, 3.7 ΔE^*_{ab} units based on a spectrophotometer was used as a clinical perceptibility limit.

All-ceramic materials address the increased demand for esthetically pleasing restorations (Anusavice [19]) because restorations with these materials can be made to match natural tooth structure accurately in terms of color, surface texture and translucency (Rosenstiel *et al.* [20]). The recommended reduction thickness for most all-ceramic crowns is generally regarded as 1.5 mm (Rosenstiel *et al.*, [20]).

Although fluorescence of direct esthetic restoratives and other related materials was determined by spectrophotometry, there have been few studies on the fluorescence of all-ceramic materials based on this method. The purpose of this study was to evaluate the fluorescence of simulatedly layered all-ceramic specimens at a clinically relevant thickness with a color measuring spectrophotometer. The null hypothesis assumed in the present study was that the fluorescence of all-ceramic specimens would be the same regardless of the type of all-ceramic material.

Materials and Methods

Specimen Preparation

Seven all-ceramic core materials were fabricated, 11 mm in diameter, following the manufacturers' instructions (Table 1). The Vita Lumin A2 (Vita Zahnfabrik, Bad Sackingen, Germany) corresponding shade was selected for all core ceramics. Thickness of specimens was controlled by grinding with a polishing machine, using a series of silicon carbide papers up to #2000, to the manufacturers' recommended thicknesses required for masking the underlying tooth (Table 1). Seven specimens were made for each material. A dentin ceramic (Vita VM7, Vita Zahnfabrik) and a high noble alloy for metal ceramic crown (BiOcclus 4, DeguDent, Hanau-Wolfgang, Germany) were used as reference core materials. Detailed procedures are reported in a previous study (Lee *et al.* [21]).

Veneer ceramics were selected for each core material (Table 2), and the combination of core and veneer ceramics is listed in Table 3. The final thickness of layered specimens was set to 1.5 mm. The shades for veneer ceramics were selected to correspond to the A2 and A3 shades in the Vita Lumin shade guide. For the grinding of the veneer ceramics, specimens were ground with sintered diamond wheels of 200-grit, 400-grit and 600-grit sequentially. The grinding procedure was performed for both sides of the specimens to adjust the final thickness. Detailed procedures are reported in a previous study (Lee *et al.* [21]).

As a fluorescence reference, fluorescence data of human dentin previously reported (Lee *et al.* [8]) was used in the present study. Dentin specimens from 10 intact human teeth were prepared after storage of the extracted teeth in 0.01% sodium azide solution. Tooth was embedded in cold curing acrylic denture resin and polished up to 2000-grit.

Table 1. All-ceramic core ceramics investigated

Type	Code	Brand name	Thickness (mm)	Batch number	Manufacturer
Slip-cast block	ICS	In-Ceram Spinell Blanks	0.5	7951	Vita Zahnfabrik, Bad Sackingen, Germany
	ICA	In-Ceram Alumina Blanks	0.5	7502	Vita Zahnfabrik
Zirconia block	AZC	ADENS Zi-Ceram	0.4	122005	ADENS, Seoul, Korea
	DIZ	Digident Digizon	0.4	22	Hint-ELS, Griesheim, Germany
	VIZ	Vita 2000 YZ Cubes	0.4	7412	Vita Zahnfabrik
Feldspathic block	MK2	Vitablocks	0.7	7920	Vita Zahnfabrik
Hot pressing	EM2	IPS Empress 2	0.8	H22609	Ivoclar Vivadent, Schaan, Liechtenstein
Sintering	VM7	Vita VM7	0.5	7550	Vita Zahnfabrik
Alloy	ALO	BiOcclus 4	0.5	10013558	DeguDent, Hanau-Wolfgang, Germany

Table 2. All-ceramic veneer ceramics investigated

Code	Shade	Brand name (shade)	Thickness (mm)	Batch number	Manufacturer
V72	A2	Vita VM7 (2M2)	1.0	7550	Vita Zahnfabrik
V73	A3	Vita VM7 (2M3)	1.0	7360	Vita Zahnfabrik
V9-1	A2	Vita VM9 (2M2)	0.8	7480	Vita Zahnfabrik
V9-1	A3	Vita VM9 (2M3)	0.8	7605	Vita Zahnfabrik
V9-2	A2	Vita VM9 (2M2)	1.1	7480	Vita Zahnfabrik
V9-2	A3	Vita VM9 (2M3)	1.1	7605	Vita Zahnfabrik
ER	A2	IPS ERIS (120)	0.7	H13505	Ivoclar Vivadent

Table 2. (Continued)

Code	Shade	Brand name (shade)	Thickness (mm)	Batch number	Manufacturer
ER	A3	IPS ERIS (210)	0.7	H03466	Ivoclar Vivadent
OM	A2	Omega 900 (2M2)	1.0	7910	Vita Zahnfabrik
OM	A3	Omega 900 (2M3)	1.0	7967	Vita Zahnfabrik

Table 3. Combinations of core and veneer ceramics to make clinically relevant specimens

Code (combined)	Core	Veneer (A2)	Code (combined)	Core	Veneer (A3)
ICS2	ICS	V7	ICS3	ICS	V7
ICA2	ICA	V7	ICA3	ICA	V7
AZC2	AZC	V9-2	AZC3	AZC	V9-2
DIZ2	DIZ	V9-2	DIZ3	DIZ	V9-2
VIZ2	VIZ	V9-2	VIZ3	VIZ	V9-2
MK22	MK2	V9-1	MK23	MK2	V9-1
EM22	EM2	ER2	EM23	EM2	ER2
VM72	VM7	V7	VM73	VM7	V7
ALO2	ALO	OM	ALO3	ALO	OM

For the measurement of layered specimens, veneer ceramic specimen was placed over the core ceramic specimen. Among the same type veneer ceramic specimens (n = 7), only one specimen that showed the most similar color coordinates to those of the average color coordinates of seven specimens was used as the veneer ceramic to reduce the deviation of layered color caused by the color deviation of veneer ceramics. When layering, a drop of optical fluid (1.5 index of refraction fluid, Cargille Lab, Cedar Grove, NJ, USA) was applied to the core ceramic specimen. Optical fluid was placed between the veneer porcelain and the core porcelain for an optical connection.

Measurement of the Fluorescence

Color and spectral reflectance of the layered specimens was measured according to the CIELAB color scale over a white standard tile (CIE L^* = 82.4, a^* = -0.1 and b^* = -0.6) on a reflection spectrophotometer (Color-Eye 7000A, GretagMacbeth Instruments Corp., New Windsor, NY, USA) with the specular component excluded (SCE) geometry. The aperture size was 3 × 8 mm, and the illuminating and viewing configuration was the CIE diffuse/8-degree geometry (CIE 22).

Color was measured relative to the xenon lamp that simulates the CIE standard illuminant D65. The UV-filter of the spectrophotometer was inserted or removed to exclude or include the UV component of illumination. Differences in color and color coordinates were calculated by the change of illuminant.

Differences in color (ΔE^*_{ab}-FL) and color coordinates (ΔL^*, Δa^* and Δb^*) by the inclusion or exclusion of the UV component were calculated, where ΔL^* is the change in lightness (CIE L^* of the UV included – that of the UV excluded), Δa^* is the change in red-green coordinate and Δb^* is the change in yellow-blue coordinate. ΔE^*_{ab}-FL was calculated with the equation: $\Delta E^*_{ab}\text{-FL} = [(\Delta L^*)^2 + (\Delta a^*)^2 + (\Delta b^*)^2]^{1/2}$, in which ΔL^* indicates the difference in lightness between the UV excluded and included measurements and so on (CIE [22]).

From the spectral reflectance values, the difference in reflectance by the inclusion and exclusion of the UV component was calculated. With the following calculations, subtraction spectra were obtained. Preliminary subtraction spectrum from 410 to 750 nm (*i.e.*, the reflectance spectrum obtained with the UV-excluded condition subtracted at each wavelength from the reflectance spectrum obtained with the UV-included condition) was obtained. To eliminate the bias in illumination by the inclusion or exclusion of the UV component, the difference in reflectance spectrum at each wavelength of the white standard tile by the inclusion or exclusion of the UV component was subtracted from the preliminary subtraction spectrum at each wavelength (Lee *et al.* [8]).

To determine whether the difference in the color coordinates (ΔL^*, Δa^* and Δb^*) and the color (ΔE^*_{ab}-FL) by the fluorescence induced by the UV component of the illuminant D65 was influenced by the type of core (9 type), the type of the veneer (5 type) and the shade of the veneer (2 type), 3-way ANOVA (analysis of variance) and Scheffe's multiple range test was performed (SPSS 12.0, SPSS, Chicago, IL, USA, $p=0.05$).

RESULTS

Differences in the color coordinates (ΔL^*, Δa^* and Δb^*) and color (ΔE^*_{ab}-FL) by the fluorescence for the A2-veneer layered specimens are presented in Figure 1, and for the A3-veneer layered specimens are in Figure 2. ΔE^*_{ab}-FL for the A2-veneer layered specimens was in the range of 0.4 (AZC2) to 4.3 (ALO2), and that for the A3-veneer layered specimens was in the range of 0.4 (AZC3) to 2.1 (ALO3).

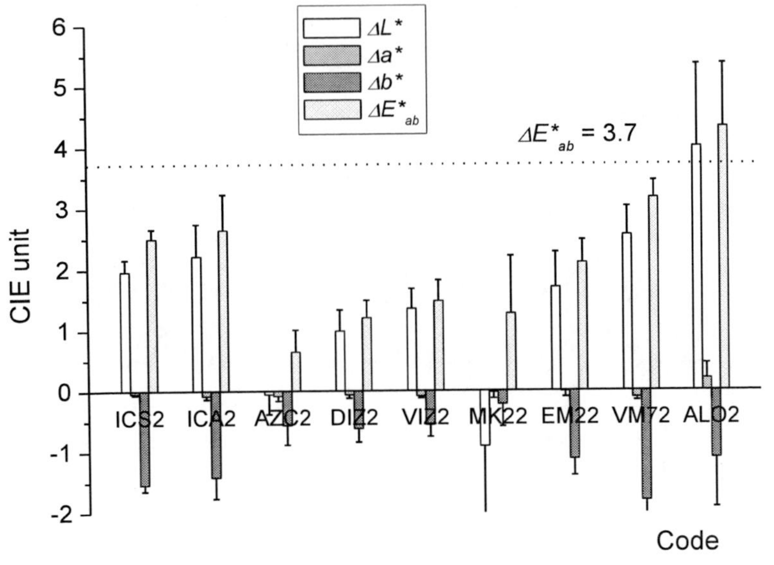

Figure 1. Difference in the color coordinates (ΔL^*, Δa^* and Δb^*) and color (ΔE^*_{ab}-FL) by the inclusion or exclusion of the UV component of the illuminant D65 for the A2-veneer layered specimens.

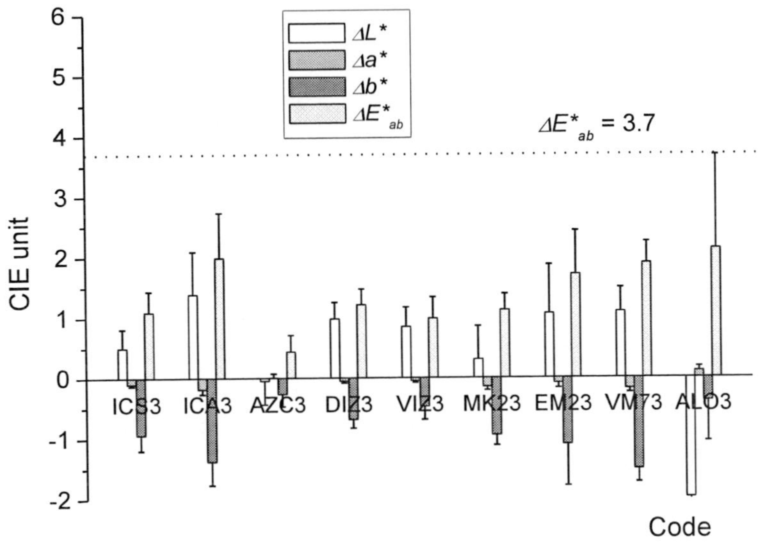

Figure 2. Difference in the color coordinates (ΔL^*, Δa^* and Δb^*) and color (ΔE^*_{ab}-FL) by the inclusion or exclusion of the UV component of the illuminant D65 for the A3-veneer layered specimens.

ΔE^*_{ab}-FL values sorted by the core material regardless of the shade of the veneer are presented in Figure 3. The range for ΔE^*_{ab}-FL was 0.5 (AZC core) to 3.2 (ALO core). ΔE^*_{ab}-FL values sorted by the veneer material regardless of the core material are presented in Fig. 4. The range for ΔE^*_{ab}-FL for the A2 veneer was 1.1 (V9-2) to 4.3 (OM) and that for the A3 veneer was 0.9 (V9-2) to 2.1 (OM), which was averaged to 1.0 (V9-2) to 3.2 (OM) for both shades.

Differences in spectral reflectance by the inclusion or exclusion of the UV-component of the illuminant D65 for ICS, ICA and VM7 core materials are listed in Figure 5, and that for EM2 and ALO core materials are listed in Figure 6. Although a clear peak was not detected in each subtraction spectrum, the difference by the UV component of the illuminant was observed.

Based on the 3-way ANOVA for the difference in the color coordinates (ΔL^*, Δa^* and Δb^*) and the color (ΔE^*_{ab}-FL), the results were as follows.

ΔL^* value was significantly influenced by the three factors of the type of core, the type of the veneer and the shade of the veneer based on 3-way ANOVA ($p<0.01$), although the thickness in each of the core and the veneer ceramics varied by the brand. Based on Scheffe's multiple comparison test by the type of core, the following homogenous subsets were observed: MK2. AZC / DIZ. ALO. VIZ. ICS. EM2 / ICS. EM2. ICA. VM7 ($p<0.05$). Based on the same test by the type of veneer, the following homogenous subsets were observed: V9-1 / V9-2. OM / OM. ER/ ER. V7 ($p<0.05$).

Δa^* value was significantly influenced by the three factors ($p<0.01$). Based on Scheffe's multiple comparison test by the type of core, the following homogenous subsets were observed: VM7. ICA. MK2. ICS / ICA. MK2. ICS. VIZ. DIZ / MK2. ICS. VIZ. DIZ. EM2. AZC / ALO ($p<0.05$). Based on the same test by the type of veneer, the following homogenous subsets were observed: V7. V9-1 / V9-1. V9-2. ER / OM ($p<0.05$). '/' is the group separation mark.

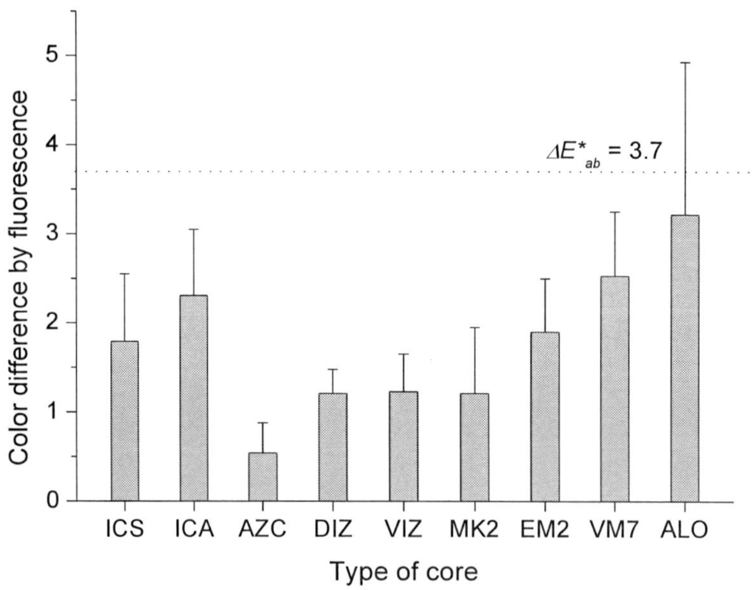

Figure 3. Color difference (ΔE^*_{ab}-FL) by the inclusion or exclusion of the UV component of the illuminant D65 sorted by the core material regardless of the shade of the veneer.

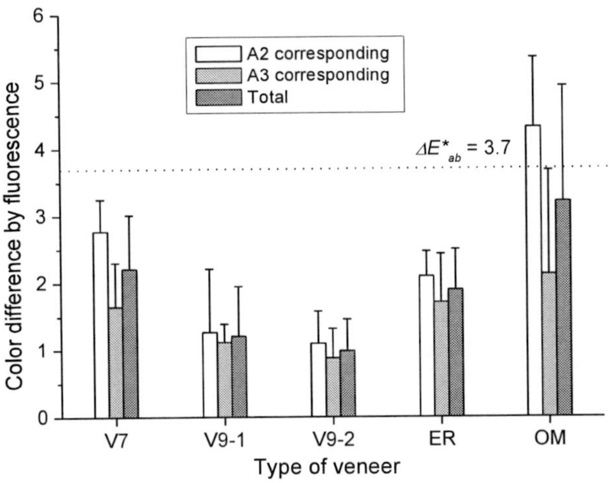

Figure 4. Color difference (ΔE^*_{ab}-FL) by the inclusion or exclusion of the UV component of the illuminant D65 sorted by the veneer material regardless of the core type.

Δb^* value was significantly influenced by the three factors ($p<0.01$). Based on Scheffe's multiple comparison test by the type of core, the following homogenous subsets were observed: VM7. ICA / ICA. ICS. EM2 / ALO. DIZ. MK2. VIZ / DIZ. MK2. VIZ. AZC ($p<0.05$). Based on the same test by the type of veneer, the following homogenous subsets were observed: V7 / ER / OM. V9-2. V9-1 ($p<0.05$).

ΔE^*_{ab}-FL value was significantly influenced by the three factors of the type of core, the type of the veneer and the shade of the veneer based on 3-way ANOVA ($p<0.01$), although the thickness in each of the core and the veneer ceramics varied by the brand. Based on Scheffe's multiple comparison test by the type of core, the following homogenous subsets were observed: AZC/ DIZ. MK2. VIZ / ICS. EM2. ICA / ICA. VM7 / ALO ($p<0.05$). Based on the same test by the type of veneer, the following homogenous subsets were observed: V9-2. V9-1 / ER. V7/ OM ($p<0.05$).

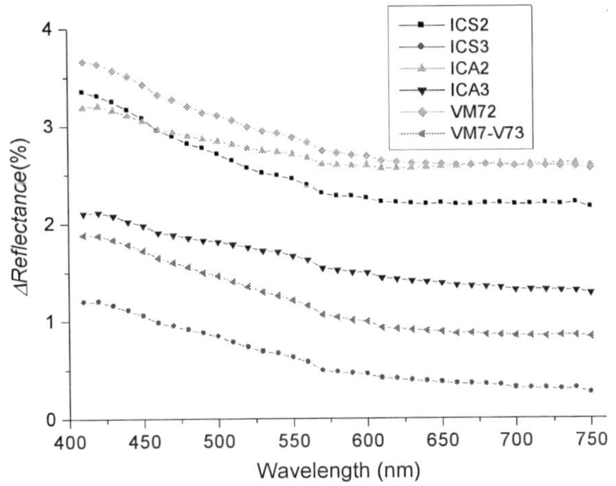

Figure 5. Difference in spectral reflectance by the inclusion or exclusion of the UV-component of the illuminant D65 (1).

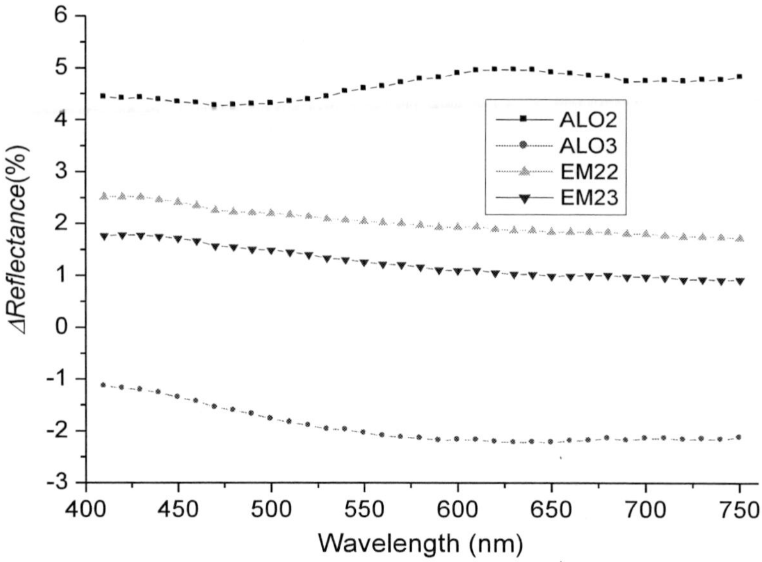

Figure 6. Difference in spectral reflectance by the inclusion or exclusion of the UV-component of the illuminant D65 (2).

DISCUSSION

The null hypothesis, the fluorescence of all-ceramic specimens would be the same regardless of the type of all-ceramic material, was rejected because ΔE^*_{ab}-FL value was significantly influenced by the three factors of the type of core, the type of the veneer and the shade of the veneer based on 3-way ANOVA. ΔE^*_{ab}-FL value of human dentin, determined with the same protocol in the previous study (Lee *et al.* [8]), was 0.73 ± 0.04 and yellow-blue coordinate difference (Δb^*) was -0.10 ± 0.03. Comparing with the results of the present study, in which ΔE^*_{ab}-FL was 0.6 to 4.3 for the A2-veneer layered ceramics and 0.4 to 2.1 for the A3-veneer layered ceramics, the color difference by the fluorescence of all-ceramics was higher than that of human dentin. However, peak pattern of all-ceramics was different from those of human dentin (Figures 5 and 6). Therefore, further study should be performed whether ΔE^*_{ab}-FL of all-ceramics would be perceived as fluorescence like that in teeth.

The CIE standard illuminant D65 represents average daylight with a correlated color temperature of approximately 6500 K (ISO [23]). The illuminant D65 contains relative spectral power of 37-69% in the wavelength range of 330-395 nm (CIE [22]); therefore, this contains a strong emission in the UV range compared to the illuminant A or F2. The difference in reflection spectra of teeth was measured between two illuminants (A and D65), and the influence of the illuminants on the color of teeth was found to be insignificant (ten Bosch and Coops [11]). Color differences of resin composites between the values measured relative to the standard illuminants A and D65, or A and C, were larger than those between D65 and C (Lee *et al.* [24]). In these previous studies, exact measurement of fluorescence should have been impossible because spectral distribution of illuminants were different in visible range as well as in UV range. Therefore, new method to determine the fluorescence using the UV portion of the illuminant D65 was developed that uses a spectrophotometer with an adjustable UV filter (Lee *et al.* [8]), which was previously introduced in the specification (ASTM [4]).

Previous studies used fluorescence spectrophotometers to determine the fluorescence of dental substances, in which single wavelength was usually used for the emission of fluorescence. To induce fluorescence of dentin, UV light of 365 nm (or 363.8 nm) was employed (Monsenego *et al.* [6]; Matsumoto *et al.* [7]). After excitation, dentin showed blue fluorescence in a peak at 440±10 nm (Matsumoto *et al.* [7]), or 430 nm (Monsenego *et al.* [6]). With the protocol of the present study, dentin showed peak intensity at 440 nm, and the subtraction spectrum (fluorescence) had a wide band form which is similar to those of previous studies (Lee *et al.* [8]). Therefore, the UV light emitted from the illuminant D65 excited the fluorescence of dentin. It should be mentioned that the use of UV component of the illuminant D65 has clinical relevance that can induce fluorescence observable under daylight condition because the ambient light is not a monochromatic light.

In the present study, color difference (ΔE^*_{ab}-FL) by the fluorescence of all-ceramic materials was 0.4 to 4.3 (Figures 1 and 2). Although almost all of these values were lower than generally considered clinically perceptible limit of 3.7 (Johnston and Kao [17]), the contribution of the fluorescent emission on the color would be different from that under UV depleted illumination. The fluorescence of teeth makes an important contribution to its appearance even though it may not be apparent in daylight.

Fluorescence of anterior restorative materials was measured previously with a spectrophotometer with a fluorescent attachment (Panzeri *et al.* [13]). The results varied for silicate cement, acrylic resin and resin composites, and resin composites showed fluorescence peaks around 450 nm. However, quantitative comparison with the results of the present study was impossible because the method was different. In dental ceramics, a fluorescent material called luminary was used to brighten dark teeth without negatively affecting the translucency (McLaren [25]). Therefore, the influence of fluorescence emission from dental ceramics on the masking effect should be studied further.

In the present study, the fluorescence of all-ceramic materials was measured with a color measuring spectrophotometer. All-ceramic materials investigated showed color difference by the fluorescence induced by the UV component of the illuminant D65.

ACKNOWLEDGMENT

This work was supported by the Korea Research Foundation Grant funded by the Korean Government (MOEHRD, Basic Research Promotion Fund; KRF-2006-311-E00091).

REFERENCES

[1] Nassau K. Color for science, art and technology. Elsevier, New York, 1998; pp. 10-11.

[2] Berns RS. Billmeyer and Saltzman's principles of color technology. 3rd ed. New York: John Wiley and Sons, 2000; pp. 10, 27-29, 83-87.

[3] American Society for Testing and Materials (ASTM). E 991-98. Standard practice for color measurement of fluorescent specimens. West Conshohocken: ASTM, 1998.

[4] ASTM. E 1247-03. Standard practice for detecting fluorescence in object-color specimens by spectrophotometry. West Conshohocken: ASTM, 2003.

[5] Spitzer D, ten Bosch JJ. The total luminescence of bovine and human dental enamel. *Calcif Tissue Res* 1976; 20: 201-208.

[6] Monsenego G, Burdairon G, Clerjaud B. Fluorescence of dental porcelain. *J Prosthet. Dent.* 1993; 69: 106-113.

[7] Matsumoto H, Kitamura S, Araki T. Autofluorescence in human dentine in relation to age, tooth type and temperature measured by nanosecond time-resolved fluorescence microscopy. *Arch. Oral Biol.* 1999; 44: 309-318.

[8] Lee YK, Lu H, Powers JM. Fluorescence of layered resin composites. *J. Esthet Restor. Dent* 2005; 17: 93-101.

[9] Wozniak WT, Moore BK. Luminescence spectra of dental porcelains. *J. Dent Res.* 1978; 57: 971-974.

[10] Lee YK, Powers JM. Metameric effect between resin composite and dentin. *Dent. Mater.* 2005; 21: 971-976.

[11] ten Bosch JJ, Coops JC. Tooth color and reflectance as related to light scattering and enamel hardness. *J. Dent Res.* 1995; 74: 374-380.

[12] Chu SJ, Devigus A, Mieleszko A. Fundamentals of color Shade matching and communication in esthetic dentistry. Chicago: Quintessence Publishing Co, Inc, 2004; p. 45.

[13] Panzeri H, Fernandes LT, Minelli CJ. Spectral fluorescence of direct anterior restorative materials. *Aust. Dent. J.* 1977; 22: 458-461.

[14] Ruyter IE, Nilner K, Moller B. Color stability of dental composite resin materials for crown and bridge veneers. *Dent. Mater.* 1987; 3: 246-251.

[15] Seghi RR, Hewlett ER, Kim J. Visual and instrumental colorimetric assessments of small color differences on translucent dental porcelain. *J. Dent. Res.* 1989; 68: 1760-1764.

[16] Douglas RD, Brewer JD. Acceptability of shade differences in metal ceramic crowns. *J. Prosthet Dent.* 1998; 79: 254-260.

[17] Johnston WM, Kao EC. Assessment of appearance match by visual observation and clinical colorimetry. *J. Dent. Res.* 1989; 68: 819-822.

[18] Douglas RD, Steinhauer TJ, Wee AG. Intraoral determination of the tolerance of dentists for perceptibility and acceptability of shade mismatch. *J. Prosthet. Dent.* 2007; 97: 200-208.

[19] Anusavice K. Philips' science of dental materials. 11th ed. St. Louis: Saunders; 2003; pp. 655-719.

[20] Rosenstiel SF, Land MF, Fujimoto J. Contemporary fixed prothodontics. 4th ed. St. Louis: Mosby, 2006; p. 774.

[21] Lee YK, Cha HS, Ahn JS. Layered color of all-ceramic core and veneer ceramics. *J. Prosthet Dent.* 2007; 97: 279-286.

[22] CIE (Commission Internationale de l'Eclairage). Colorimetry - Technical Report. CIE Pub. No.15, 3rd ed. Vienna, Austria: Bureau Central de la CIE; 2004.

[23] International Standardization Organization (ISO). CIE standard illuminant for Colorimetry. ISO 10526: 1999(E), CIE S 005-1998.

[24] Lee YK, Lim BS, Kim CW, Powers JM. Color characteristics of low-chroma and high translucency dental resin composites by different measuring modes. *J. Biomed Mat. Res., Appl. Biomat.* 2001; 58: 613-621.
[25] McLaren EA. Luminescent veneers. *J. Esthet Dent.* 1997; 9: 3-12.

In: Clinical Dentistry
Editor: Scardina Giuseppe Alessandro

ISBN: 978-1-61122-354-5
© 2011 Nova Science Publishers, Inc.

Chapter 9

MICRO-MECHANICAL INTERLOCKING AND CHEMICAL BONDING OF SELF-ETCHING ADHESIVES AT THE RESIN-TOOTH HARD TISSUE INTERFACES[§]

***Baiping Fu*[*1,2], *Ling Bi*[1] *and Matthias Hannig*[2]**

[1]Department of Stomatology, No. 1 Hospital affiliated to Medical College, Zhejiang University, Hangzhou, 310003, China

[2]Clinic of Operative Dentistry, Periodontology and Preventive Dentistry, Saarland University, Homburg/Saar, Germany

ABSTRACT

Purpose: The aim of this review is to elucidate the relationship of micro-mechanical interlocking and chemical bonding of self-etching adhesives at the resin-tooth hard tissues interfaces.

Methods: Instrumental analysis is widely used for detection of surface chemistry. Electron microscopy is used to analyze the interfaces between adhesives and tooth surface. This paper critically reviews the recent research on the interaction of the self-etching primers/adhesives and some carboxylic acids with tooth hard tissues/ hydroxyapatite, and the interfaces of resin-tooth hard tissues.

Clinical Significance: Some self-etching adhesives have been proven to provide chemical bonding to hydroxyapatite. Thus, self-etching adhesives possess a high possibility to form a tight micro-mechanical interlocking at the tooth hard tissue-resin interfaces. However, the clinical performance of the self-etching adhesives such as bond durability, marginal adaptation, and sealing capacity or the potential to reduce post-operative hyper-sensitivity depends on the individual self-etching adhesive system used,

---

[§] A version of this book was also published as a chapter in *International Journal of Clinical Dentistry, Volume 1, Issue 3*, published by Nova Science Publishers, Inc. It was submitted for appropriate modifications in an effort to encourage wider dissemination of research.

[*] Corresponding Author: Prof. Baiping Fu, Department of Stomatology, No. 1 Hospital aff. to Medical College, Zhejiang University, Qingchun Road 79, Hanghou 310003, China. Tel: 0086-571-87236338, 0086-571-85924253. Fax: 0086-571-86560107. Email address: baiping_fu@yahoo.com

the operator's/dentist's clinical technique, the chemical stability of the adhesives system itself and its chemical bonding to tooth hard tissues.

Keywords: chemical bonding, micro-mechanical interlocking, carboxylic acids, self-etching adhesives.

Enamel, Dentin, and Hydroxyapatite

The main inorganic component of the human hard tissues is apatite --- a natural mineral. Synthetic hydroxyapatite (HA) is extensively studied as a biomaterial due to its close chemical resemblance of the natural mineral [1]. Human enamel contains about 96wt% of a nano-crystalline, oriented, inorganic material, which is closely related to hydroxyapatite. The remainder consists of heterogeneous proteinaceous materials (~1%) and water (3.9%). The chemical composition of the mineral component of dentine and cementum is rather similar to enamel [2]. Dentin is about 20% organic, 70% inorganic, and 10% aqueous by weight [3,4]. Hydroxyapatite crystallites in the sound enamel are 160 nm long, 40~70 nm wide and 30 nm thick, whereas hydroxyapatite crystallites in the dentin are 20 nm in length, 18~20 nm in width, and 35 nm in diameter [3,4]. The organic materials in the dentin are approximately 95% collagen, and 5% non-collageneous proteins. The crystallites in the dentin are embedded in a collagenic fibril network, whereas the crystallites within the enamel are highly oriented in prisms [3,4].

Bonding to Enamel

A main goal in restorative dentistry is the tight and durable seal between the tooth hard substance and the restorative materials. In 1955, Buonocore reported etching of the enamel with 85% phosphoric acid in order to facilitate microretentive adhesion of acrylic resins to the enamel surface [5]. Since then, phosphoric acid has become one of the most important acids in the field of adhesive dentistry [5-8]. Phosphoric acid or some water-soluble carboxylic acids can dissolve the mineral of human hard tissues---hydroxyapaptite, and produce calcium phosphate/carboxylate and calcium hydrogen phosphate [9,10]. Phosphoric/carboxylic acid etching extracts the calcium from the enamel substrate, causes partial demineralization of the enamel surfaces, and produces micro- and nano-porosities on the enamel surfaces (Figure 1). Subsequently, these micro- and nano-porosities on the enamel surfaces are refilled with a low-viscosity resin (Figure 2). The micro- and nano-mechanical interlocking at the enamel-resin interfaces is the main retentive force for the resin restorations [8,11-13]. Under clinical conditions, enamel bonding is successfully achieved after the enamel etching with 30~40% phosphoric acid, rinsing with water, air-drying, and subsequent application and polymerization of a low-viscosity hydrophobic resin [8,12].

Besides phosphoric acid, maleic acid is used as an etchant prior to application of bonding agents. Similar bond strengths were recorded when 10% maleic acid etching was compared to 37% phosphoric acid etching [14]. The bond strengths of enamel etched with maleic acid were time dependent [15], in other words, the longer the etching time, the greater the bond strengths. The reports on malic acid as an etchant in dental literature are limited [16,17], however, the malic acid was often studied as a dietary acid for tooth erosion [18].

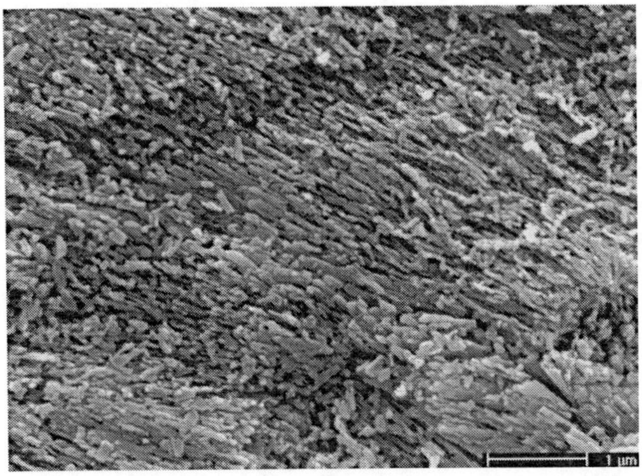

Figure 1. The enamel surface was etched with 15% citric acid for 30 s. The micro- and nano- porosities were exposed among the enamel hydroxyapatite crystallites after removal of smear layer (original magnification=20,000 fold, bar= 1 μm).

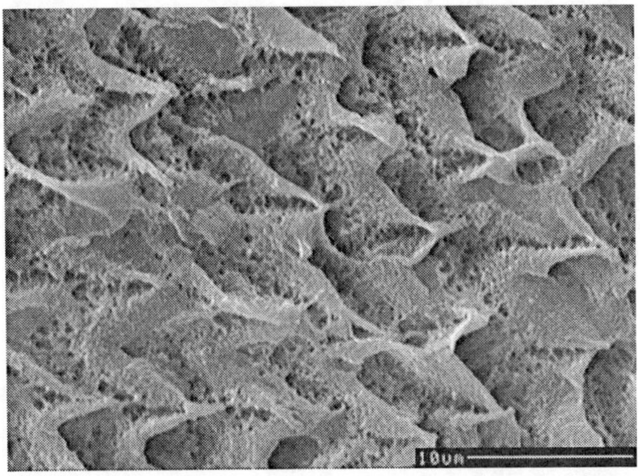

Figure 2. SEM pictures of resin tags. The resin tags formed within human enamel that was acid-etched and applied with a conventional hydrophobic resin--Heliobond (Ivoclar Vivadent, Liechtenstein) revealed honeycomb-like etching pattern (original magnification=2,870 fold, bar= 10μm).

Bonding to Dentin

In contrast to the well-established resin-to-enamel bonding, achievement of a durable bonding between resin materials and dentin is still a challenge in restorative dentistry [19]. After bur preparation, the dentinal surfaces are covered by a so-called smear layer consisting of bur-prepared debris. The dentin etching was thought to widen the orifices of the dentinal tubules and provoke the dental pulp till a strong dentin bond strength was obtained after the dentin was etched with 40% phosphoric acid [19]. Acid etching and water-rinsing of the bur-prepared dentin surface cause the removal of the smear layer and demineralization of the human dentin surfaces, expose the collagen fibrils encapsulated by dentin hydroxyapatite crystallites, and open the dentinal tubules (Figure 3). Nakabayashi et al. in 1982 were the first who found that the monomers penetrate through the exposed collagenic networks into the demineralized dentinal surface, and are polymerized in situ to form a hybrid layer at the interfaces of resin-dentin restorations [20]. Since then, it is thought that the dentin adhesion is mainly based on the hybrid layers of the micro-mechanical interlocking at the resin-dentin interfaces [20-24].

The exposed collagen networks on the demineralized dentin surfaces will collapse without water support, if the etched dentin surfaces are completely dried by air blow (Figure 4). The collapsed fibril layer on the conditioned dentin surface can hinder the monomers from permeating into the demineralized dentin [25-30].

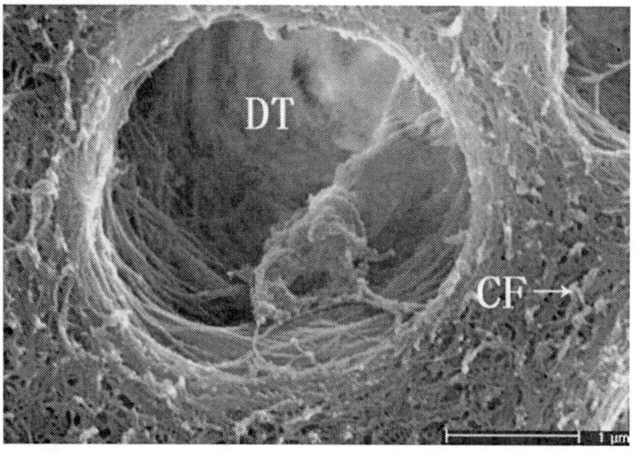

Figure 3. The dentin surface was etched with 5% malic acid for 15 s, dried with a serial of alcohol and critical point dried. The removal of dentin smear layer revealed exposure of the collagen fibrils and the patent dentinal tubules. DT: Dentinal tubule, CF: Collagen fibrils (original magnification=20,000 fold, bar= 1 μm).

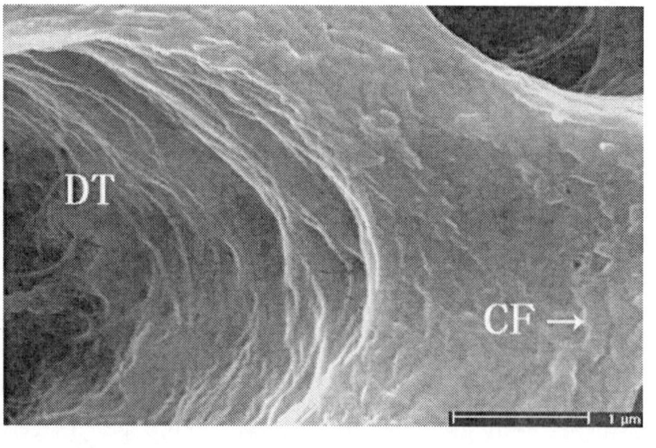

Figure 4. The dentin surface was etched with 15% citric acid, and dried in air, suggesting that the collagen fibrils between the patent dentin tubules collapsed due to water evaporation. DT: Dentinal tubule, CF: Collagen fibrils (original magnification=20,000 fold, bar= 1 μm).

Therefore, Kanca in the early 1990s proposed the wet/moist-bonding technique that involved the following application steps. The dentin surfaces were etched, water-rinsed, gently air-dried for 3~5 s, subsequently primed with hydrophilic primers, and applied with hydrophobic bonding resin [25].

With subsequent development of self-etching adhesive systems, it is not necessary to use phosphoric acid etching prior to the application of the self-etching primers [13,31,32].

Contrary to the wet/moist-bonding technique, Tay et al. in 2007 proposed a new concept for hydrophobic dentin bonding or ethanol-wetting bonding [33,34]. This concept indicates that ethanol replacement of water-saturated/hydrogenated demineralized dentin produced wider interfibrillar spaces, more extensive shrinkage of collagen fibrils and narrower hybrid layer.

Self-Etching Adhesives

The non-resin-impregnated demineralized dentin layer between the hybrid layer and the intact dentin becomes the weakest zone in the resin-dentin interfaces, [35-37] and is susceptible to hydrolytic degradation [32]. Concerning the problem of incomplete diffusion of dental monomers into the demineralized dentin as well as simplification of the clinical application procedures, self-etching adhesive systems were introduced in the early 1990s. A self-etching primer containing Phenyl-P (2-methacryloxyethyl phenyl hydrogen phosphate) was manufactured in the early 1990s [38]. The self-etching primers can partly decalcify the tooth substrates, permeate simultaneously into the intact enamel and dentin, and be in situ polymerized [13,31,32,38-40]. The self-etching primers eliminate the acid-etching and water-rinsing steps, and simplify the clinical application procedure [13,31,32,38,39]. The self-etching primers contain some acidic functional groups --- water-soluble carboxylic acid, derivatives of carboxylic acid, phosphoric acid esters, and phosphonic acid esters [41]. The water-soluble carboxylic acid and the phosphoric group of phosphoric acid esters possess an enamel etching ability [31,42] (Figure 5). The reaction of phosphoric acid esters with hydroxyapatite produces calcium salts of phosphoric acid esters [42,43] (Figure 6).

Due to the treatment with self-etching primers, the tooth surfaces/substrates are partly decalcified and dissolved in the self-etching primers. Subsequently, gentle air-blow will cause vaporization of the primer solvents and some dissolved tooth mineral components in the primer solvents will re-deposit within the de-mineralized dentin collagenic networks and the de-mineralized enamel surfaces/substrates.

Covalent bonding between the dentin and the bonding agents was not found in an early FTIR (Fourier Transformed Infrared Spectroscopy) photoacoustic spectroscopy study [44]. More interestingly, scanning transmission electron microscopy and energy-dispersive spectroscopy analysis revealed that a sulfur-labeled HEMA (thiolated HEMA or 2-hydroxyethylthiomethycrylate; HETMA) primer could completely penetrate into the demineralized dentin zone resulting from etching with 10-3 solution (citric acid + ferric chloride) or maleic acid, and keep an intimate contact with the underlying non-demineralized dentin [45]. However, phase separation at the dentin-adhesive interfaces was found by means of a histo-chemical staining and micro-Raman spectroscopic analysis [46], and by micro-morphological observations [47-50].

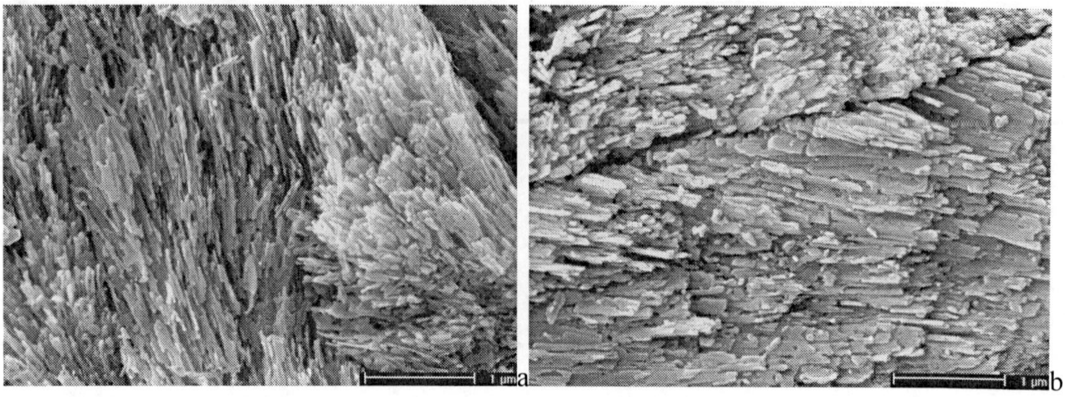

Figure 5. The enamel surface was rubbed with Prompt-L-pop (a) (3M ESPE, Germany) or Clearfil Protect Bond (b) (Kuraray Co. Japan) for 30 s, rinsed with water for 30 s, and dried with a series of alcohol. The SEM pictures revealed a weak etching pattern---the individual enamel crystallites were exposed and the matrix around enamel prisms was decalcified more deeply than the enamel prisms (original magnification=20,000 fold, bar= 1 μm).

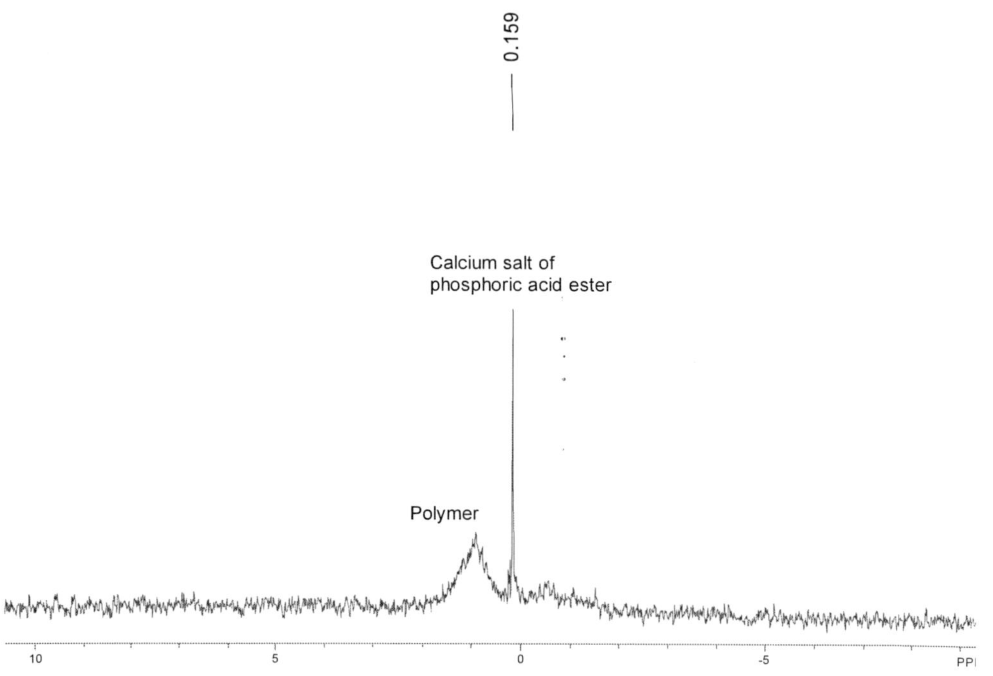

Figure 6. Spectrum of ^{31}PMNR The solid material of the reaction of Prompt L-pop with HA was separated, washed with 10 ml de-ionized water for three times, dried and analyzed with ^{31}P MNR in $CDCl_3$. The spectrum revealed calcium salts of phosphoric acid esters and polymer.

The incomplete micro-emulsion of adhesives' compositions/ingredients was attributable to the phase separation [51], revealing that variables of oil in water and water in oil or vice versa exist not only in the hydrophilic domain, but also in the hydrophobic domain (Figure 7). These phase separation phenomena strongly interfere with the polymerization of the adhesive layer, and, thus, have detrimental effects on the resin-tooth hard tissue interfaces.

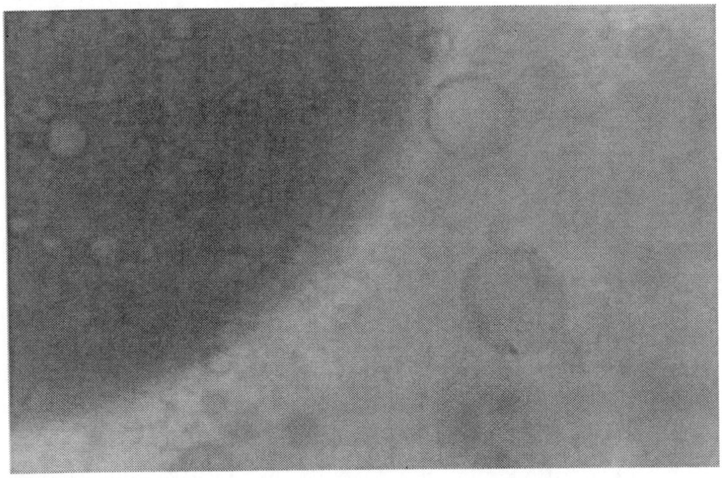

Figure 7. Light Microscopy of a mixture of Prime and Bond NT (Dentsply, Germany) added with 0.5% methylene blue. A hydrophilic domain in dark blue and a hydrophobic area in light blue suggested the inhomogeneous micro-emulsion of the primer and bonding/adhesive components. (original magnification=100 fold).

The smear layer contains bur-prepared debris, and the weak smear layer is not removed by the self-etching primers. The inherent weakness will interfere with the adherence of self-etching primer-adhesive systems to enamel/dentin substrates. Therefore, the coarse (#180 grit) smear layer results in a lower tensile bond strength of self-etching priming agents to dentin than the smooth (#600 grit) smear layer [52]. Clinically, the fine grit diamond bur is strongly recommended to prepare the tooth prior to the application of the self-etching adhesive systems [13].

The recent self-etching primers containing the carboxylic acids, carboxylic derivatives, or the phosphoric acid esters are designed and manufactured on the basis of the formation of the hybrid layer at the dentin-resin interfaces [20,39,53,54]. These functional groups react with the enamel/dentin substrates [13]. Therefore, the prolongation of the priming time will increase the thickness of the hybrid layer [53]. The aggressiveness of the self-etching primers is quite different, which is also correlated with the thickness of the hybrid layer [54]. However, the thickness of the hybrid layer is not directly correlated with the dentin bond strength [22,24,39,53-56].

Recently, Sano's group [57] proposed a nanointeraction zone at the resin-dentin interface, indicating that the bonded interfaces produced by some self-etching adhesives were extremely thin (300 nm or less), the dentin surface was slightly demineralized, and the collagen fibrils of the dentin substrate were still coated by hydroxyapatite.

Chemical Bonding and Micro-Mechanical Interlocking

The chemical bonding, especially the covalent bond, might be expected to reveal a more durable bond strength than the mechanical bonding and interlocking [58]. Chemical bonding does eliminate any unnecessary preparations in the sound tooth hard tissues in order to get a sufficient mechanical retention [59].

Previous studies on the kinetics of demineralization have indicated that demineralization of the tooth surface is affected by the acidic conditioner's pH and counterion [60-62]. Most interestingly, for maleic acid, the ability of demineralization positively correlates to the proton concentration, while for citric acid, a negative correlation has been reported [61,62].

If the solubility of carboxylic acids such as itaconic acid and benzoic acid is too low in water, the acid-base reaction with HA is difficult to take place. The chemical reaction of HA with itaconic acid or benzoic acid was not detected by FTIR spectra according to our unpublished data. In other words, the FTIR spectra of the solid materials separating from the reaction products of HA with itaconic acid or benzoic acid were the same as HA's spectra. The FTIR spectra of the filtrate separating from the reaction products of HA with itaconic acid or benzoic acid correspond well with the spectra of the carboxylic acids themselves. These findings are consistent with the previous morphological obseravation indicating that the enamel etched with benzoic acid did not reveal any distinct surface changes [63]. Inversely, if the calcium carboxylate such as calcium acrylate has very high solubility in water, the acid can only decalcify HA and will not adhere to the HA surfaces according to our unpublished preliminary data. These phenomena are completely consistent with the adhesion-decalcification concept (AD concept) introduced by Yoshida et al. (2001) [64]. In detail, whether the carboxylic acids either adhere to or decalcify HA depends on the dissolution rate of the respective calcium carboxylate in the solution of the carboxylic acids themselves, regardless of concentration and pH.

After self-etching primers reacted with HA particles, the primers, the HA particles and the reaction products of them were analyzed by FTIR. After FTIR spectra of the reaction products of the primer and HA were subtracted by those of the primer, there still existed the self-etching primer's characteristic stretching bands (Figure 8). After the HA disks were treated with the self-etching primer (Prompt L-pop) and thoroughly water-sprayed, the typical stretching bands of the primer such as carbonyl groups, the double bond, as well as of HA such as the phosphoric groups were found on HA disk surfaces (Figure 9). If HA disks were treated with the primer component of adhesive containing carboxylic acid, ATR (Attenuated Total Reflectance) spectra revealed not only the typical stretching bands of the self-etching primers ($\nu_{C=O}$, $\nu_{C=C}$) and HA ($\nu_{P\text{-}O}$, $\nu_{P=O}$), but also stretching bands of carboxylic salts (Figure 10). This finding indicated that the self-etching priming agents reveal chemical adsorption on the HA particle surfaces.

The phosphor-31 of the solid materials of the reaction products of self-etching adhesives containing phosphoric acid esters revealed a broad peak and several sharp peaks, suggesting the existence of polymer of phosphoric acid esters and calcium salts of phosphoric acid esters on the HA surfaces [42]. (Figure 6, 11). This observation might imply chemical adhesion of the phosphoric acid esters onto the hydroxyapatite surfaces.

Evidence of the inter- and intra-crystallite hybridization at the enamel-resin interfaces was recently found after the enamel surfaces were conditioned with self-etching primers [13]. The individual hydroxyapatite crystallites were intimately encapsulated in the self-etching adhesive systems at a nanometer level [13]. The absence of nano-gaps indicates that the chemical reaction of the self-etching primers with tooth hard tissues is concomitant with the physiosorption/chemisorption of the self-etching primers onto HA.

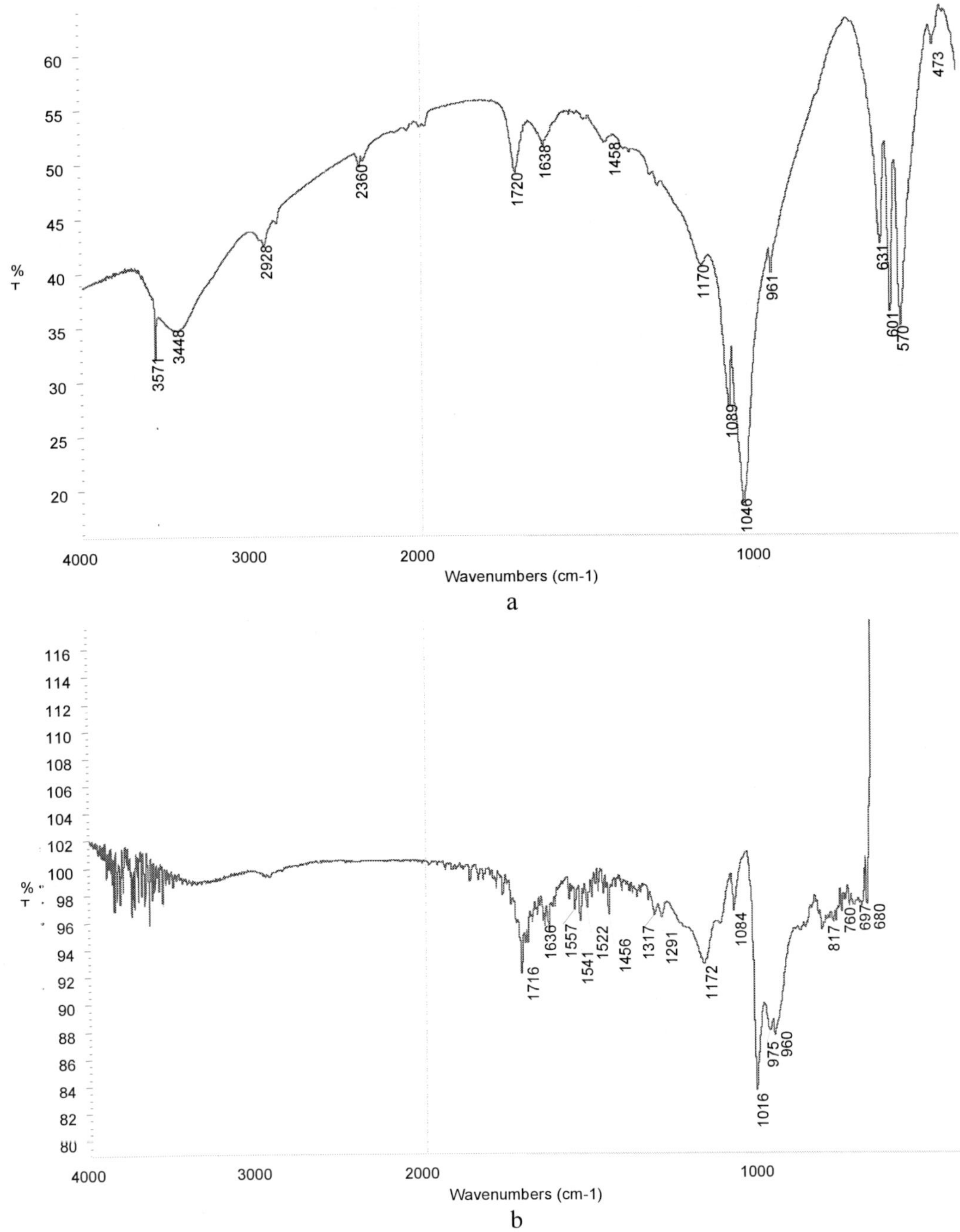

Figure 8. Primer-subtracted FTIR Spectra There still existed the typical bands of the self-etching primers (a: Clearfil Liner Bond 2v (CLB 2v, Kuraray Co., Japan); b: Promt L-pop (3M ESPE, Germany)) such as carbonyl group ($\nu_{C=O}$ at 1720, 1716 cm^{-1})), double bonds ($\nu_{C=C}$ at 1738, 1736 cm^{-1}) etc., and of HA such as the phosphoric groups (ν_{P-O} at 1089, 1084 cm^{-1},$\nu_{P=O}$ at 1046, 1016 cm^{-1}) after the spectra of the reaction products of HA with the primers were subtracted by the spectra of the corresponding primer.

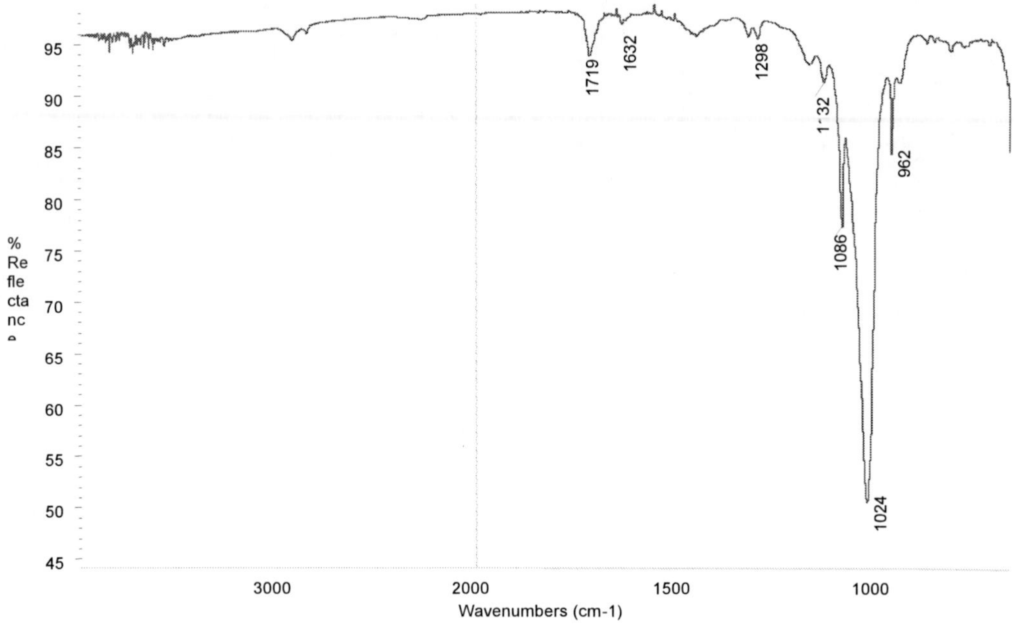

a

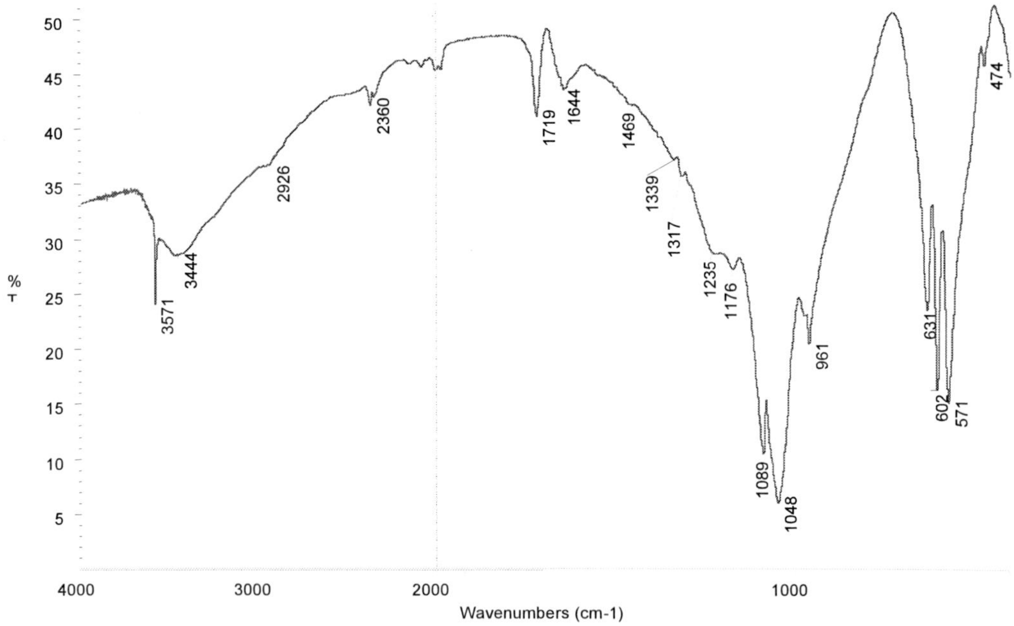

b

Figure 9. ATR Spectra on the HA surfaces primed with CLB 2v primer (a) or Prompt L-pop (b). There were the stretching bands of the carbonyl group ($\nu_{C=O}$ at 1719 cm^{-1}), double bond ($\nu_{C=C}$ at 1732, 1744 cm^{-1}) and the phosphoric groups ($\nu_{P\text{-}O}$ at 1086, 1089 cm^{-1},$\nu_{P=O}$ at 1026, 1048 cm^{-1} (a, b), as well as the separate hydroxyl groups (ν_{OH} at 3571, 3444 cm^{-1})(b).

Although the chemical bonding at the interfaces of the resin-tooth hard tissues/hydroxyapatite was found by many researchers [9,10,42,64,65], it is not possible to indicate how much contribution of the chemical bonding/adhesion at the resin-tooth hard tissues is made in comparison to the mechanical bond strength.

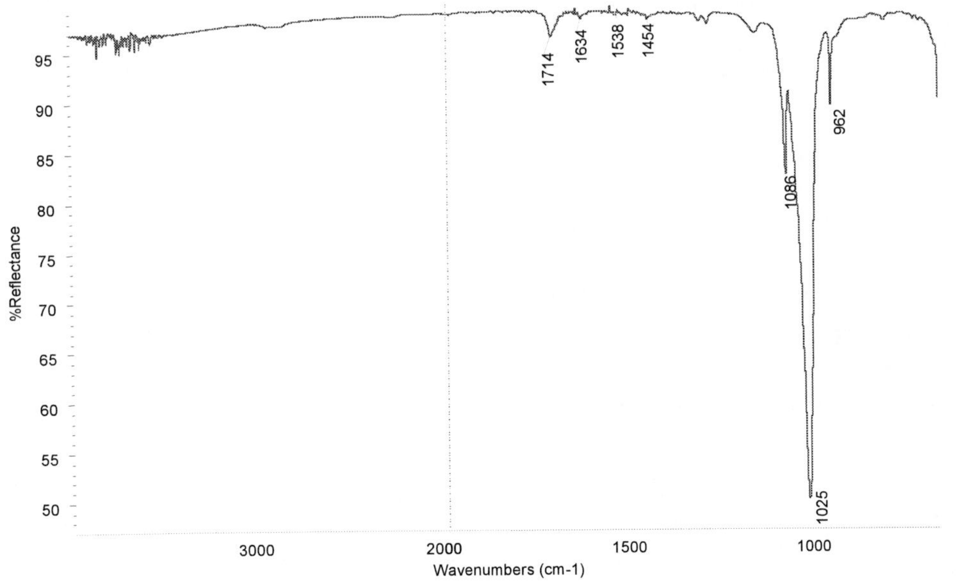

Figure 10. ATR Spectrum on the HA surface primed with Syntac primer (Ivoclar Vivadent, Liechtenstein). There were the weak stretching bands of carboxylic salts (ν^{as}_{COO-} at 1538 cm^{-1}, ν^{s}_{COO-} at 1454 cm^{-1}), besides the stretching bands of the carbonyl group ($\nu_{C=O}$ at 1714 cm^{-1}), double bonds ($\nu_{C=C}$ at 1734 cm^{-1}) and the phosphoric groups ($\nu_{P\text{-}O}$ at 1086 cm^{-1}, $\nu_{P=O}$ at 1025 cm^{-1}).

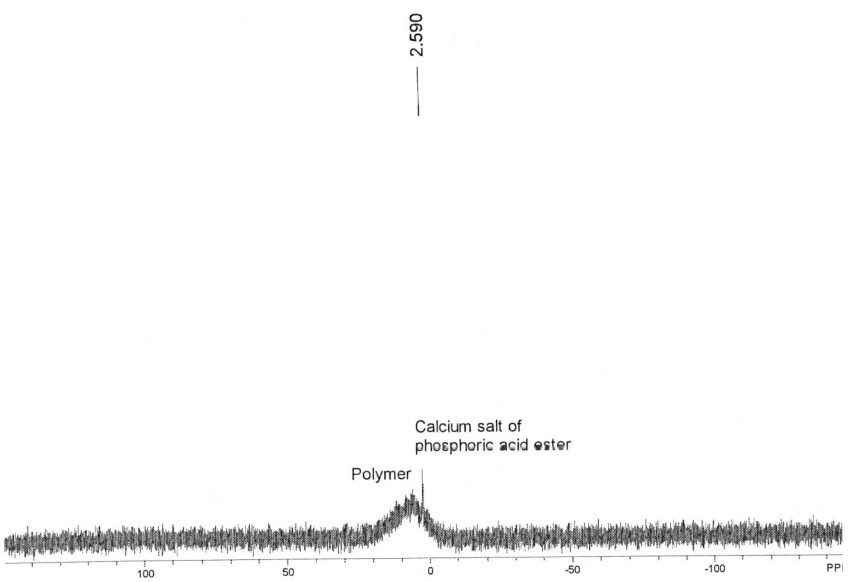

Figure 11. Spectrum of ^{31}PMNR The solid materials of the reaction product of CLB 2v primer (Clearfil Liner Bond 2v, Kuraray Co., Japan) with HA was separated, washed with 10 ml de-ionized water 3 times, dried and analyzed with ^{31}P MNR in $CDCl_3$. The spectrum revealed calcium salts of phosphoric acid esters and polymer.

The mechanical bond strength at the resin-tooth hard tissues depends on the quality of the hybrid layer, and not on the quantity (thickness) of the hybrid layer. What is the real meaning of the quality of the hybrid layer? It has not explained yet how the quality of the hybrid layer determines the mechanical bond strength in detail.

The relationship of the micro-mechanical interlocking and chemical bonding at the enamel-resin interface is supposed as following:

The mechanical bond strength depends on 1) the quality of the hybrid layer that depends on a) the hermetic seal between the resin-tooth hard tissues, and b) the strength of the enamel substrate and resin tags, and 2) co-polymerization of the adhesives and composite resin. The resin tags are mixtures of the dental adhesives and partly demineralized enamel hydroxyapatite crystallites --- the adhesives and their enclosed partial demineralization of the enamel hydroxyappatite crystallites (Figure 12).

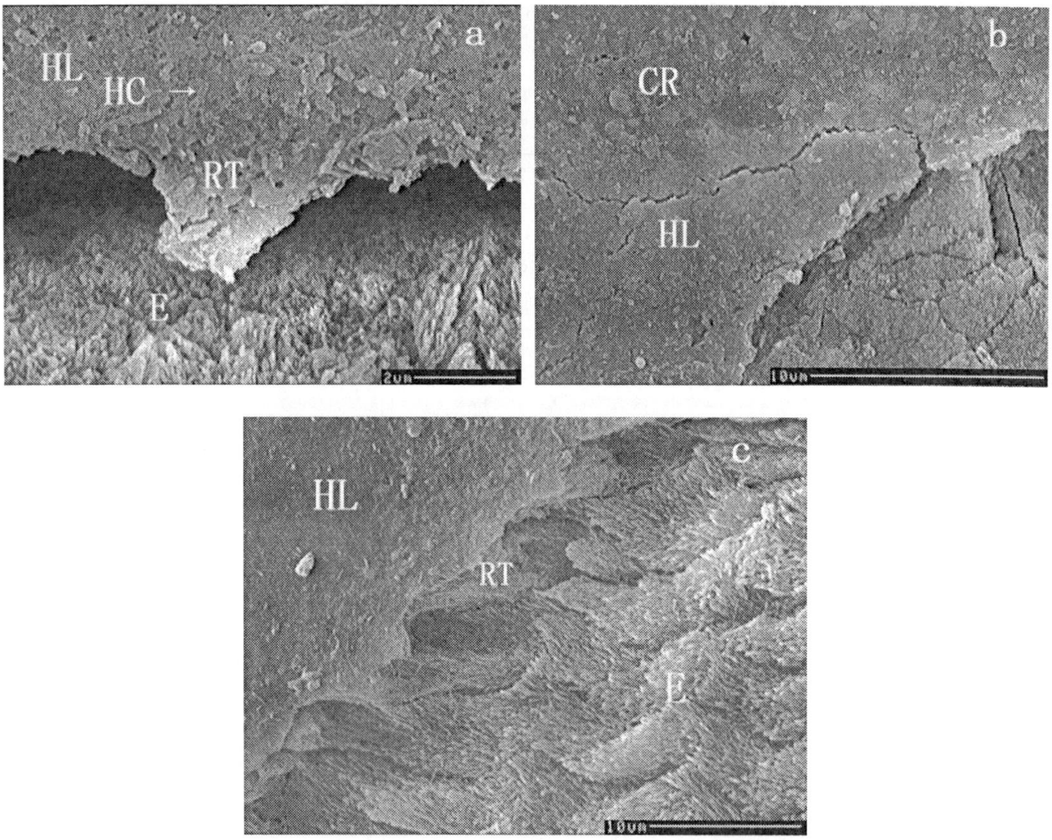

Figure 12. Micro-morphology of resin-enamel interfaces. The sectioned surfaces of the enamel-resin (Clearfil SE Bond, Clearfil AP-X, Kuraray Co. Japan (a, b); Prime and Bond NT, Dentsply, Germany (c)) were etched with 37.5% phosphoric acid for 3 s (a, c) or not etched (b). The partly demineralized enamel hydroxyapaptite crystallites were enclosed in the hybrid layer (HL). There is a gap between the HL and intact enamel (a). No gap was found on the etched (c) and un-etched (b) sectioned surfaces of the enamel-resin interface (b). E: enamel, HL: hybrid layer, RT: resin tag, CR: composite resin, HC: hydroxyapatite crystallites (original magnification=10,400 (a), 4,960 (b), 2,930 (c); bar= 2 (a), 10 (b, c) μm).

The hermetic seal at the interfaces between resin and enamel is associated with the chemical bonding of dental adhesives to enamel, and the chemo-physical (affinity) of dental adhesives to enamel. If the strength of resin tags is low, the micro-mechanical interlocking at the resin-tooth interface is weak, too. If the resin tags are too strong, the substrate strength of the enamel becomes weak, and the micro-mechanical interlocking is weak, too. If the both strengths of resin tags and enamel substrate are strong, the micro-mechanical interlocking is strong. In other words, the mechanical bond strength mainly depends on the appropriate ratio of resin tags to enamel substrate in the hybrid layer. The chemical bonding at the enamel-resin interface only exists along the micro-interlocking interface between resin and enamel. In theory, chemical bonding achieves a higher bond strength than mechanical bond. Phosphoric acid esters have been proven to bind chemically to hydroxyapatite [42,43], however, the mechanical bond strength of self-etching adhesives was not superior to the other non-chemical bonding adhesives [66]. The bond strengths of dental adhesives depend on the individual dental adhesive used [66] and operator's clinical technique [67]. Therefore, we conclude that the minimum or small contribution of chemical bonding of self-etching adhesives is related to the immediate mechanical bond strength between resin and the tooth surface at the micro-mechanical interlocking interfaces. However, long-term enamel bond strength is dependent on the chemical stability of chemical bonding between adhesives and enamel, and adhesives themselves [41]. Moreover, the acidic functional monomers weakened the primed enamel substrate (Figure 12a) between the hybrid layer and the intact enamel. This might be one of the reasons that the self-etching adhesives sacrifice the bond durability for the simplification of clinical procedure/performance [66].

The chemical bonding of dental adhesives to the dentin substrate is much more complicated than that to enamel because dentin contains near 20% collagen in weight. Up to now, no direct evidence of chemical bonding to dentin collagen was found.

According to the present hypothesis, the process of the chemical reaction (decalcification), chemical bonding, and micro-mechanical interlocking can be described as two stages:

Stage 1: The decalcification or chemical reaction is dominated in the moment that tooth hard tissues are treated with self-etching primers containing either carboxylic acids or phosphoric acid esters. The surfaces of tooth hard tissues are roughened by demineralization of the smear layer and penetration of the primer into the substrate of tooth hard tissues (Figure 13,14).

Stage 2: A saturated or over-saturated solution is reached on the HA surfaces after HA reacts with self etching primers, and subsequently the solvents are clinically vaporized by air-drying. In this moment, the balance of the chemical reaction is achieved and simultaneously the chemical adsorption between carboxylic acids/phosphoric acid esters and HA surfaces takes place by means of ionic bonds [9,10,42,43,60,64,65]. Considering that there are many hydrogen-bonding-groups (COOH, OH, etc.) in carboxylic acids, self-etching primers and HA, the adsorption also is dependent on the presence of hydrogen-bonding groups and hydrophobic moieties (hydrocarbon chains or rings) [60]. The nano- and micro-mechanical interlocking at the resin-tooth hard tissues is formed when the adhesives are polymerized. The phenomena of adsorption are shown in Figure 15.

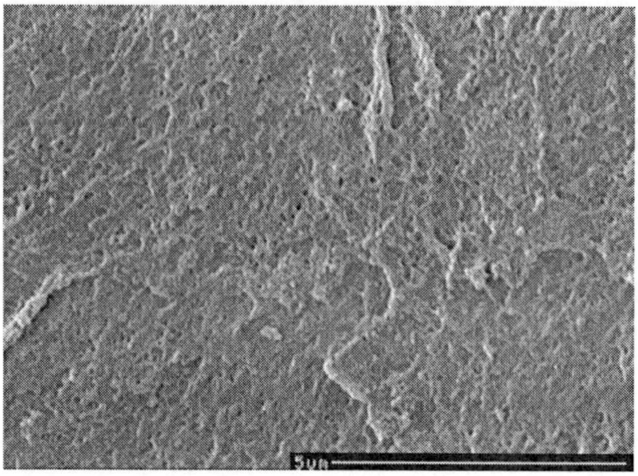

Figure 13. Resin tags. The resin tags at human enamel surface after treatment with Xeno III (Dentsply, Germany) revealed that the adhesive penetrated into the enamel substrate and formed an indistinct etching pattern (original magnification=10,100 fold, bar= 5 μm).

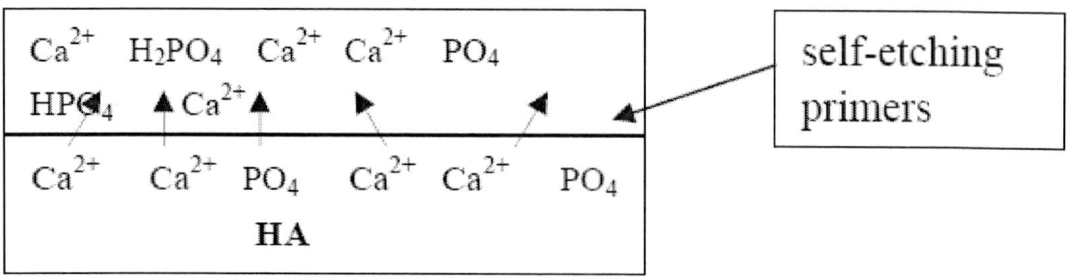

Figure 14. The chemical reaction takes place immediately when HA is treated with self-etching primers containing either carboxylic acids or phosphoric acid esters. Hence, HA is decalcified at first.

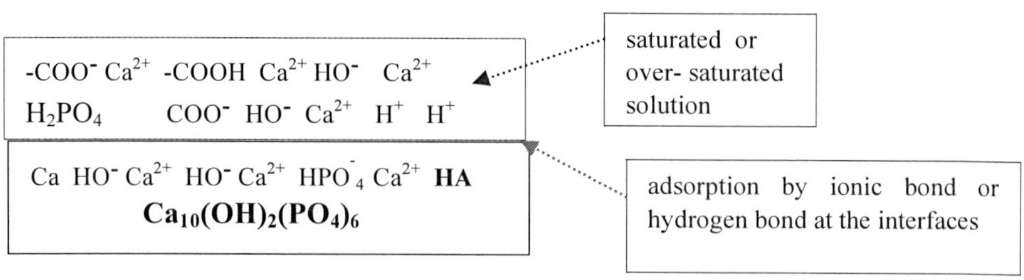

Figure 15. When the balances of the chemical reaction of HA with self-etching primers containing carboxylic acids or phosphoric acid esters are reached, the chemical adsorption (ionic bond and hydrogen bond) takes place among them. The micro-mechanical interlocking at the interfaces of resin-tooth hard tissues is formed when the adhesives is polymerized.

Conclusions

The self-etching adhesives containing carboxylic acids or phosphoric acid esters decalcify hydroxyapatite immediately when they get in contact with HA or tooth hard substances. Hence, when the balance of the chemical reaction among them is achieved after vaporization of the primers'/adhesives' solvents, the chemical adsorption takes place by means of ionic bond and hydrogen bond between the self-etching primers and HA. Nano- and micro-mechanical interlocking of self-etching adhesives is formed at the interfaces of resin-tooth hard tissues when adhesives are polymerized. Hence, the self-etching adhesives reveal a high ability to form a strong interlocking at the tooth-resin restoration interfaces.

References

[1] McConnell D. Crystal chemistry of hydroxyapatite. Its relation to bone mineral. *Arch Oral Biol.* 1965; 10:421-31.

[2] McAinsh TF, ed. *Physics in medicine and biology encyclopedia.* Volume I. Pergamon press, Oxford, 1986; 254-256.

[3] Thylstrup A, Fejerskov G. *Textbook of clinical cariology*, 2nd ed, Munksgaard, Copenhagen, 1994;112-115.

[4] Craig RG. Restorative dental materials, 10th ed, Mosby, St. Louis, 1997; 140.

[5] Buonocore MG. A simple method of increasing the adhesion of acrylic filling materials to enamel surfaces. *J. Dent. Res.* 1955; 26:95-110.

[6] Retief DH. A comparative study of three etching solutions: effects on enamel surface and adhesive-enamel interface. *J. Oral Rehabil.* 1975; 2:75-96.

[7] Rochette AL. A ceramic restoration bonded by etched enamel and resin for fractured incisors. *J. Prosthet. Dent.* 1975; 33:287-293.

[8] Swift EJ Jr., Perdigao J, Heymann HO. Bonding to enamel and dentin: A brief history and state of the art, 1995. *Quintessence Int* 1995; 26:95-110.

[9] Fu B, Yuan JQian W, Shen QSun X, Hannig M. Evidence of chemisorption of maleic acid to enamel and hydroxyapatite. *Eur. J. Oral Sci.* 2004; 112:362-367.

[10] Fu B, Shen QQian W, Sun X, Hannig M. Interfacial interaction of tartaric acid with hydroxyapatite and enamel. *J. Mater. Sci. Mater. Med.* 2005; 16:827-31.

[11] Buonocore MG, Matsui A, Gwinnett AJ. Penetration of resin dental materials into enamel surfaces with reference to bonding. *Arch. Oral Biol.* 1968; 13:61-70.

[12] Raney JT. Air abrasion: an emerging standard of care in conservative operative dentistry. *Dent. Clin. North Am.* 2002; 46:185-209.

[13] Hannig M, Bock H, Bott B, Hoth-Hannig W. Inter-crystallite nano-retention of self-etching adhesives at enamel imaged by transmission electron microscopy. *Eur. J. Oral Sci.* 2002; 110:464-470.

[14] Barkmeier WW, Erickson RL. Shear bond strength of composite to enamel and dentin using Scothchbond multi-purpose. *Am. J. Dent* 1994; 7:175-179.

[15] Triolo PT, Swift EJ Jr, Mudgil A, Levine A. Effects of etching time on enamel bond strengths. *Am. J. Dent* 1993; 6:302-304.

[16] Prati C, Montanari G, Biagini G, Fava F, Pashley DH. Effects of dentin surface treatments on the shear bond strength of Vitrabond. *Dent. Mater* 1992; 8:21-26.

[17] Fu B, Shen Q, Qian W, Hannig M. Decalcification of and chemisorption to hydroxyapatite by malic and tartaric acids. *J. Dent. Res.* 2003; 82:192 (Abstract 1440).

[18] Hughes JA, West NX, Parker DM, van den Braak MH, Addy M. Effects of pH and concentration of citric, malic and lactic acids on enamel, in vitro. *J. Dent.* 2000; 28:147-52.

[19] Fusayama T, Nakamura M, Kurosaki N, Iwaku M. Non-pressure adhesion of a new adhesive restorative resin. *J. Dent. Res.* 1979; 58 :1364-1370.

[20] Nakabayashi N, Kojima K, Masuhara E. The promotion of adhesion by the infiltration of monomers into tooth substrates. *J. Biomed. Mater Res.* 1982; 16:265-273.

[21] Wang T, Nakabayashi N. Effect of 2-(methacryloxy)ethyl phenyl hydrogen phosphate on adhesion to dentin. *J. Dent Res.* 1991; 70:59-66.

[22] Nishiyama N, Suzuki K, Asakura T, Nakai H, Yasuda S, Nemoto K. The effects of pH on N-methacryloyl glycine primer on bond strength to acid-etched dentin. *J. Biomed. Mater Res.* 1996; 31:379-384.

[23] Bouillaguet S, Gysi P, Wataha JC, Ciucchi B, Cattani M, Godin C, Meyer JM. Bond strength of composite to dentin using conventional, one-step, and self-etching adhesive systems. *J. Dent.* 2001; 29:55-61.

[24] Miyasaka K, Nakabayashi N. Combination of EDTA conditioner and Phenyl-P/HEMA self-etching primers for bonding to dentin. *Dent. Mater* 1999; 15:153-157.

[25] Kanca J 3rd. Resin bonding to wet substrate. I. Bonding to dentin. *Quintessence Int* 1992; 23:39-41.

[26] Kanca J 3rd. Improving bond strength through acid etching of dentin and bonding to wet dentin surfaces. *J. Am. Dent. Assoc.* 1992; 123:35-43.

[27] Pashley DH, Ciucchi B, Sano H, Horner JA. Permeability of dentin to adhesive agents. *Quintessence Int* 1993; 24:618-631.

[28] Fusayama T. Total etch technique and cavity isolation. J Esthet Dent 1992; 4:105-109.

[29] Gwinnett AJ. Moist versus dry dentin: its effect on shear bond strength. *Am. J. Dent.* 1992; 5:127-129.

[30] Gwinnett AJ, Dickerson WG, Yu S. Dentin bond shear strength and microleakage for Syntac/Heliomolar: a comparison between the manufacturer's and total etch technique. *J. Esthet Dent.* 1992; 4:164-168.

[31] Hannig M, Reinhardt KJ, Bott B. Self-etching primer vs. phosphoric acid: An alternative concept for composite-to-enamel bonding. *Oper. Dent.* 1999; 24:172-180.

[32] Tay FR, Pashley DH. Dental adhesives of the future. *J. Adhes. Dent.* 2002; 4:91-103.

[33] Pashley DH, Tay FR, Carvalho R, Rueggeberg FA, Agee K, Carrilho M, Donnelly A. From dry bonding to water-wet bonding to ethanol-wet bonding. A review of the interactions between dentin matrix and solvated resins using a macromodel of the hybrid layer. *Am. J. Dent* 2007; 20:7-21.

[34] Tay FR, Pashley DH, Kapur RR, Carrilho MR, Hur YB, Garrett LV, Tay KC. Bonding BisGMA to dentin--a proof of concept for hydrophobic dentin bonding. *J. Dent. Res.* 2007; 86:1034-9.

[35] Van Meerbeek B, Inokoshi S, Braem M, Lambrechts P, Vanherle G. Morphological aspects of the resin-dentin interdiffusion zone with different dentin adhesive systems. *J. Dent. Res.* 1992; 71:1530-1540.

[36] Van Meerbeek B, Dhem A, Goret-Nicaise M, Braem M, Lambrechts P, VanHerle G. Comparative SEM and TEM examination of the ultrastructure of the resin dentin interdiffusion zone. *J. Dent Res*. 1993; 72:495-501.

[37] Eick JD, Gwinnett AJ, Pashley DH, Robinson SJ. Current concepts on adhesion to dentin. *Crit Rev. Oral Biol. Med.* 1997; 8:306-335.

[38] Watanabe I, Nakabayashi N, Pashley DH. Bonding to ground dentin by a Phenyl-P self-etching primer. *J. Dent. Res.* 1994; 73:1212-1220.

[39] Hannig M, Reinhardt KJ, Bott B. Composite-to-dentin bond strength, micromorphology of the bonded dentin interface and marginal adaptation of Class II composite resin restorations using self-etching primers. *Oper. Dent.* 2001; 26:157-165.

[40] Hannig M, Fu B. Effect of air abrasion and resin composite on microleakage of class V restorations bonded with self-etching primers. *J. Adhes. Dent*. 2001; 3:265-272.

[41] Moszner N, Salz U, Zimmerman J. Chemical aspects of self-etching enamel-dentin adhesives: A systematic review. *Dent. Mater.* 2005; 21:895-910.

[42] Fu B, Sun X, Qian W, Shen Q, Chen R, Hannig M. Evidence of Chemical bonding to hydroxyapatite by phosphoric acid esters. *Biomaterials* 2005; 26: 5104-5110.

[43] Fukegawa D, Hayakawa S, Yoshida Y, Suzuki K, Osaka A, Van Meerbeek B. Chemical Interaction of phosphoric acid ester with hydroxyapatite. *J. Dent. Res*. 2006; 85:941-944.

[44] Spencer P, Byerley TJ, Eick JD, Witt JD. Chemical characterization of the dentin/adhesive interface by Fourier transform infrared photoacoustic spectroscopy. *Dent. Mater* 1992; 8:10-15.

[45] Eick JD, Robinson SJ, Byerley TJ, Chappell RP, Spencer P, Chappelow CC. Scanning transmission electron microscopy/energy-dispersive spectroscopy analysis of the dentin adhesive interface using a labeled 2-hydroxyethylmethacrylated analogue. *J. Dent. Res.* 1995; 74:1246-1252.

[46] Spencer P, Wang Y, Walker MP, Wieliczka DM, Swafford JR. Interfacial chemistry of the dentin/adhesive bond. *J. Dent. Res*. 2000; 79:1458-1463.

[47] Tay FR, Gwinnett JA, Wei SH. Micromorphological spectrum from overdrying to overwetting acid-conditioned dentin in water-free acetone-base, single-bottle primer/adhesives. *Dent. Mater* 1996; 12:234-244.

[48] Tay FR, Gwinnett JA, Wei SH. The overwet phenomenon in two-component acetone-based primers containing aryl amine and carboxylic acid and monomers. *Dent. Mater* 1997; 13:118-127.

[49] Tay FR, Gwinnett JA, Wei SH. Relation between water content in acetone/alcohol-based primer and interfacial ultrastructure. *J. Dent.* 1998; 26: 147-156.

[50] Tay FR, Gwinnett JA, Wei SH. Micromorphological spectrum of acid-conditioned dentin following the application of a water-based adhesive. *Dent. Mater.* 1998; 14:329-38.

[51] Fu B, Shen Y, Wang H, Hannig M. Sealing ability of dentin adhesivers/desensitizer. *Oper Dent.* 2007, 32:496-503.

[52] Koibuchi H, Yasuda N, Nakabayashi N. Bonding to dentin with a self-etching primer: the effect of smear layers. *Dent. Mater* 2001; 17:122-126.

[53] Nakabayashi N, Saimi Y. Bonding to intact dentin. *J. Dent. Res*. 1996; 75:1705-1715.

[54] Tay FR, Pashley DH. Aggressiveness of contemporary self-etching systems. I: Depth of penetration beyond dentin smear layers. *Dent. Mater.* 2001; 17:296-308.

[55] Hashimoto M, Ohno H, Kaga M, Sano H, Endo K, Oguchi H. Fractured surface characterization: wet versus dry bonding. *Dent. Mater.* 2002; 18:95-102.

[56] Suzuki K, Nishiyama N, Nemoto K, Torii Y, Inoue K. Effect of n-methacryloyl amino acid applications on hybrid layer formation at the interface of intertubular dentin. *J. Dent. Res.* 1998; 77:1881-1888.

[57] Koshiro K, Sidhu S, Inoue S, Ikeda T, Sano H. New concept of resin-dentin interfacial adhesion: The nanointeraction zone. *J. Biomed. Mater. Res. Part B: Appl. Biomater.* 2006; 77B:401-408.

[58] Alis SA, Williams DF. The characteristics and performance of dentine bonding agents. *Clin. Mater.* 1993; 14:243-254.

[59] Laswell HR, Welk DA. Rational for designing cavity preparations. *Dent. Clinic. North Am.* 1985; 29:241-249.

[60] Misra DN. Interaction of citric acid with hydroxyapatite: surface exchange of ions and precipitation of calcium citrate. *J. Dent. Res.* 1996; 75:1418-1425.

[61] Marshall GW Jr, Inai N, Wu-Magidi IC, Balooch M, Kinney JH Tagami J, Marshall SJ. Dentin demineralization: effects of dentin depth, pH and different acids. *Dent. Mater.* 1997; 13:338-343.

[62] Breschi L, Gobbi P, Mazzotti G, Falconi M, Ellis TH, Stangel I. High resolution SEM evaluation of dentin etched with maleic and citric acid. *Dent. Mater.* 2002; 18:26-35.

[63] Zimehl R, Hannig M. Adsorption onto tooth enamel-the biological interface and its modification. *Progr. Colloid. Polym. Sci.* 2001; 117:42-46.

[64] Yoshida Y, Van Meerbeek B, Nakayama Y, Yoshioka M, Snauwaert J, Abe Y, Lambrechts P, Vanherle G, Okazaki M. Adhesion to and decalcification of hydroxyapatite by carboxylic acids. *J. Dent. Res.* 2001; 80:1565-1569.

[65] Yoshida Y, Van Meerbeek B, Nakayama Y, Snauwaert J, Hellemans L, Lambrechts P, Vanherle G, WakasaK. Evidence of chemical bonding at biomaterial-hard tissue interfaces. *J. Dent. Res.* 2000; 79: 709-714.

[66] De Munck J, Van Landuyt K, Peumans M, Poitevin A, Lambrenchts P, Braem M, Van Meerbeek B. A critical review of the durability of adhesion to tooth tissue: Methods and Results. *J. Dent. Res.* 2005; 84:118-132.

[67] Van Meerbeek B, Van Landuyt K, De Munck J, Hashimoto M, Peumans M, Lambrechts P, Yoshida Y, Inoue S, Suzuki K. Technique-sensitivity of contemporary adhesives. *Dent. Mater. J.* 2005; 24:1-13.

In: Clinical Dentistry
Editor: Scardina Giuseppe Alessandro

ISBN: 978-1-61122-354-5
© 2011 Nova Science Publishers, Inc.

Chapter 10

APICAL STATUS OF ENDODONTICALLY TREATED TEETH IN A GERMAN POPULATION AS RADIOGRAPHED BETWEEN 1989-91 AND 1999-2001[#]

Claudia Barthel*[*1], *Yevgeni Victorov*[2], *Andreas Roloff*[3], *Christian Scheifele*[3], *Wolfgang Raab*[1] *and Stefan Zimmer*[1]

[1]Heinrich-Heine-University Duesseldorf,
Department of Operative and Preventive Dentistry and Endodontics
[2]Charité Humboldt University Berlin,
Department of Operative and Preventive Dentistry and Endodontics
[3]Charité Humboldt University Berlin, Germany,
Department of Oral Surgery and Radiology

ABSTRACT

The aim of this study was to assess the prevalence of apical lucencies in a German population, radiographed between 1989 -1991 ("Group 1990") and 1999 - 2001 ("Group 2000").

Twelve hundred and forty-seven panoramic images were evaluated by two observers which were calibrated prior to evaluation. Numbers of endodontic treatments, apical lucencies, and quality of root fillings were registered. Relations between apical status and quality of root canal filling as well as quality and presence of coronal seal were statistically calculated with χ^2 test.

In group 1990, 5.2% of all teeth were endodontically treated (ET); 41.2% of these showed apical lucencies. In group 2000, 5.8% were ET and 49.1% showed apical lucencies. The quality of root fillings had decreased within ten years. In group 1990, the

---

[#] A version of this book was also published as a chapter in *International Journal of Clinical Dentistry, Volume 1, Issue 2*, published by Nova Science Publishers, Inc. It was submitted for appropriate modifications in an effort to encourage wider dissemination of research.

[*] Corresponding author: Prof. Dr. Claudia R. Barthel, Building 18.13. Department of Operative and Preventive Dentistry and Endodontics, Heinrich-Heine-University, Moorenstr. 24. D- 40225 Duesseldorf, Germany. Phone: +49-211 8119716. Fax: +49-211-8119244. Email: claudia.barthel@med.uni-duesseldorf.de

quality of coronal seal had no significant impact on the radiological status of apices, whereas in group 2000, unacceptable coronal fillings were significantly more often associated with apical lesions. The presence of a coronal filling and a good root filling had in both groups a significant positive impact on the apical status of ET teeth.

Clinical Significance

In endodontically tretated teeth, the presence of a coronal restoration seems to be associated with significantly fewer apical lesions. Therefore, it is recommended after endodontic treatment to place a definitive restoration as soon as possible.

Introduction

Success or failure of endodontically treated teeth can only be determined by clinical and radiological means. The possible outcome may be investigated in longitudinal studies. For evaluation of such studies, a number of success criteria have been defined by different authors. A very strict definition of success would be complete absence of clinical and radiological signs of apical periodontitis. Some authors used these criteria as definition of success; in addition, a slightly widened periodontal ligament (PDL) around extruded material would also be accepted (Sjögren et al. 1990; Strindberg 1956). Other authors added a decreased size of apical lesion in the follow-up radiograph to their definition of success (Matsumoto et al. 1987; Morse et al. 1983; Seltzer et al. 1963).

Such longitudinal studies may demonstrate how much success can be achievable under certain conditions. In contrast to this, cross-sectional studies will show the actual status of root canal therapy in a certain population. However, they do not consider the course of time. A widened PDL, which formerly may have been a large apical lesion will not be recognized as healing lesion but just as a lesion.

The prevalence of periapical radiolucency in endodontically treated teeth ranges from 20 to 38% in Scandinavian studies and between 31 and 61% in North American studies (Buckley and Spangberg 1995; Eriksen et al. 1995; Hansen and Johansen 1976; Ray and Trope 1995). In German studies, these numbers range between 46 and 61% (Klimek et al. 1995; Weiger et al. 1997).

To observe the development of the status of root canal therapy within a country or district, the repetition of a cross-sectional study after a certain amount of time may be informative. Petersson detected a slight improvement in the quality of root canal treatment between 1974 and 1985, however, the average number of apical lesions did not decrease in these years (Petersson 1993). Eckerbom et al. also detected a slight improvement in the quality of root canal treatment in a Swedish population after 5 to 7 years, whereas the apical health had only improved marginally (Eckerbom et al. 1983). Kirkevang et al. examined two Danish populations in 1974 and in 1997 and found a clear enhancement in the technical quality of root canal treatment (Kirkevang et al. 2001a). They stated, however, that the two compared populations showed too much basic differences which prevented a clear assessment of any impact on the disease frequencies.

In recent years the term "coronal leakage" has come into focus after many in vitro studies showed that bacteria could bypass root fillings within days or weeks after obturation (Barthel et al. 1999; Torabinejad et al. 1990). Knowing that the etiology of apical periodontitis is the presence of bacteria (Sundqvist 1976) and assuming that bacteria can penetrate root canal fillings so easily, the question arises how success rates of over 90% can be achieved clinically (Sjögren et al. 1990). The answer seems to be the quality of the coronal restoration as shown by Ray and Trope (Ray and Trope 1995). Opposed to this, Ricucci et al. doubted the impact of the quality of the coronal restoration on the periapical status of endodontically treated teeth after their in vivo investigation (Ricucci et al. 2000).

The aim of the present study was to determine the prevalence of apical lucencies in a German population as radiographed between 1989 and 1991 and between 1999 and 2001. In addition, the number and technical quality of root fillings was to be assessed. Secondarily, the impact of the radiological appearance or presence of a coronal restoration on the presence or absence of apical lesions in endodontically treated teeth was to be investigated.

Materials

Five hundred panoramic images as taken between 1989 and 1991 (Group 1990) and 742 panoramic images as taken between 1999 and 2002 (Group 2000) were used for this cross-sectional study. The radiographs were performed with an Orthophos CD unit (Siemens, Bensheim, Germany) on Kodak T-Mat G Films (Kodak, Stuttgart, Germany) at the patient's initial appointment in the former Dental Clinic North of the Free University, now Dental Clinic of the Charité, Berlin, Germany. One observer (AR) evaluated the 1990 group and another observer (YV) evaluated the 2000 group. Prior to evaluation the two observers were calibrated and the inter- and intra-observer reliability was tested with κ-test. The radiographs were regarded in a darkened room on an illuminated backlight screen. The marginal light was blinded out with a black stencil.

The age of the patients was recorded and all present teeth were counted. The numbers of apical radiolucencies were gathered as well as the numbers of endodontically treated teeth (ET). An apical lucency was judged as present, if the width of the apical PDL was at least 2-3 times wider than the marginal PDL of the same or an adjacent sound tooth. A tooth was regarded as endodontically treated, if a radioopaque material was detected somewhere in or throughout the entire root canal system. In all ET teeth and in all teeth with apical lucencies, the quality of the coronal restoration was judged. A coronal filling was entitled as "acceptable", if there was no translucency detectable between the filling and the tooth at the mesial or distal margin and if the filling was not broken. It was entitled as "unacceptable" if the coronal filling was missing, incomplete or with marginal gaps or signs of primary or secondary caries. All these judgements were assessed on the basis of the radiographs.

To judge the quality of the root canal fillings, several parameters were investigated.

A root filling had a "correct length" if it ended 0-2 mm from the radiological apex, otherwise it was labelled as root filling with "incorrect length", which included too long or too short fillings. The homogeneity of the root canal fillings was also judged and they were entitled as "homogenous" if no voids were detectable within or at the margins of root fillings. Otherwise they were labelled as "not homogenous". Furthermore, procedural errors such as zip, ledge and perforation were recorded. To find out whether there was a context between the quality of root fillings and the presence of apical lucencies, all ET which showed either "incorrect length" and/or appeared "not homogenous" and/or with a procedural error, were called "poor" root fillings. Root fillings with correct length, homogeneity and absence of procedural errors were entitled as "good" root fillings.

To detect significant differences between teeth with and without apical lucencies, χ^2-test was calculated with SPSS12.0.

Results

The intraobserver liability for the Group 1990 was 0.83, and 0.86 for the Group 2000 The liability between the two observers was 0.92.

In Group 1990, 11,961 teeth were counted. 5.2% of these were endodontically treated (ET). 6.0% of all teeth showed apical radiolucencies. 41.2% of all ET teeth showed apical lucencies.

In Group 2000, 17948 teeth were counted, 5.8% of these were ET. 6.3% of all teeth were associated with an apical lesion. 49.9% of the ET showed apical lucencies.

The numbers of patients and numbers of teeth related to the age distribution can be seen in Tables 1 and 2.

Table 1. Age distribution related to number of patients, teeth, endodontically treated teeth and apical lucencies

	Nr. and % of patients		Nr. and % of teeth	
Age (years)	Group 1990	Group 2000	Group 1990	Group 2000
<20	27 (5.4%)	36 (4.9%)	809 (6.8%)	1102 (6.1%)
20-29	170 (34.0%)	137 (18.5%)	4983 (41.7%)	4087 (22.8%)
30-39	99 (19.8%)	118 (15.9%)	2541 (21.2%)	3257 (18.1%)
40-49	72 (14.4%)	156 (21.0%)	1508 (12.6%)	3740 (20.8%)
50-59	64 (12.8%)	130 (17.5%)	1219 (10.2%)	2845 (15.9%)
60-69	41 (8.2%)	111 (15.0%)	617 (5.2%)	2105 (11.7%)
70-79	20 (4.0%)	44 (5.9%)	248(2.1%)	677 (3.8%)
80-89	7 (1.4%)	10 (1.3%)	36 (0.3%)	136 (0.8%)
Total	500 (100%)	742 (100%)	11961(100%)	17949 (100%)
	Nr. and % of endodontically treated teeth		Nr. and %of apical lucencies	
Age (years)	Group 1990	Group 2000	Group 1990	Group 2000
<20	24 (3.9%)	7 (0.7%)	27 (3.8%)	15 (1.3%)
20-29	171 (27.8%)	114 (10.9%)	196 (27.2%)	169 (15.0%)
30-39	113 (18.3%)	160 (15.3%)	149 (20.7%)	130 (11.6%)
40-49	115 (18.3%)	257 (24.6%)	122 (16.9%)	260 (23.1%)
50-59	91 (14.8%)	250 (23.9%)	109 (15.1%)	249 (22.2%)
60-69	67 (10.9%)	163 (15.6%)	75 (10.4%)	198 (17.6%)
70-79	32 (5.2%)	76 (7.3%)	36 (5.0%)	83 (7.4%)
80-89	3 (0.5%)	19 (1.8%)	6 (0.8%)	20 (1.8%)
Total	616 (100%)	1046 (100%)	720 (100%)	1124 (100%)

Table 2. Percentage of endodontically treated teeth(ET), overall apical lucencies and ET with apical lucencies per age group

Group 1990			
Age (years)	% of teeth with ET per age group	% of teeth with apical lucencies per age group	% of ET with apical lucencies per group
<20	3.0	3.3	41.7
20-29	3.4	3.9	32.7
30-39	4.4	5.9	38.9
40-49	7.6	8.1	44.3
50-59	7.5	8.9	47.3
60-69	10.9	12.2	37.3
70-79	12.9	14.5	50.0
80-89	8.3	16.7	66.7
Group 2000			
Age (years)	% of teeth with ET per age group	% of teeth with apical lucencies per age group	% of ET with apical lucencies per group
<20	0.6	1.4	42.9
20-29	2.8	4.1	56.1
30-39	4.9	4.0	36.9
40-49	6.9	7.0	47.9
50-59	8.8	8.8	49.6
60-69	7.7	9.4	51.5
70-79	11.2	12.3	43.4
80-89	14.0	14.7	47.4

In the Group1990, 36.6% of all ET were incisors and canines, 33.1% were premolars and 30.4% molars. In the Group 2000, 31.9% were incisors and canines, 32.7% premolars and 35.4% molars.

Quality of Fillings

The quality of root fillings, i.e. the numbers of teeth with correct length, good homogeneity and absence of procedural errors for both groups can be seen in table 2. The overall quality of root fillings in the Group 1990 was “poor” in 37.7% of the cases whereas in the Group 2000, it was ”poor” in 55.4% of the cases.

The quality of the coronal fillings was acceptable in 82.5% in the 1990 Group, in the 2000 Group it was only in 47.0% acceptable.

For the 1990 Group, the quality of the coronal filling shortly missed statistical significant influence on the status of the apical tissues ($p=0.091$), however, if coronal fillings were missing, significantly more apical lucencies could be detected in ET ($p<0.0001$). Significantly more apical lesions were also found, if the quality of the root filling was poor ($P<0.0001$). In the 2000 group, significantly more apical lesions were associated with ET with unacceptable coronal fillings ($p<0.0001$) or with poor root canal fillings ($p<0.0001$) or if the coronal filling was missing ($p<0.0001$).

Table 3. Quality of root fillings and coronal fillings as seen in groups 1990 and 2000

	Group 1990		Group 2000	
Homogeneity of root filling (%)	homogenous	not homogenous	homogenous	not homogenous
	71.3	28.7	69.9	30.1
Length of root filling (%)	correct	not correct	correct	not correct
	42.8	57.2	54.3	45.7
Procedural errors (%)	not detectable	detectable	not detectable	detectable
	81.6	18.4	82.6	17.4
Overall quality of root filling (%)	good	poor	good	poor
	62.3	37.7	44.6	55.4
Quality of coronal filling (%)	acceptable	unacceptable	acceptable	unacceptable
	82.5	17.5	47.0	53.0

The prevalence of apical lesions in all examined teeth did not increase significantly between1990 and 2000. In contrast to this, the quality of the root canal fillings and the coronal fillings decreased significantly within the ten years ($p<0.0001$). The prevalence of ET increased within this time span ($p=0.012$), same as the numbers of ET which were associated with apical lesions ($p=0.001$).

Discussion

Although the evaluated patients were radiographed at the Dental School, they had not been treated there before having their panoramic images taken. The radiographs were performed at their initial appointment and it had not been assessed where and by whom they had been treated formerly. It may therefore be assumed that the patients came mainly from dental practitioners in the Berlin area. Although the catchment area was the same for the Group 1990 and the Group 2000, the patients were not the same in 1990 and 2000. It may thus be more correct to talk about two examined populations rather than one. In former cross-sectional studies, different study designs have been used. Some authors evaluated radiographs only (Kirkevang et al. 2001b; Kirkevang et al. 2000; Tronstad et al. 2000), others appointed the patients and investigated them clinically and radiographically (Dugas et al. 2003; Hommez et al. 2002).

In some studies, radiographs from full mouth examinations (Hommez et al. 2002; Kirkevang et al. 2001a; Tronstad et al. 2000), in others panoramic images were used (Hülsmann et al. 1991; Klimek et al. 1995). In the present study – knowing their disadvantages of fuzziness and superimposition of bone structures – panoramic images were used for evaluation, because the routine protocol of the Dental School at that time did not intend for a full mouth status but rather an panoramic overview at the initial appointment. Therefore, some endodontically treated teeth had to be excluded from statistical analysis because their shape or length was not clearly distinguishable. This may have been avoidable if a full mouth status would have been used. The panoramic image did also not allow any further distinction of the apical status of teeth as suggested by Ørstavik et al. (PAI-Score) (Ørstavik et al. 1986).

In the present study, 5.2% of all teeth or 5.8% respectively were endodontically treated, this lies within the range of the international literature (between 2.3% and 13%, (de Cleen et al. 1993; Eckerboom et al. 1989). There are studies, in which up to 21.5% of all examined teeth were endodontically treated. These studies, however, were restricted to a population of "elderly" patients and therefore do not represent the entire age spectrum (Imfeld 1991; Soikkonen 1995). In this study, an apical pathology could be observed in 6.0% of all teeth or 6.3% respectively, the ET, however, showed apical lesions in 40.1% or 49.1% of the cases. In the literature, these numbers range between 3% and 7% (apical lesions in all teeth) (de Moor et al. 2000; Kirkevang et al. 2000) and between 25% and 61% (apical lesions in ET) (Ödesjö et al. 1990; Weiger et al. 1997).

Within the observation period of ten years, there was no significant increase of apical lesions if all teeth were regarded. In contrast to Scandinavian studies (Eriksen et al. 1988; Kirkevang et al. 2001a), the quality of treatment (root filling, coronal filling) had not improved over ten years in the present study.

An explanation for this may be the relatively short observation period. Eriksen et al. evaluated their population between 1973 and 1993 and Kirkevang et al. between 1974 and 1998. Another factor of influence may be the fact, that within these ten years, many new practices have been opened in the area of the Dental Clinic after the Berlin Wall has been removed, resulting in a possible shift of patients. The proportion of patients with general health risks and thus less attention for their teeth and worse dental care may have increased, whereas the average patient remained outside in the general practices. Furthermore, for the 1990 group, it was a routine protocol in the Dental Clinic to perform a panoramic image in every patient entering the Clinic for any kind of treatment. This was established as preventive screening device for possible pathology in the jaw region. Later on, panoramic images were taken only if needed for diagnostic purposes. Overall, a certain selection bias due to these factors cannot be excluded.

Another explanation for the decrease of quality of coronal fillings may be that an increasing number of composite restorations have been inserted in the late nineties, with different degrees of radioopacity and thus maybe evaluability.

A secondary goal of this study was to examine, whether the radiological appearance of the coronal filling had an impact on the apical status of ET. In 1995, Ray and Trope posed this question the first time and found a significant correlation between poor coronal fillings and the presence of apical lesions in ET (Ray and Trope 1995). Kirkevang et al. and Dugas et al. were able to confirm this coherence in 2000 and 2003, respectively (Dugas et al. 2003; Kirkevang et al. 2000). In contrast to this, Tronstad et al. did not find such correlation, but rather a correlation between the technical quality of root fillings and the status of apical tissues (Tronstad et al. 2000). The question is whether a radiological evaluation of coronal restorations is sufficient, since it only reflects two dimensions of the restoration, i.e., the mesial and distal parts of fillings can be judged but not the buccal and oral areas. Hommez et al. investigated coronal fillings clinically and did not find that the quality of fillings had an impact on the apical status of ET (Hommez et al. 2002). Interestingly and in contrast to this, they did find a significant correlation to the apical status if they used the radiological appearance of coronal fillings. In the present study, there was no such correlation detected in the 1990 group, only the quality of root fillings had an impact on the apical status of root filled teeth. In the group 2000, both, a good quality of coronal restoration as well as good quality of the root fillings were found to be associated with significantly less apical lesions in ET. In both groups, however, the ET showed significantly more apical lucencies if the coronal filling was completely missing.

It may be concluded that the prevalence of apical lucencies has remained similar within the ten years of observation. In contrast to this, the number of apical lesions in ET has increased and the quality of root fillings and coronal restorations as observed radiologically has decreased. Whether the quality of coronal restoration has an impact on the apical status of ET can not finally be stated, since the results were not conform between groups 1990 and 2000. However, the presence of a coronal restoration seems to be associated with significantly less apical lesions in ET.

References

Barthel CR, Moshonov J, Shuping G, Ørstavik D. Bacterial leakage versus dye leakage in obturated root canals. *Int. Endod. J.* 1999; 32: 370-375.

Buckley M, Spångberg LSW. The prevalence and technical quality of endodontic treatment in an american subpopulation. *Oral Surgery Oral Medicine Oral Pathology Oral Radiology and Endodontics* 1995; 79: 92-100.

de Cleen MJ, Schuurs AH, Wesselink PR, Wu MK. Periapical status and prevalence of endodontic treatment in an adult Dutch population. *Int. Endod. J.* 1993; 26: 112-119.

de Moor RJG, Hommez GMG, De Boever JG, Delme KI, Martens GE. Periapical health related to the quality of root canal treatment in a Belgian population. *Int. Endod. J.* 2000; 33: 113-120.

Dugas NN, Lawrence HP, Teplitzsky PE, Pharoah MJ, Friedman S. Periapical health and treatment quality assessment of root-filled teeth in two Canadian populations. *Int. Endod. J.* 2003; 36: 181-192.

Eckerbom M, Andersson J-E, Magnusson T. A longitudinal study of changes in frequency and technical standard of endodontic treatment in a Swedish population. *Endod. Dent. Traumatol.* 1989; 5: 27-31.

Eriksen H, Bjerntness E, Orstavik D. Prevalence and quality of endodontic treatment in an urban adult population in Norway. *Endod. Dent. Traumatol.* 1988; 4: 122-126.

Eriksen HM, Berset GP, Hansen BF, Bjertness E. Changes in endodontic status 1973-93 among 35-year olds in Oslo, Norway. *Int. Endod. J.* 1995; 28: 129-132.

Hansen BF, Johansen JR. Oral roentgenologic findings in a Norwegian urban population. *Oral Surg. Oral Med. Oral Pathol.* 1976; 41: 261-266.

Hommez GMG, Coppens CRM, De Moor RJG. Periapical health related to the quality of coronal restorations and root fillings. *Int. Endod. J.* 2002; 35: 680-689.

Hülsmann M, Lorch V, Franz B. Untersuchung zur Häufigkeit und Qualität von Wurzelfüllungen. *Deutsche Zahnärztliche Zeitung* 1991; 46: 296-299.

Imfeld TN. Prevalence and quality of endodontic treatment in an elderly urban popilation of Switzerland. *J. Endod.* 1991; 17: 604-607.

Kirkevang LL, Hörsted-Bindslev P, Ørstavik D, Wenzel A. A comparison of the quality of root canal treatment in two Danish subpopulations examined 1974-75 and 1997-98. Int Endod J 2001a; 34: 607-612.

Kirkevang LL, Hörsted-Bindslev P, Ørstavik D, Wenzel A. Frequency and distribution of endodontically treated teeth and apical periodontitis in an urban Danish population. *Int. Endod. J.* 2001b; 34: 198-205.

Kirkevang LL, Ørstavik D, Hörsted-Bindslev P, Wenzel A. Periapical status and quality of root fillings and coronal restorations in a Danish population. *Int. Endod. J.* 2000; 33: 509-515.

Klimek J, Kockapan C, Borchert J. Häufigkeit und Qualität von Wurzelkanalfüllungen in den Jahren 1983 und 1991. *Dtsch Zahnärztl* Z 1995; 50: 154-156.

Matsumoto T, Nagai T, Ida K, Ito M, Kawai Y, Horiba N, Sato R, Nakamura H. Factors affecting successful prognosis of root canal treatment. *J. Endod.* 1987; 13: 239-242.

Morse DR, Esposito JV, Pike C, Furst ML. A radiographic evaluation of the periapical status of teeth treated by the gutta-percha-eucapercha endodontic method: a one-year follow-up study of 458 root canals. Part III. *Oral Surg. Oral Med. Oral Pathol.* 1983; 56: 190-197.

Ödesjö B, Hellden L, Salonen L, Langeland K. Prevalence of previous endodontic treatment, technical standard and occurrence of periapical lesions in a randomly slelcted adult, general population. *Endod. Dent. Traumatol.* 1990; 6: 265-272.

Ørstavik D, Kerekes K, Eriksen HM. The periapical index: a scoring system for radiogrphic assessment of apical periodontitis. *Endod. Dent. Tramatol.* 1986; 2: 20-34.

Petersson K. Endodontic status of mandibular premolars and molars in Swedish adults. A repeated cross-sectional study in 1974 and 1985. *Endod. Dent. Traumatol.* 1993; 9: 185-189.

Ray HA, Trope M. Periapical status of endodontically treated teeth in relation to the technical quality of the root filling and the coronal restoration. *Int. Endod. J.* 1995; 28: 12-18.

Ricucci D, Gröndahl K, Bergenholtz G. Periapical status of root-filled teeth exposed to the oral environment by loss of restoration or caries. *Oral Surg. Oral Med. Oral Pathol. Oral Radiol. Endod.* 2000; 90: 354-359.

Seltzer S, Bender I, B, Turkenkopf S. Factors affecting successful repair after root canal therapy. *Journal of the American Dental Association* 1963; 53: 651-662.

Sjögren U, Hagglund B, Sundqvist G, Wing K. Factors affecting the long-term results of endodontic treatment. *J. Endod.* 1990; 16: 498-504.

Soikkonen KT. Endodontically treated teeth and preiapical findings in the elderly. *Int. Endod. J.* 1995; 28: 200-203.

Strindberg L. The dependence of the results of pulp therapy on certain factors. An analytic study based on radiographic and clinical follow-up examination. *Acta Odontol. Scand* 1956; 14: 1-175 (Suppl 121).

Sundqvist G. *Bacteriologic studies of necrotic pulps*. University of Umeå 1976, Umeå.

Torabinejad M, Ung B, Kettering JD. In vitro bacterial penetration of coronally unsealed endodontically treated teeth. *J. Endod.* 1990; 16: 566-569.

Tronstad L, Asbjørnsen K, Døving L, Pedersen I, Eriksen HM. Influence of coronal restorations on the periapical health of endodontically treated teeth. *Endod. Dent. Traumatol.* 2000; 16: 218-221.

Weiger R, Hitzler S, Hermle G, Löst C. Periapical status, quality of root canal fillings and estimated endodontic treatment needs. *Endod. Dent. Traumatol.* 1997; 13: 69-74.

In: Clinical Dentistry
Editor: Scardina Giuseppe Alessandro

ISBN: 978-1-61122-354-5
© 2011 Nova Science Publishers, Inc.

Chapter 11

PREVALENCE OF SELF-REPORTED XEROSTOMIA IN 50- AND 60-YEAR-OLD SUBJECTS#

Ann-Katrin Johansson[*] [a], *Anders Johansson*[b], *Lennart Unell*[c] *and Gunnar E. Carlsson*[d]

[a]Department of Clinical Dentistry - Cariology
University of Bergen, Norway
[b]Department of Clinical Dentistry - Prosthodontics
University of Bergen, Norway
[c] Department of Oral Public Health, Malmö University, Malmö
Sweden and Consultant, Örebro County Council, Örebro, Sweden
[d] Department of Prosthetic Dentistry, University of Gothenburg
Göteborg, Sweden

ABSTRACT

Purpose: To study age and gender differences regarding xerostomia in 50- and 60-year-old subjects. It was hypothesized that the prevalence would be higher in women and among older subjects.

Methods: Identical questionnaires were sent to all subjects born in 1942 and 1952 living in two Swedish counties (N=17138). The final response rate was 72.8 %. Responses regarding day- and nighttime xerostomia were analyzed.

Results: The prevalence of "often dry mouth" ranged from 6.9 % in 50 year old men to 16.0 % in 60-year-old women. Xerostomia was more common at age 60 compared to 50 and more common in women compared to men. Approximately twice as many subjects perceived "often dry mouth" at nighttime compared to daytime. Logistic

A version of this book was also published as a chapter in *International Journal of Clinical Dentistry, Volume 1, Issue 2*, published by Nova Science Publishers, Inc. It was submitted for appropriate modifications in an effort to encourage wider dissemination of research.

* Correspondence: Ann-Katrin Johansson Department of Clinical Dentistry – Cariology, University of Bergen Årstadveien 17, 5009 Bergen, Norway Email: Ann-Katrin.Johansson@iko.uib.no Telephone: +47 55586699 (Business)

regression showed that xerostomia was associated to impaired general and oral health. The hypothesis that xerostomia was higher in women and among the older subjects was confirmed.

Clinical significance: The dramatic increase of self-reported xerostomia between age 50 and 60, especially among women, needs to be considered in the management of this age group.

INTRODUCTION

The subjective feeling of dry mouth, or xerostomia, is common. It is well documented that both salivary gland hypofunction and xerostomia increase with age and occur more often in women than in men [1,2]. Hyposalivation may increase the occurrence and severity of oral diseases, for example dental caries and dental erosion [3-5]. However, xerostomia is not always related to salivary gland hypofunction and decreased salivary flow rate [1,6]. There is strong evidence that the main causes are systemic diseases and daily medication [7-10]. It has recently been demonstrated that the discomfort caused by dry mouth has an impact on oral health-related quality of life [11-13].

The prevalence of xerostomia has been studied over several decades, but much remains unanswered about the epidemiology of dry mouth [14]. It was reported that the prevalence varied from 12% to 39% in representative epidemiological samples. A more recent systematic review reported an even greater variation in prevalence, ranging from 1% to 65% [15]. In this review, the studies were mainly conducted in Scandinavia and in elderly people; none in subjects younger than 18 years. A Swedish study on a large sample (> 3000 subjects ranging from 20 to 80 years of age) found that a mean of 21% of the men and 27% of the women reported xerostomia. The prevalence was 17% and 21% among the 20-year-old men and women and 32% and 39% among the 80-year olds [8]. A recent study from New Zealand presented prospective data on 26-year-old subjects followed up to age 32. The prevalence of xerostomia was 10% without gender difference and higher among those taking medications [10].

With respect to the inconclusive results of the epidemiological studies and the scarcity of findings in middle-aged people this study tries to explore the prevalence of xerostomia in a large population sample of 50- and 60-year-old subjects. It was hypothesized that the prevalence of reported mouth dryness would be higher in women than in men, as well as higher among the 60-year-old than the 50-year-old subjects.

MATERIALS AND METHODS

Population and Response Rate

In 2002, a questionnaire was mailed to all 50- and 60-year-old subjects in two Swedish counties, Örebro and Östergötland (N=17,138; n50=8,878; n60=8,260). Individuals not responding within two weeks were given a reminder by letter. If still not answering, a new questionnaire was sent. The final response rate was 72.8% (n=12,468) with some age and gender variation (50-year-olds =70.2%, 60-year-olds =75.5%).

Analysis of Non-Response

The non-response has been analyzed previously in part of the sample. For the total group born in 1942 and 1952 only gender, age and county of the non-responders could be analyzed. There was no significant difference between non-respondents as regards to county. In the total population there were 50.6% men and 49.4% women. However, there was an overrepresentation of women who answered the questionnaire, i.e. 46.2% men and 53.8% women ($P < 0.001$). The response rate for those born in 1942 (60-year-olds) was significantly higher than those born in 1952 (50-year-olds) ($P < 0.01$). Previous analyses of the non-response performed on those born in 1942 demonstrated some minor deviation from a random distribution, e.g., an over-representation of women and individuals with low education and fewer teeth [16]. Thus, some caution is advisable in interpreting the data.

Questionnaire

The questionnaire comprised 53 questions, with altogether 123 items. The questions were divided into socio-economic conditions (e.g. age, gender, occupation), general health (e.g., physician visits, tobacco habits, drug consumption), and oral conditions (e.g., satisfaction with teeth and dental appearance, oral problems, oral hygiene habits, number of teeth).

This study has focused on answers to two questions regarding perceived mouth dryness, in the daytime and at night, respectively. Both questions had four response alternatives (yes often, yes sometimes, no seldom, no never).

The complete questionnaire design, originally used in a study of 50-year-old subjects in 1992, has previously been described [17]. Descriptions of risk factors associated with symptoms of temporomandibular disorders of these subjects and on two cohorts of 50 year-olds, both in 2002, have also been published [18,19].

Statistical Methods

All statistical analyses were performed using the Statistical Package for Social Sciences (SPSS, Release 15; SPSS Inc., 233 S. Wacker Drive, Chicago, Illinois 60606, USA) on an IBM Personal Computer. A Mann-Whitney U-test was used for testing differences between age 50 and 60 and gender.

In the logistic regression analysis (Forward Conditional Method), the dependent variable was dichotomized as 1. those who never experienced dry mouth, and 2. those who reported that they had dry mouth often at night- or daytime. Those who had the answer alternatives "Yes sometimes" and "No seldom" were thus excluded from the analysis. For the selection of the independent variables, a Spearman correlation analysis was first performed between the dependent variable (1 = never dry mouth; 2 = often dry mouth) and all recorded variables (n=72). Numerous significant correlations were exhibited.

From the groups of variables that were interrelated, one representative variable was chosen for the final selection. Thus, 23 independent variables from the demographic, social, general and oral health domains, all showing significant ($P < 0.001$) correlation in the bivariate test, were included in the logistic regression analysis (Table 1).

Table 1. Dichotomization of independent variables (description 1 and 2) used in the stepwise logistic regression models

Variable	Description 1	Description 2
Gender	Man	Woman
Birth year	1952	1942
Working hours	Full-time	Less than full-time
Place of birth	Sweden	Outside Sweden
Education	University	High school/elementary/lower school
Healthy	Yes/on the whole	No/absolutely not
Use of medicine last 2 weeks	Yes	No
Smoking	Daily	Not daily
Alcohol	Alcohol every week	Less than weekly
Chewing ability	Very good	Rather good/not so good/bad
Toothache	During the last year	More than 1 year ago
Teeth changed position	Yes	No
Number of teeth	All or almost all remaining	Many missing and no teeth
Removable complete or partial denture	Yes	No
Burning mouth	No problems	Some problems/rather many/great problems
Taste changes	— ″—	— ″—
TMJ pain	— ″—	— ″—
Difficulty wide opening	— ″—	— ″—
Bruxism	— ″—	— ″—
Gum bleeding	— ″—	— ″—
Bad mouth smell	— ″—	— ″—
Dental restorations	— ″—	— ″—

RESULTS

There were marked and highly significant age and sex differences regarding reported mouth dryness (Figure 1 and Table 2).

Table 2. Distribution (%) of answers among 50- and 60-year-old subjects to the questions "Does your mouth usually feel dry at daytime" and "Does your mouth usually feel dry at nighttime" with four response alternatives. The responses to the two questions are compounded and the answer reporting the highest level of mouth dryness is presented

	60 yr	50 yr		60 yr	50 yr
	Men	Men		Women	Women
Answer	n=3058	n=2818		n=3228	n=3275
Yes, often	8.9	6.9	P1<0.001	16.0	9.5
Yes, sometimes	32.4	27.3	P2<0.001	36.2	30.8
No, seldom	33.5	37.0	P3<0.01	24.9	30.9
No, never	25.3	28.8	P4<0.001	22.9	28.8

P1= denotes the difference between 50 and 60 in men; P2 = Denotes the difference between 50 and 60 in women; P3= denotes the difference between men and women at age 50; P4= denotes the difference between men and women at age 60 (Mann-Whitney U-test).

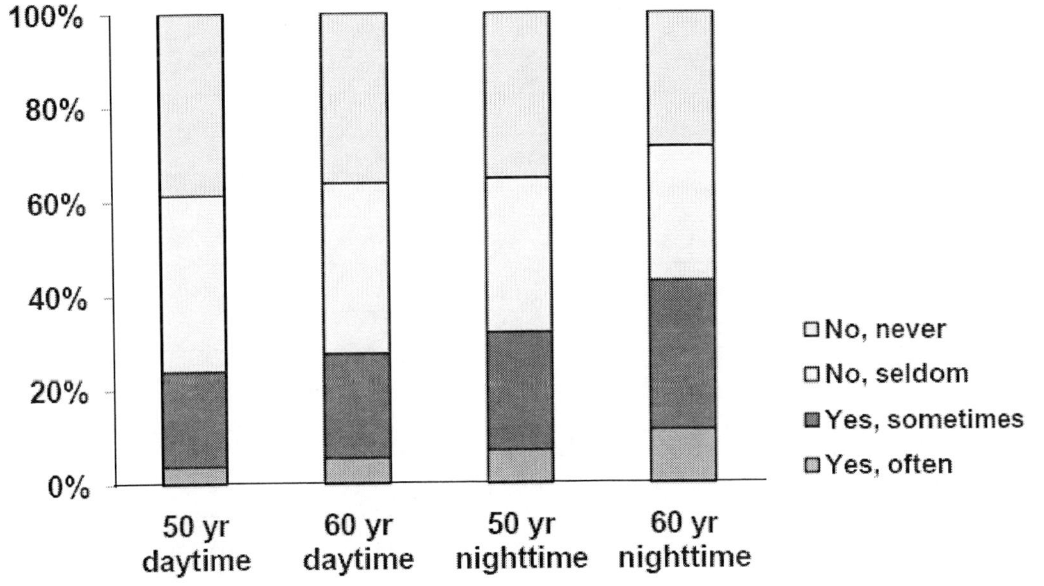

Figure 1. Distribution (%) of answers among 50- and 60-year-old subjects to the questions "Does your mouth usually feel dry at daytime" and "Does your mouth usually feel dry at nighttime" with four response alternatives.

The prevalence was higher in women than in men both at age 50 and age 60. In both genders, the prevalence was higher at age 60 than at age 50, both for mouth dryness in the daytime and at night. The difference between age 50 and 60 for often experienced xerostomia day or night was much greater in the women (9.5% to 16.0%) than in the men (6.9% to 8.9%; Table 2). Approximately twice as many subjects perceived frequent dry mouth at night compared to in daytime, both among women and men.

Logistic Regression Analysis

Among the 23 independent variables included in the analysis, 11 were highly significantly ($P < 0.001$) associated with the dependent variable. The differences regarding age and gender reported above were corroborated in the regression analysis (Table 3). Burning mouth showed the highest odds ratio (OR) 4.1. The variables taste changes, impaired general health, and use of medicine during the last two weeks, as well as impaired chewing ability and difficulty with wide opening of the mouth exhibited OR above 2. Daily smoking and bad mouth smell showed OR just below 2.

Table 3. Logistic regression model (Forward Conditional Method) presenting independent variables highly significantly associated with the dependent variable ($P < 0.001$). Dependent variable 1=never dry mouth (n=3281), 2= often dry mouth night- or daytime (n=1300). OR = Odds ratio, CI=Confidence interval

	OR	95 % CI for OR	
		Lower	Upper
60 year old	1.8	1.5	2.2
Female gender	1.5	1.3	1.9
Not feeling healthy	2.5	2.0	3.1
Medicine usage last 2 weeks	2.1	1.7	2.6
Daily smoking	1.9	1.5	2.4
Impaired chewing ability	2.2	1.8	2.7
Burning mouth	4.1	2.7	6.5
Taste changes	2.5	1.8	3.6
Difficulty wide opening	2.0	1.5	2.7
Bruxism	1.5	1.2	1.9
Bad mouth smell	1.9	1.5	2.3

Discussion

The results of the study were in line with the hypotheses. Thus it was found that the prevalence of reported mouth dryness was higher among the 60-year-old subjects than among the 50-year-old subjects as well as higher in women than in men. It is difficult to compare the present prevalence figures with those published in the literature because of the great variation in the presentation of data [15]. One reason for the varying results is the different methods used in collecting the data, for example the wording of questions of measuring dry mouth symptoms [14]. The prevalence presented by Nederfors et al. [8] was based on the question "Does your mouth usually feel dry?". They found that 19% of the men at age 50 and 28% at age 60 answered affirmatively. The corresponding figures in women were 25% and 36%, respectively. Our results were based on a similar question but divided into daytime and night dryness, to be answered with one of four alternatives. Our results are smaller when focusing on the answer "Yes often", but higher when combining "Yes often" and "Yes sometimes" (Figure 1 and Table 2). Another comparison of interest is the prevalence of dryness of the mouth in 70-year-old subjects. To the question "Does your mouth feel distinctly dry?" 16% of the men and 25% of the women answered positively [7].

It is well established that the prevalence of xerostomia increases with age. This knowledge is mainly based on cross-sectional studies and there is a paucity of longitudinal investigations. It has been suggested that we need more prospective cohort studies, so that our knowledge of the natural history of dry mouth is enhanced [14].

An interesting finding related to the two questions on day and nighttime dryness was that xerostomia was experienced approximately twice as often at night than during the day. This seems to correspond to clinical observations but has not been directly reported in the cited studies.

Reported xerostomia was associated with several independent variables according to the logistic regression analysis (Table 3). Some of the associations indicate that dry mouth may be part of impaired general and oral health, which may explain its impact on the quality of life [11-13]. The significant association with use of medicine are in line with results of several studies [7-10,20].

The strong associations between xerostomia and burning mouth, taste changes and para- and dysfunction of the masticatory system corroborate earlier findings and demonstrate the complexity of these conditions [18,21,22]. Smoking has been considered a risk factor for dry mouth [14]. The present results (OR 1.9) support this opinion.

The results of this study should be of interest as it is based on a large population sample, which can be considered representative of 50- and 60-year-old subjects in Sweden.

Conclusions

The prevalence of self-reported day- and nighttime xerostomia was higher at age 60 than at age 50. Women reported mouth dryness more often than men did in both age groups. Mouth dryness was associated with several variables related to impaired general and oral health.

Acknowledgment

This study was supported from Örebro and Linköping County Council, Sweden.

REFERENCES

[1] Nederfors T. Xerostomia: prevalence and pharmacotherapy. With special reference to beta-adrenoceptor antagonists. *Swed. Dent. J. Suppl.* 1996; 116: 1-70.

[2] Osterberg T, Birkhed D, Johansson C, Svanborg A. Longitudinal study of stimulated whole saliva in an elderly population. *Scand. J. Dent. Res.* 1992; 100: 340-345.

[3] Younger H, Harrison T, Streckfus C. Relationship among stimulated whole, glandular salivary flow rates, and root caries prevalence in an elderly population: a preliminary study. *Spec. Care Dentist* 1998; 18: 156-63.

[4] Risheim H, Arneberg P, Birkhed D. Oral sugar clearance and root caries prevalence in rheumatic patients with dry mouth symptoms. *Caries Res.* 1992; 26: 439-444.

[5] Jarvinen VK, Rytomaa II, Heinonen OP. Risk factors in dental erosion. *J. Dent. Res.* 1991; 70: 942-947.

[6] Narhi TO. Prevalence of subjective feelings of dry mouth in the elderly. *J. Dent. Res.* 1994; 73: 20-25.

[7] Osterberg T, Landahl S, Hedegard B. Salivary flow, saliva, pH and buffering capacity in 70-year-old men and women. Correlation to dental health, dryness in the mouth, disease and drug treatment. *J. Oral Rehabil.* 1984; 11: 157-170.

[8] Nederfors T, Isaksson R, Mornstad H, Dahlof C. Prevalence of perceived symptoms of dry mouth in an adult Swedish population--relation to age, sex and pharmacotherapy. *Community Dent. Oral Epidemiol.* 1997; 25: 211-216.

[9] Narhi TO, Meurman JH, Ainamo A. Xerostomia and hyposalivation: causes, consequences and treatment in the elderly. *Drugs Aging* 1999; 15: 103-116.

[10] Murray Thomson W, Chalmers JM, John Spencer A, Slade GD, Carter KD. A longitudinal study of medication exposure and xerostomia among older people. *Gerodontology* 2006; 23: 205-213.

[11] Locker D. Dental status, xerostomia and the oral health-related quality of life of an elderly institutionalized population. *Spec. Care Dentist* 2003; 23: 86-93.

[12] Baker SR, Pankhurst CL, Robinson PG. Utility of two oral health-related quality-of-life measures in patients with xerostomia. *Community Dent. Oral Epidemiol.* 2006;34:351-62.

[13] Ikebe K, Matsuda K, Morii K, Wada M, Hazeyama T, Nokubi T, Ettinger RL. Impact of dry mouth and hyposalivation on oral health-related quality of life of elderly Japanese. *Oral Surg. Oral Med. Oral Pathol. Oral Radiol. Endod.* 2007; 103: 216-222.

[14] Thomson WM. Issues in the epidemiological investigation of dry mouth. *Gerodontology* 2005; 22: 65-76.

[15] Orellana MF, Lagravere MO, Boychuk DG, Major PW, Flores-Mir C. Prevalence of xerostomia in population-based samples: a systematic review. *J. Public Health Dent.* 2006; 66: 152-158.

[16] Stahlnacke K, Soderfeldt B, Unell L, Halling A, Axtelius B. Perceived oral health: changes over 5 years in one Swedish age-cohort. *Community Dent. Oral Epidemiol.* 2003; 31: 292-299.

[17] Unell L. On oral disease, illness and impairment among 50-year-olds in two Swedish counties. *Swed. Dent. J.* 1999 Suppl; 135: 1-45.

[18] Johansson A, Unell L, Carlsson GE, Söderfeldt B, Halling A. Risk factors associated with symptoms of temporomandibular disorders in a population of 50- and 60-year old subjects. *J. Oral Rehabil.* 2006: 33: 473-481.

[19] Unell L, Johansson A, Carlsson GE, Halling A, Söderfeldt B. Changes in reported orofacial symptoms over a ten-year period as reflected in two cohorts of fifty-year-old subjects. *Acta Odontol. Scand.* 2006; 64: 202-208.

[20] Thomson WM, Chalmers JM, Spencer AJ, Slade GD. Medication and dry mouth: findings from a cohort study of older people. *J. Public Health Dent.* 2000; 60: 12-20.

[21] Grushka M, Sessle BJ. Burning mouth syndrome. *Dent. Clin. North Am.* 1991; 35: 171-184.

[22] Bergdahl J, Anneroth G. Burning mouth syndrome: literature review and model for research and management. *J. Oral Pathol. Med.* 1993; 22: 433-438.

In: Clinical Dentistry
Editor: Scardina Giuseppe Alessandro

ISBN: 978-1-61122-354-5
© 2011 Nova Science Publishers, Inc.

Chapter 12

CRANIOFACIAL ANTHROPOMETRY: THE PAST OR THE FUTURE IN EVALUATION OF THE CRANIOFACIAL PHENOTYPE[#]

***Erika Nagle**[*1]**, Uldis Teibe**[2]**, Dzintra Kažoka**[3]** and Ieva Grīnfelde**[4]*

Riga Stradiņš University, [1]Department of Medical Biology and Genetics
[2]Department of Medical Physics
[3]Institute of Anatomy and Anthropology
[4]Clinic of Medical Genetics, Children's Clinical University Hospital

ABSTRACT

Purpose: This study was aimed to analyze the anthropometric measurements of parents who have a child with nonsyndromic orofacial cleft to determine deviations in craniofacial morphology.

Methods: Measurements (total of nine) characterizing head and face were taken from parents who have children with clefts and healthy Latvia residents as controls. As a reference group we have used established standards of North American whites.

Results: Statistical analysis showed significant differences ($p<0.05$) between the cleft parents, controls, and the reference group for four measurements in males and for six measurements in females. This suggests that craniofacial morphology in parents of children with clefts is distinctive from that observed in healthy individuals.

Clinical significance: Anthropometry could be useful in clinical practice as objective approach to evaluate changes in the craniofacial region.

[#] A version of this book was also published as a chapter in *International Journal of Clinical Dentistry, Volume 1, Issue 2*, published by Nova Science Publishers, Inc. It was submitted for appropriate modifications in an effort to encourage wider dissemination of research.

[*] Address correspondence to Erika Nagle, Department of Medical Biology and Genetics, Riga Stradiņš University, Latvia, Dzirciema Street 16, Riga, LV-1007 Latvia. E-mail address: erikanagle@gmail.com

INTRODUCTION

The purpose of this study was to analyze the anthropometric measures of parents who have a child with nonsyndromic orofacial cleft and compare them to controls and the reference group in order to determine deviations in craniofacial morphology among parents of cleft children.

It is well known that head and face by anthropometric approach have been studied for centuries. Early studies were based mainly on comparison of facial differences among people from different geographical areas, races and with different social background. Today anthropometry has broad scientific and practical uses, especially in medicine. The diagnosis of many dysmorphic syndromes is based on measurements taken from a patient and compared with normal individuals, and deviations from normative values are evaluated. For instance, anthropometry of the face could be used to characterize morphology of the syndrome. Thus skull, face and ears of the patients with the unilateral form of lateral facial dysplasia were examined for the purpose of contributing to the morphology of this syndrome [1]. It was also found that craniofacial measurements could differentiate individuals with and without prenatal alcohol exposure [2, 3]. Anthropometric analysis was used to characterize the facial phenotype of patients with Smith-Magenis syndrome [4]. It was noted [5] that craniofacial measurement data can help in early diagnosis of multisystem disorder – Noonan syndrome. Early diagnosis of this relatively common disorder would result in better use of treatment therapies (therapeutic approaches). Anthropometry as an objective methodology for craniofacial assessment was used to avoid misdiagnosis in patients with Holt-Oram syndrome [6]. Several researchers [7] have used anthropometric approach describe the phenotype more precisely of sickle cell disease patients. Craniofacial anthropometric measurements with respect to orofacial clefts have been widely studied [8,9,10]. Distinct craniofacial features in phenotypically healthy parents have been reported [11]. The aim of this study was to determine are there differences in several craniofacial parameters between parents who have a child with orofacial cleft and individuals with negative family history regardless clefts. Nowadays craniofacial anthropometrics along with the advanced molecular techniques has become an important tool used by genetic counsellors and reconstructive surgeons. The data from this study suggest craniofacial anthropometry still has and in future will have a place in clinical practice to quick evaluation of genotypes at higher risk to produce child with anomalies.

MATERIALS AND METHODS

In this study the subjects were parents who had children with nonsyndromic facial clefts and healthy Latvia residents as a control group. Criterion for cleft parent group – child born with cleft lip alone, cleft lip and palate, cleft palate alone. Criteria for control group were as follows: Latvia resident, normal craniofacial configuration, no history of craniofacial abnormalities in the family. A total 201 subjects (57 fathers with cleft children, 67 mothers with cleft children, 39 control males and 38 control females) were studied. The individuals participating in the study were informed about the nature of the study and informed agreement was received. As a reference group we have used established standards of North American whites [12].

GPM Anthropological Instruments, Siber Hegner & Co.AG were used for taking measurements. Measurements were performed at the Institute of Stomatology Riga Stradiņš University, Department of Medical Biology and Genetics Riga Stradiņš University, and at University of Daugavpils. Landmarks and measurements between them used in this study are shown in Table 1. A subject was asked to sit upright in resting position for measurements. For identification of landmarks and measuring techniques we have followed instructions given by Farkas LG (personal communication) and guidelines described by Kolar JC, Salter ME [13]. Measurements were evaluated separately for males and females in both study groups and in the reference group, because of well known sexual dimorphism of the craniofacial region.

Table 1. Landmarks and measurements

Landmark	Measurement
zy – *zygion*	zy-zy – maximum facial breadth
go – *gonion*	go-go – mandible breadth
al – *alare*	al-al – nose width
ch – *cheilion*	ch-ch – labial fissure width
en – *endocanthion*	en-en – intercanthal width
ex – *exocanthion*	ex-ex – biocular width
tr – *trihion*	tr-gn – physiognomial face height
gn – *gnation*	
n – *nasion*	n-gn – morphological face height
gn – *gnation*	
n – *nasion*	n-sn – nose height
sn – *subnasale*	

All measurements were processed by SPSS (11.0). Means, standard deviations and t-test were used for evaluating the differences between cleft, control and reference groups.

RESULTS

Anthropometric measurements of 201 subjects were obtained. The total 9 measurements were compared in different study groups (control males and females, cleft fathers and mothers and in the reference group). Landmarks and measurements are shown in Table 1. Mean values and standard deviations of the measurements are shown in the Tables 2 and 3. All measurements are given in millimetres. Statistically significant differences between cleft parents, controls, and the reference group for 5 measurements characterizing the face were obtained.

Table 2 shows measurements of the face of males (reference group, control Latvia, cleft fathers). Higher values in cleft fathers when compared with the reference group and control group were observed in maximum facial breadth (*zy-zy*) and mandible breadth (*go-go*). In contrary we observed that biocular width (*ex-ex*) in cleft group is smaller in comparison with reference and control groups. Cleft fathers showed also shorter noses (*n-sn*), although significant only in comparison with the Latvia control. and smaller labial fissure width (*ch-ch*), but only in comparison with the reference group. Other measurements showed tendency in reduced values in cleft group in comparison with the reference group and controls (*tr-gn, en-en*), but these differences are not significant.

Table 3 represents results of face measurements in females. Reference group, Latvia control, and cleft group were compared. In females almost all measurements are significant different between cleft mothers, reference group, and Latvia control. Results are similar to those obtained in males.

Table 2. Craniofacial measurements (mm) in reference group, Latvia control and cleft group (males)

	Reference group		Control Latvia		Clefts		Difference between reference group and clefts	Difference between control Latvia and clefts
	Mean	SD	Mean	SD	Mean	SD		
zy-zy	137.1	4.3	133.1	9.8	143.6	6.8	S	S
go-go	97.1	5.8	105.4	6.3	111.9	8.3	S	S
tr-gn	187.5	8.1	187.3	7.3	185.9	10.3	NS	NS
n-gn	121.3	6.8	124.1	6.0	121.9	7.0	NS	NS
en-en	32.9	2.7	29.1	3.0	28.3	3.0	NS	NS
ex-ex	89.4	3.6	106.3	5.8	85.3	4.7	S	S
n-sn	53.0	3.5	58.7	5.4	52.3	5.6	NS	S
al-al	34.7	2.6	35.3	3.2	35.4	3.6	NS	NS
ch-ch	53.3	3.3	50.8	3.7	51.0	7.1	S	NS

NS – not significant; S – significant.

Table 3. Craniofacial measurements (mm) in reference group, Latvia control and cleft group (females)

	Reference group		Control Latvia		Clefts		Difference between reference group and clefts	Difference between control Latvia and clefts
	Mean	SD	Mean	SD	Mean	SD		
zy-zy	129.9	5.3	122.4	8.0	133.7	6.5	S	S
go-go	91.1	5.9	96.9	7.5	102.7	5.3	S	S
tr-gn	172.5	7.5	177.0	7.9	172.9	8.2	NS	S
n-gn	111.8	5.2	117.6	6.2	110.1	5.3	S	S
en-en	31.6	2.4	26.6	2.4	28.1	2.5	S	S
ex-ex	86.8	4..0	100.6	6.0	82.0	3.7	S	S
n-sn	48.9	2.6	56.7	5.7	48.4	3.2	NS	S
al-al	31.4	1.9	32.8	2.7	32.4	2.6	NS	NS
ch-ch	49.8	3.2	46.5	3.4	48.5	4.2	S	S

NS – not significant; S – significant.

Higher values in cleft group were obtained in maximum facial breadth (*zy-zy*) and mandible breadth (*go-go*). Biocular width (*ex-ex*), morphological facial height (*n-gn*), physiognomical face height (*tr-gn*) as well as nose height (*n-sn*) is smaller in cleft group.

Nevertheless it should be noted, that difference in the value *tr-gn* if to compare with reference group is higher but not significant. Several facial measurements when compared in cleft, reference group and Latvia control were not as uniform as expected, for instance, intercanthal width (*en-en*), labial fissure width (*ch-ch*) showed higher values if clefts were compared with Latvia controls, but lower – with the reference group.

DISCUSSION

The purpose of this study was to analyze the anthropometric measures of cleft parents and compare them to controls and the reference group. Our results presented in Tables 2 and 3 are supported by data observed by other authors [14, 15] that craniofacial measurements in cleft parents if compared with the same measurements of phenotypically normal individuals are different. Of the nine measurements compared, the two horizontal ones (*zy-zy, go-go*) showed higher and statistically significant ($p< 0.05$) values in cleft group if compared with controls and the reference group in both sexes. Results in respect to mandible breadth in our study showed similar results as in other author's reports [15, 16]. However some other researchers have reported lower values of this dimension in cleft mothers in comparison with control females [14]. Other horizontal measurements such as (*ex-ex*) in cleft fathers and mothers group were found in lower values than in controls and reference group. Nevertheless in some horizontal measurements only subtle deviations (not significant) were observed. This refers to the nose width (*al-al*) in both sexes. Some differences are not easy interpreted, because results are no uniform. Intercanthal width (*en-en*) showed different results in males and females. In males differences between cleft fathers, controls and the reference group were found to be unremarkable, but in females significant differences were observed in study groups. If this distance (*en-en*) in females was compared between cleft group and controls – cleft group showed higher values, but if compared with the reference group – lower values. Mouth width (*ch-ch*) tended to show lower values in cleft parents if compared with the reference group, but higher – if compared with controls, but in control males this association is not significant. Other measurements (*tr-gn, n-gn, n-sn*) were used to characterize vertical dimensions of the face. General tendency observed in vertical dimensions was reduced values with respect to clefts compared with controls, on a cleft and control group bases in females we can conclude that vertical dimensions are reduced in cleft group. Similar tendency, but not significant was observed in male group also. Some researchers have reported smaller facial dimensions in mothers of cleft children [15], and that individuals at risk for having child with clefts can be recognized through reduced facial height [8]. Results in reference group in comparison with cleft parent group are no uniform. Some dimensions (*n-gn*) show higher, some other (*tr-gn, n-sn*) lower values. In male group these differences are not significant, except of nose length compared between cleft and control group. In female reference group differences in the vertical dimensions when compared with clefts are not equipollent. Physiognomial face height is increased but not significant in cleft group, but morphological face height – decreased. Nose length is also decreased, but not significant. Overall the analysis of the anthropometric data for this study in respect of differences between clefts, controls and the reference group was found to be remarkable. The lack of differences in some measurements between the clefts, controls and reference group could be result of the population peculiarity with respect to craniofacial complex or/and because of subjective element in measuring technique. Comparison of cleft parent data with the controls and established norms of the North American whites offered possibility to evaluate deviations of face morphology in cleft parents in the most objective way.

CONCLUSIONS

1. Results of this study suggest that craniofacial morphology is different in parents who have children with nonsyndromic orofacial clefts if compared with control individuals (negative family history concerning the clefts).
2. Comparison of anthropometric data between cleft parents controls from the same population and the reference group could strongly suggest that deviations in craniofacial complex in cleft parents have overall tendency.
3. Such data offer possibility to evaluate the phenotype of the face in cleft parent in a very objective manner.

ACKNOWLEDGMENTS

We wish to thank all participants, especially parents of cleft children, students of the University of Daugavpils and Riga Stradiņš University, and Institute of Stomatology Riga Stradiņš University for support of our investigations.

REFERENCES

[1] Farkas LG, James JS. Anthropometry of the face in lateral facial dysplasia: the unilateral form. *Cleft Palate J.* 1977 Jul; 14(3):193-9.

[2] Moore ES, Ward RE, Jamisson PL, et al. The subtle facial signs of prenatal exposure to alcohol: an anthropometric approach. *J. Pediatr*. 2001 Aug: 139(2):215-9.

[3] Naidoo S, Chikte U, Laubscher R, et al. Fetal Alcohol Syndrome: Anthropometric and Oral Health Status. *J. Contemp. Dent. Pract*. 2005 Nov; 6(4):1-15.

[4] Allanson JE, Greenberg F, Smith ACM. The face of Smith-Magenis syndrome: a subjective and objective study. *J. Med. Genet*. 1999; 36:394-397.

[5] Okada M, Sasaki N, Kaihara Y, et al. Oral findings in Noonan syndrome: report of a case. *Journal of Oral Science*. 2003; 45(2):117-121.

[6] Allanson JE, Newbury-Ecob RA. Holt-Oram syndrome: is there a "face"? *Am. J. Med. Genet*. 2003 May 1; 118 A(4):314-8.

[7] Kaimbo Wa Kaimbo D, Ngiyulu Makuala R, Tshilolo Mwepu L, et al. Outer orbital distance, inner canthal distance and interpupillary distance, proptosis in children with homozygous sickle cell disease. *Bull. Soc. Belge Ophtalmol.* 2000; 275:33-37.

[8] Ward RE, Bixler D, Jamison PL. Cephalometric evidence for a dominantly inherited predisposition to cleft lip-cleft palate in a single large kindred. *Am. J. Med. Genet.* 1994; 50:57-62.

[9] Mossey PA, Arngrimsson R, McColl J, et al. Prediction of liability to orofacial clefting using genetic and craniofacial data from parents. *J. Med. Genet.* 1998; 35:371-8.

[10] Yoon YJ, Perkiomaki MR, Tallents RH, et al. Transversal craniofacial features and their genetic predisposition in families with nonsyndromic unilateral cleft lip and palate. *Cleft Palate Craniofac J.* 2004; 41:256-61.

[11] Perkiomaki MR, Yoon YJ, Tallents RH, et al. Association of Distinct Craniofacial features in Nonsyndromic Cleft Lip and Palate Family members. *Cleft Palate Craniofac J.* 2003; 40:397-402.

[12] Farkas LG, Katic MJ, Forrest CR. International Anthropometric Study of Facial Morphology in Various Ethnic Groups/Races. *J. Craniofac Surg.* 2005 Jul; 16(4):615-46.

[13] Kolar JC, Salter ME. *Craniofacial anthropometry: practical measurement of the head and face for clinical, surgical and research use.* Sprinfield, IL: Charles C Thomas publisher; 1997.

[14] Suzuki A, Takenoshita Y, Honda Y, et al. Dentocraniofacial Morphology in Parents of Children with Cleft Lip and/or Palate. *Cleft Palate Craniofac J.* 1999; 36: 131-8.

[15] Alemran SE, Fatani E, Hassanain JE. Craniofacial variability in parents of children with cleft lip and cleft palate. *J. Clin. Pediatr. Dent.* 1999; 23:337-41.

[16] Mossey PA, McColl J, O`Hara M. Cephalometric features in the parents of children with orofacial clefting. *Br. J. Oral Maxillofac. Surg.* 1998; 36:202-12.

In: Clinical Dentistry
Editor: Scardina Giuseppe Alessandro

ISBN: 978-1-61122-354-5
© 2011 Nova Science Publishers, Inc.

Chapter 13

ENDODONTIC TREATMENT OF A FUSED MAXILLARY LATERAL INCISOR AND A SUPERNUMERARY TOOTH: A CASE REPORT

Rodrigo Sanches Cunha[1]*, Vivian Allendorf[1], Carlos Eduardo Fontana[1], Rogério de Castilho Jacinto[¥], Eduardo Rodrigues Fregnani[1] and Carlos Eduardo da Silveira Bueno[1]

[1]Centre for Dental Research, São Leopoldo Mandic, Campinas. Brazil
[¥]Dental School of Piracicaba, State University of Campinas, UNICAMP, Piracicaba, Brazil

ABSTRACT

Fusion is currently defined as a developmental anomaly that occurs due to an union of two or more adjacent teeth during morphodifferentiation of the dental germs. The [#]present case reports the endodontic treatment of a fused maxillary lateral incisor and supernumerary tooth. A 12-year-old girl had an excessively large anterior tooth. The endodontic therapy was carried out, so the patient could receive a surgical therapy to remove the supernumerary tooth and orthodontic treatment to correct the malocclusion. Electronic apex locator, rotary instrumentation and thermo-mechanical obturation were used under the direct view of a dental operating microscope.

Keywords: dental anatomy; fusion; tooth abnormalities; endodontology.

* Corresponding author: Rodrigo Sanches Cunha, Rua Aglair Buratto Villas Boas, 508 - apto. 61 C, Campinas, São Paulo - Brazil, Zip Code: 13087-725, Phone/Fax: - 0055-19-32965335, e-mail: rscunha@dglnet.com.br

A version of this book was also published as a chapter in *International Journal of Clinical Dentistry, Volume 1, Issue 3*, published by Nova Science Publishers, Inc. It was submitted for appropriate modifications in an effort to encourage wider dissemination of research.

Clinical Significance: This case report is unique and brings complete information regarding endodontic management of fused teeth.

Introduction

Fusion and gemination have been reported as being the same developmental anomaly and known as double teeth [1,2]. However, in most cases a diagnosis can be made with the clinical and radiographical aspects. In cases of fusion, the crowns are united by enamel and/or dentine, but there are two roots or two root canals in a single root. It has been showed that fusion may be from two normal teeth or from one tooth of the normal series and a supernumerary tooth [3]. It is not always possible to differentiate between gemination and a case in which there has been fusion between a normal tooth and supernumerary tooth [4]. The correct etiology of this anomaly is not yet well established, even though many theories have been proposed to explain it. According to Neville *et al* [5] fusion occurs due to the union of two separated tooth germs with a resulting formation of a joint tooth with the confluence of dentin. Fusion predominantly occurs in incisors and canines and their frequency is very rare in molars [6]. Due to its abnormal crown shape and size, the tooth presents an unaesthetic shape with excessive mesiodistal width and irregular morphology and periodontal problems [7,8]. Therefore, the approach is usually multidisciplinary. The field of endodontics has seen vast improvements in technology and techniques over the latest years. The use of advanced equipment such as apex locators and rotatory systems, new endodontic techniques, improved materials and surgical operating microscope have enhanced the ability to attain consistent clinical results and to treat cases with clinical anomalies [9]. This paper reports the endodontic therapy of a fused maxillary lateral incisor with a supernumerary tooth in which a contemporary endodontic approach was used to achieve success.

Case Report

A healthy 12-year-old female Caucasian was referred to the Endodontic team from São Leopoldo Mandic Centre for Dental Research - Campinas, Brazil for evaluation and root canal treatment of the left maxillary lateral incisor as part of a multidisciplinary treatment (Figure 1). The patient presented a chief cosmetic complaint of an excessively large anterior tooth, although there was no symptom history. The oral hygiene condition was good, and the intraoral soft tissues were free of pathological signs. Clinical examination revealed the presence of an abnormally large left maxillary permanent lateral incisor. Clinical and radiographic findings lead us to the diagnosis of fusion between the lateral maxillary incisor and a supernumerary tooth (Figure 2). A multidisciplinary treatment plan was proposed and accepted by the patient parents. This included the root canal therapy and subsequently, hemisection and the surgical removal of the supernumerary tooth, so that the orthodontic therapy could take place to correct the spacing and alignment problems. Anesthesia was administered by using 4% Articaine with 1:100,000 of epinephrine (DFL, Rio de Janeiro, R.J, Brazil) Access cavity was prepared using a Dental Operating Microscope (D F Vasconcelos, São Paulo, Brazil) and a rubber dam was applied and disinfected with 2% chlorhexidine.

After the initial radiographic examination, the access was performed with high-speed stainless steel burs No. 1557 (KG-Sorensen, Barueri, SP, Brazil), under continuous water spray irrigation. Working length was determined with an apex locator (Root ZX, J. Morita Europe GmbH, Dietzenbach, Germany). The root canals were copiously irrigated with 5.25 % sodium hypochlorite solution. Cleaning and shaping were carried out by the Crown-Down technique with Protaper system (Dentsply-Maillefer, Ballaigues, Switzerland). This was performed up to file F3 for lateral incisor canal, and up to file F2 for the supernumerary canal. After canal preparation, the canal was irrigated with 17% EDTA for three minutes followed by irrigation with 5.25% sodium hypochlorite, then dried and were obturated by the use of the hybrid thermo-mechanic technique with AH Plus sealer (Dentsply-De Trey, Konstanz, Germany) and immediately after, the access cavities were sealed with a bonded composite restoration. Figure 3 shows the final X-ray after root canal therapy.

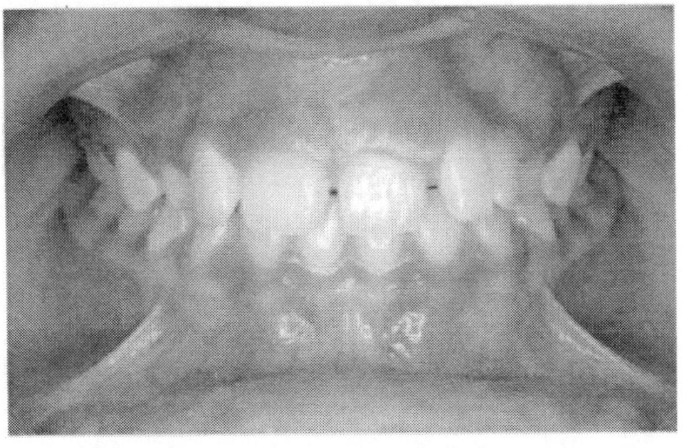

Figure 1. Clinical view of fusion between left lateral maxillary incisor and a supernumerary tooth.

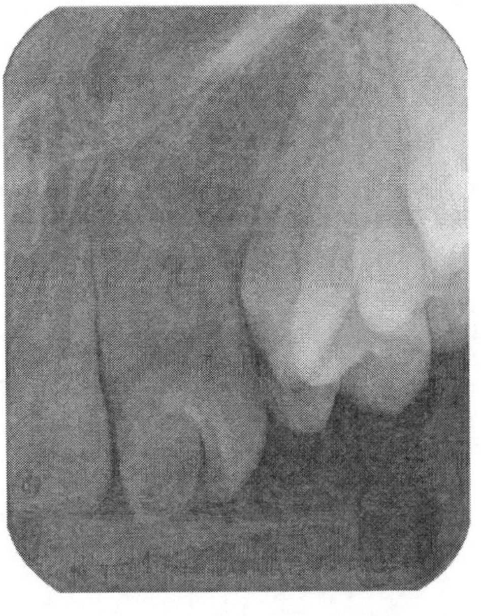

Figure 2. Radiographic view of fusion between left lateral maxillary incisor and a supernumerary tooth.

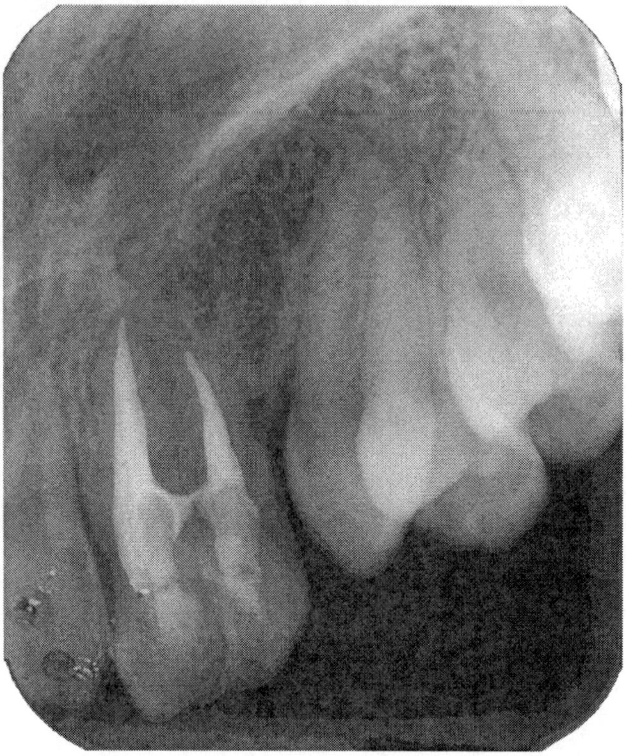

Figure 3. Final radiograph after root canal therapy.

Discussion

Two teeth may be fused either by their crown and root or only by the roots. Root canals may also be separated or shared [4]. In the present case, two distinct root canal systems were present and pulp chamber communication between the supernumerary tooth and the permanent left maxillary lateral incisor were evident in both radiographs. The abnormal shape and size of the fused crown caused a space and occlusion problem and impossibility to the complete eruption of the permanent canine. Therefore, due to aesthetic and orthodontic reasons the teeth hemisection and further supernumerary extraction were indicated. The endodontic treatment was performed before surgery in order to prevent pulp exposure, which could lead to a necrosis of the pulpal tissues [10]. According to the literature, the endodontic treatment of fused teeth can be accomplished when their pulp are integrated by a pulp chamber or when a communication exists between both root canals [11]. Plank *et al* [12] performed the hemisection before the endodontic treatment, which affected the outcome of the clinical case. Owing to this fact, in our case, the endodontic treatment was demanded firstly. Differently from the case reported by Indra *et al* [7], the present case was accomplished by using some contemporary endodontic apparatus. The operatory microscope was used to locate the canals providing higher visual magnification and better lightening [13]. As the tooth presented a shape abnormality, the use of an apex locator to precisely detect the foramen, which is not frequently located in the radiographic vertex, and determine the working length was also important [14]. Irrigation was performed with 5.25% sodium hypochlorite in order to obtain better dissolution of the pulp tissue located between both roots (isthmus), where mechanical shaping could not have reached [15]. The root canal filling with a gutta-percha thermo-plastic technique was associated with a highly fluid root canal sealer. This allowed the whole system obturation, including the communication area between both canals. Moreover, it is well know that a definitive bonded restoration immediately after endodontic therapy is essential to avoid coronal microleakage and contamination of the canals [16].

Conclusion

This case reports the endodontic therapy of fused teeth as a part of a multidisciplinary approach. The aesthetic and orthodontic reasons and the possibility of the hemisection and surgical removal of the supernumerary tooth lead us to the indication of the endodontic treatment of the element #10 and the fused supernumerary. The use of advanced endodontic equipment and techniques improved the quality, providing a full sealing of the anatomical complexities of the case.

References

[1] Hagman FT. Anomalies of form and number, fused primary teeth, a correlations of the dentitions. *J. Dent. Child* 1988; 55: 359-361.

[2] Killian CM, Croll TP. Dental twinning anomalies: The nomenclature enigma. *Quintessence Int* 1990; 21: 571-76.

[3] Yücel AÇ, Güler E. Nonsurgical endodontic retreatment of geminated teeth: A Case Report. *J. Endod.* 2006; 32: 1214-16.

[4] Shafer WG, Hine MK, Levy BM. Developmental disturbances of oral and paraoral structures. In: Shafer WG, Hine MK, Levy BM, editors. *A text book of oral pathology*. Philadelphia: W.B. Saunders; 1993. p.38 –9.

[5] Neville BW, Damm DD, Allen CM, Bouquot JE. Abnormalities of teeth. In: Neville BW, Damm DD, Allen CM, Bouquot JE, editors. *Oral and Maxillofacial Pathology*. Oxford: W.B. Saunders Company; 2002. p.74.

[6] Tsesis J, Steinbock N, Rosenberg E, Kaufmari AY. Endodontic treatment of developmental anomalies in posterior teeth: Treatment of geminated/fused teeth report of two cases. *Int. Endod. J.* 2003; 36: 372- 9.

[7] Indra, R, Srinivasan MR, Farzana H, Karthikeyan K. Endodontic Management of a fused maxillary lateral incisor with a supernumerary tooth: A Case Report. *J. Endod.* 2006; 32: 1217-9.

[8] Kim E, Jouu Y T. A Supernumerary tooth fused to the facial surface of a maxillary permanent central incisor: Case Report. *J. Endod* 2000; 26: 45-8.

[9] Duke ES. Technology may significantly improve endodontic therapy. *Compend. Contin. Educ. Dent.,* 2005; 26: 408-10.

[10] O'Reilly PMR. Structural and radiographic evaluation of four cases of tooth fusion. *J. Endod.* 1989; 15: 442-6.

[11] Stillwell KD, Coke JM. Bilateral fusion of the maxillary central incisors to supranumerary teeth: report of a case. *J. Am. Dent. Assoc.* 1986; 112: 62-4.
[12] Plank BS, Randall OR, Leuy AR. A fused central incisor. Periodontal considerations in comprehensive treatment. *J. Periodont.* 1985; 56: 21-4.
[13] Yoshioka T, Kobayashi C, Suda H. Detection Rate of Root Canal Orifices with a Microscope. *J. Endod.* 2002; 28: 452-3.
[14] Herrera M, Abalos C, Planas AJ, Llamas R. Influence of apical constriction diameter on root ZX apex locator precision. *J. Endod*. 2007; 33: 995-8.
[15] 15.Zehnder M. Root Canal Irrigants. *J. Endod*. 2006; 32: 389-98.
[16] Galvan RR, West LA, Liewehr FR, Pashley DH. Coronal microleakage of five materials used to create an intracoronal seal in endodontically treated teeth. *J. Endod*. 2002; 28: 59-61.

In: Clinical Dentistry
Editor: Scardina Giuseppe Alessandro

ISBN: 978-1-61122-354-5
© 2011 Nova Science Publishers, Inc.

Chapter 14

EFFECT OF THREE DIFFERENT SEALERS ON THE SEALING ABILITY OF TWO OBTURATION TECHNIQUES[#]

Mina Zarei*[*1] and Shariar Shahriari[2]

[1]Dept of Endodontics, Member of Dental Research Center,
Faculty of Dentistry. Mashad University of Medical Sciences , Iran
[2]Dept of Endodontics, Faculty of Dentistry,
Hamedan University of Medical Sciences, Iran

INTRODUCTION

Success in endodonitc treatment based on diagnosis, treatment plan, debridement, sterilization and obturation [1]. In an early radiographic study of success and failure, Ingle indicated nearly 60% of treatment failures were due to incomplete obturation [2]. In reality, creating a fluid-tight apical, lateral and coronal seal is necessary to prevent recontamination and long-term clinical success [3].

Several root filling materials and techniques have been developed with purpose of obtaining a tight root canal seal. Most techniques employ a core material and sealer, and a wide variety of root canal sealers are available for obturation of the root canal system.

Over all many studies on the obturation of root canals indicated that most fillings do not completely fill the root canal systems [4-6].

[#] A version of this book was also published as a chapter in *International Journal of Clinical Dentistry, Volume 1, Issue 4*, published by Nova Science Publishers, Inc. It was submitted for appropriate modifications in an effort to encourage wider dissemination of research.

[*] Correspondence to: Dr.Mina Zarei, Dept of Endodontics, Faculty of Dentistry. Mashad University of Medical Sciences, Iran Mail Address: P.O.Box: 91735-984,Mashad, Iran. Tel:+98 511 8829502-11. Fax: :+98 511 8829500 E.Mail:zareim@mums.ac.ir

Lateral and vertical compaction is two common methods for obturation. There are many studies about stress generation with in the canal form these two methods [7, 8], and their sealing ability [9-11].

Mendoza et al. compared sealing ability of two different obturation techniques, they concluded that warm vertical compaction, provide better apical seal in canine teeth of dogs compared to heated lateral techniques, with fewer complications [11].

Many studies showed that thermafil obturators achieved seals comparable to lateral compaction [12, 13].

Gernhardt et al. evaluated lateral and vertical condensation and thermafil and presented that thermafil and warm vertical condensation achieved seals with low dye penetration [14].

Reader et al. evaluated filling of the lateral and main canals using root canal obturation techniques, they found that flow of gutta and sealer was more in vertical and lateral techniques respectively [9]. Yared compared the quality of coronal seal between these two techniques after removing coronal gutta and found better seal with vertical condensation independently of gutta removal technique [15]. In addition Taylor et al showed removal of smear layer and the use of AH26 and and vertical condensation obturation; reduce coronal leakage [16].

Jayalatha et al compared sealing ability of three different root canal sealers (seal apex AH26 and ZnOE) and showed that AH26 has the maximum sealing ability followed by seal apex and ZnOE [17].

Suprabha and colleagues evaluated the apical leakage of AH26/silverfree and Tubliseal using methylene blue penetration and showed superior sealing ability of AH26(18).

Studies had shown more sealing ability of resin based sealers like AH26 or AH plus versus ZnOE or Ca (OH) 2 based sealers [19-22].

Some investigation have shown that sealing ability of Ca(OH)2 based sealers is more than AH26 and less than ZnOE sealers [23,24].

The aim of this study was to compare apical sealing ability of AH26 Apexit, pure ZnOE using lateral and vertical condensation.

Methods and Materials

In this randomized preclinical trial study 120 extracted one rooted maxillary human teeth with straight canals, without any crack were used. The size of the foramen was not greater than file #20.In all samples crowns were resected with a high speed diamond bur and the length determined 12mm. The working length was visually determined 1mm shorter than anatomic apical foramen. The canals cleaned and shaped by the crown-down technique with profile rotary instruments (Dentsply-TulsaDental,Tulsa ,OK) up to MAF # 35 (2%).

The canals were irrigated with 3 ml of 5.25% Nalco (Golrang, Tehran, Iran) between each file. At last smear layer was removed by application of 17% EDTA (Asiachimiteb, Teran, Iran) followed by 5.25% Nalco and distilled water. The teeth were then randomly divided into 6 experimental groups of 18 teeth and 2 controls of 6 teeth The canals in experimental groups obturated as bellow:

Group A, and negative control: gutta percha (Ariadent, Tehran, Iran) + AH26 sealer (Dents ply, De, Trey, German) by lateral condensation.
Group B: gutta percha +AH26 by vertical condensation
Group C: gutta percha + Apexit(vivadent, schaan, liechtenstein) by lateral condensation
Group D: gutta percha + Apexit (vertical condensation)
Group E: gutta percha + ZOE (lateral condensation)
Group F: gutta percha + ZOE (vertical condensation)

The samples were incubated in 100% humidity in an incubator at 37 °C for 72h to allow the obturation materials to set.

The root surfaces of experimental groups' were coated with 2 layer of nail polish (Etude, France) except for 2mm from the apex and in negative control all the root surfaces were covered

In positive control the canals obturated with a single cone without any sealer and the roots were not covered with nail polish

All of the roots were submerged in methylene blue dye for 48 hours and then split longitudinally. Linear apical dye penetration was assessed blindly by 3 examiners using a stereomicroscope (Olympus, Tokyo, Japan) to 0.1mm accuracy. The mean score was calculated. Finally, the data were analyzed with ANOVA and Tukey test at a significant level of $P<0.05$.

RESULTS

The negative leakage control demonstrated no dye penetration, while the positive leakage control showed dye penetration along the entire root canal.

The mean linear dye leakage of all groups is shown in table 1 and figure 1. Analysis of variance revealed significantly less dye leakage for AH26+ vertical condensation than the other groups($P=0.0004$).

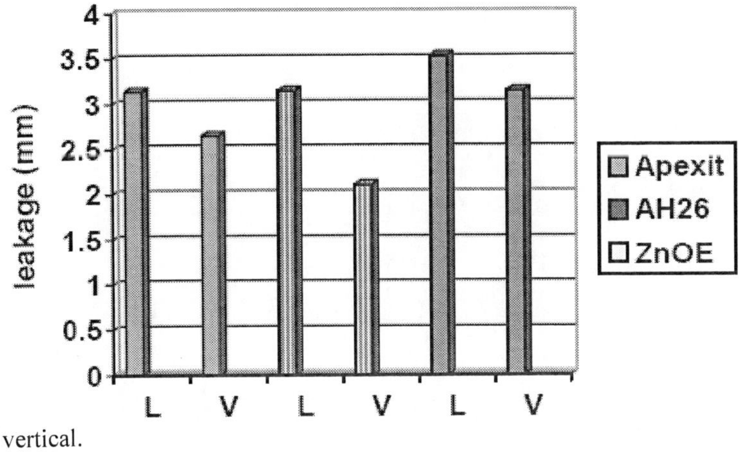

L= Lateral; V= vertical.

Figure 1. The mean leakage value in experimental groups.

Table 1. Mean leakage (mm) and SD in all groups

Sealer	Group	N	Mean (mm)	SD
AH26	V	18	2.11	0.81
	L	18	3.15	1.22
Apexit	V	18	2.26	1.14
	L	18	3.14	0.71
ZnOE	V	18	3.15	0.75
	L	18	3.54	0.97

Regardless the obturation technique the mean leakage between AH26 (2.63) and ZnOE (3.49) was statistically significant (Tukey test, P=0.01).

ZnOE groups had the most leakage but the sealing ability of AH26 and Apexit showed no significant difference(Figure 2).

Sealing ability of vertical condensation was significantly higher than lateral obturation technique (T.Test, P=0.001) (Figure 3).

In all groups apical leakage in vertical condensation was less than lateral obturation technique.

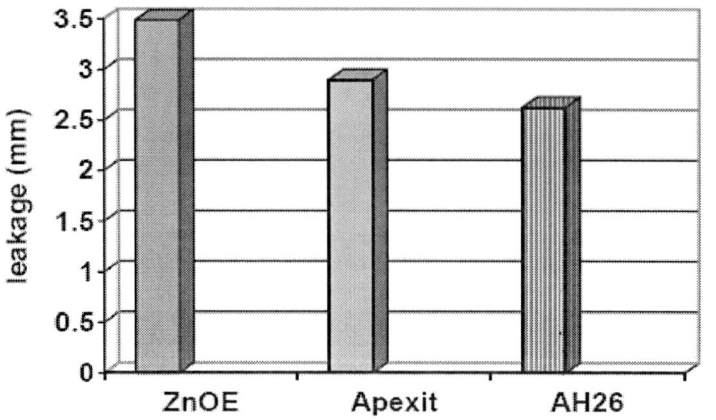

Figure 2. Mean leakage value regardless of obturation technique.

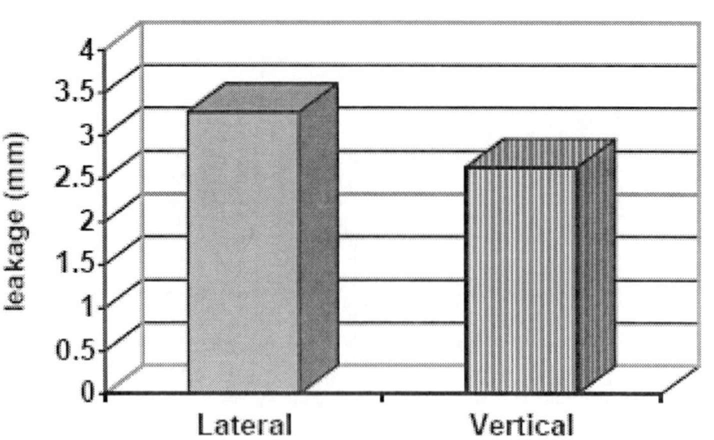

Figure 3. Mean leakage value regardless of sealer type.

DISCUSSION

Cold lateral compaction and warm vertical condensation are the most widely methods for root canal obturation. This study was designed to compare apical sealing ability of rhree root canal sealers by these methods.

In this study to minimize the variables such as anatomical variations, canal size and diameter of apical foramen, all samples were chose of the same teeth and prepared up to the same MAF.

Methylene blue dye was used as the leakage tracer like Rajput et al. [23].

Dalta and colleagues showed that the dye penetrates voids better than isotopes and reveals microlumina in obturated root canal spaces greater depth than most other tracing materials [25]. Three examiners measured dye leakage levels in order to eliminate or reduce possible bias and evaluator error.

In this study three kinds of sealer a resin base sealer (AH26) a Ca(OH)2 base sealer (Apexit) and pure ZnOE were use to compare their sealing ability. There are many studies that show sealing ability of resin based sealers significantly better than the other kind of sealers[21-23].

Suprabha and his colleagues compared AH26/silverfree with Tubliseal and showed superior sealing ability of AH26 [18].

In another study Miletic et al compared Apexit ,AH plus, AH26 and Diaket and concluded that the Apexit had more leakage, than resin based sealers, in their study the method of obturation was lateral condensation [21]. Jayalatha et al study compared the sealing ability of three root canal sealers (AH26, ZnOE and Seal apex) by bacterial and dye penetration leakage, their results showed that AH26 has the maximum sealing ability followed by Seal apex and ZnOE [17].

The results of the present study showed that ZnOE sealer in both lateral and vertical obturation techniques had the most leakage and Apexit and AH26 had the less, respectively. These results were in agreement with other studies [19, 21].

The more sealing ability of AH26, in both techniques may be due to its bond strength and adhesive properties [26-28] and more solubility of ZnOE and Apexit sealers .

This investigation showed a significantly better sealing ability of vertical condensation than lateral condensation. As Aqrabawi [24] and Farzaneh et al. [29] mentioned in their studies, this may be explained by the ability of warm gutta –percha when compacted to flow into the lateral canals, thus providing better seal.

Gernhardt [14], Mendoza [11] and Reader [9] had similar results in their studies and concluded that vertical compaction achieved seal with low dye penetration. In an other study lateral condensation presents higher leakage after one month[30], how ever the present study showed the efficacy of AH26 and vertical condensation obturation as other studies but to assess the outcome of treatment its needed to repeat micro leakage measurement after a long time.

Conclusion

Sealing ability of AH26 sealer especially using vertical condensation technique, is better than Apexit or ZnOE.

References

[1] Cohen S, Hargreaves KM. *Pathways of the pulp*. 9th ed. Canada:Mosby Inc; 2006. P.358-9.

[2] Ingle JI,Backland LK. Endodontics. 5th ed. London: Hamilton BC Deker; 2002. p.572.

[3] Siqueira JF Jr. Strategies to treat infected root canals. *J. Calif. Dent. Assoc*. 2001; 29: 825-37.

[4] Brayton SM, Davis SR, Goldman M. Gutta-percha root canal fillings. *Oral Surg. Oral Pathol. Oral Radiol. Endod*. 1973; 35: 226.

[5] Seltzer S. Endodontology. Biologic considerations. In: *Endodotnic procedures*. New York: Mc Graw-Hill; 1971.p. 381.

[6] Trope M, Debelian GJ. Endodontics manual for the general dentist.1 st ed.Germany:Quntesencepublishingco,LTD;2005.P.58.

[7] Gimlin DR,Parr CH,Aquirre-Ramirez G.. A comparison of stresses produced during lateral and vertical condensation using engineering model. *J. Endod*. 1986; 12: 235-41.

[8] Wollard RR. Brough SO,Maggio J,Seltzer S. Scanning electron microscopic examination of root canal filling materials. *J. Endod.* 1976; 2: 98-110.

[9] Reader CM, Himel VT,Germain LP,Hoen MM. Effect of three obturation techniques on the fillings of lateral canals and the main canal. *J. Endod*.: 1993; 19: 404-8.

[10] Froes JA,Horta HG,da Silveria AB. Smear layer influence on the apical seal of four different obturation techniques. *J. Endod*. 2000; 26: 351-4.

[11] Mendoza KA. Manfra Marreta S. Siegel AM, Stapleton BL, Wiggs RB, Klippert LS. Comparison of two heated gutta percha and sealer obturation techniques in canine teeth of dogs. *J. vet. Dent.* 2000; 17: 69-74.

[12] Schafer E, Olthoff G. Effect of three different sealers on the sealing ability of both thermafil obturators and cold laterally compacted Gutta-percha. *J. Endod.* 2002; 28: 638-42.

[13] Kontakiotis E, Chaniotis A, Georgopoulou M. fluid filtration evaluation of 3 obturation techniques. *Guintessence Int*. 2007; 38: e 410-6.

[14] Gernhandt CR, Kruger T, Bekes K, Schaller HG. Apical sealing ability of epexy resin based sealers used with root canal obturation techniques based on warm gutta-percha compared to cold lateral condensation. *Quintessence Int*. 2007; 38: 229-34.

[15] Yared GM, Bou Dagher F, Machtou P. Influence of the removal of coronal gutta on the seal of the root canal obturation. *J. Endod.* 1997; 23: 146-8.

[16] Taylor JK, Jeansonne GB, Leman KR. Coronal leakage effect of smear layer obturation technique and sealer. *J. Endod*. 1997; 23: 508-12.

[17] Jayalatha NS, Kuriakose S, Saradaevi KL. Comparison of sealing ability of three different root canal sealers and invitro study. *J. Indian soc. pedod. prev. Dent.* 1998; 16: 122-7.

[18] Suprabha BS, Sudha P, Vidya M. A comparative evaluation of sealing ability of root canal sealers. *Indian J. Dent. Res*. 2002; 13: 31-6.

[19] Limkang walmongkol S, Abbort PV, Sandler AB. Apical dye penetration with four root canal sealers and gutta-percha using longitudinal sectioning. *J. Endod.* 1992; 18: 535-9.

[20] Siqueira JF Jr, rocas In, valois CR. Apical sealing ability of five endodontic searers. *Aust. Endod. J.* 2001; 27: 33-5.

[21] Miletic I, Ribaric SP, Karlovic Z, Jukic S, Bosnjak A, anic I. apical leakage of five root canal sealers after one year of storage. *J. Endod*. 2002; 28: 431-2.

[22] Adanir N, Cobankara FK, Bell S. Sealing properties of different resin-based root canal sealers. *J. Biomed. Mater. Res. B Appl. Biomater*. 2006; 77: 1-4.

[23] Rajput JS, Jin RL, Pathak A. An evaluation of sealing ability of endodontic materials as root canal sealers. *J. Indian Soc. Pedod. Prev. Dent*. 2004; 22: 1-7.

[24] Agrabawi JA. Out come of endodontic treatment of teeth filled using lateral condensation versus vertical compaction (schilder's techniques). *J. Contemp. Dent. Pract.* 2006; 15: 7: 17-24.

[25] Dalta DM, Spangberg LS. Comparison of apical leakage in root canals obturated with various gutta-percha techniques using a dye vaccum tracing method. *J. Endod.* 1994; 20: 315-9.

[26] Orstavik D. Eriksen HM, Beyer olsen EM. Adhesive propertves cand leakage of root canal selers. Invitro. *Int. Endod. J.* 1983; 16: 59-63.

[27] Tagger M, Tagger E, Tjan A, Bakland LK. Mealurment of adhesion of endodontic sealers to dentin. *J. Endod*. 2002; 28: 351-4.

[28] Wennberg A, Orstavik D. Adhesion of root canal sealers to bovin dentin and gutta-percha . *Int. Endod. J*. 1990; 23: 13-19.

[29] Forzaneh M, Pbitbol S, W\Lawrence H. the Toronto stud. Out come of mitial endodontic treatment phose II. *J. Endod.* 2003; 29: 296(abstract).

[30] Pommel L, Comps J. Invitro apical leakage of system B compared with other filling techniques. *J. Endod*. 2001; 27: 449-51.

In: Clinical Dentistry
Editor: Scardina Giuseppe Alessandro

ISBN: 978-1-61122-354-5
© 2011 Nova Science Publishers, Inc.

Chapter 15

ROLE OF SOLUBLE CD14 LEVELS IN GINGIVAL CREVICULAR FLUID IN PERIODONTAL HEALTH AND DISEASE[#]

A. R. Pradeep*, V. Yashoda, Shikha Chowdhry and Swati Pradeep
Department of periodontics, Government Dental college and hospital, Bangalore-560002, Karnataka, India

ABSTRACT

Background: Recently, the study has shown negative correlation between the severity of the periodontal disease and sCD14 levels. However there are no reports correlating the levels of sCD14 in health, disease and after treatment of periodontitis. The present study was designed to explore further in understanding the role played by sCD14 in the pathogenesis of periodontal disease and also to gain insight into the levels of sCD14 in health, disease and after treatment of periodontitis affected individuals.

Methods: Age (29-39yrs) and sex matched (30 males and 30 females) sixty subjects were recruited and divided into 4 groups consisting of 20 subjects in each group based on clinical attachment loss (CAL) and radiological parameters (bone loss); healthy (group I), gingivitis (group II), periodontitis (group III) and after treatment of group III (groupIV) and GCF was collected. The sCD14 levels were determined by ELISA. Results were analyzed statistically.

Results: The sCD14 was detected in all 60 subjects tested for and values varied greatly among the subjects within the group. The mean concentration of sCD14 in GCF was observed to be highest in group I i.e., 1652.50 pg/µl (900-2300pg/µl) and lowest in group III i.e., 828.70 pg/ µl (213-1400 pg/ µl). The mean sCD14 concentrations of group II (1019.35 pg/µl ± 243.06) and group IV (1172.7 pg/µl ± 216.93) fell between the

---

[#] A version of this book was also published as a chapter in *International Journal of Clinical Dentistry, Volume 1, Issue 4*, published by Nova Science Publishers, Inc. It was submitted for appropriate modifications in an effort to encourage wider dissemination of research.

* Corresponding Author: Dr. Pradeep A.R. MDS, Professor and head, Department of periodontics, Government dental college and hospital, Bangalore-560002. Karnataka, India. Email: periodontics_gdc@yahoo.co.in (e mail to be published)

highest and lowest values. This suggests negative correlation between CAL and GCF sCD14 concentrations.

Conclusions: Currently, as our data shows inverse relationship between the levels of sCD14 and the clinical parameters like CAL and GI scores, which indicate the inflammatory conditions of the periodontal tissue, we speculate that sCD14 could be used as an inflammatory biomarker. However carefully controlled longitudinal, population-based studies are needed to verify this possibility.

Keywords: Soluble CD14, gingival crevicular fluid, analysis, periodontitis, clinical attachment loss, pathogenesis.

INTRODUCTION

Periodontal diseases, a series of infections of the periodontal tissues which eventually can lead to loss of teeth, are form of aberrant inflammation resulting from a complex biofilm of friendly commensal and periodontopathic bacteria and their products triggering the human inflammatory response [1]. The cell wall components of the pathogens, especially lipopolysaccharide (LPS) of Gram-negative bacteria, are attributed to be the virulence factor that causes the periodontal destruction [2]. Both vertebrates and invertebrates have evolved complex mechanisms to respond to infection with Gram-negative bacteria and the response is characterized by initiation of various defense mechanisms that rely on recognition of LPS [3].

CD14 is a 55kDa glycoprotein existing in a membrane form (mCD14) and soluble form (sCD14), [4] is responsible for innate recognition of bacteria by host cells. Both forms function to enhance activation of cells by lipopolysaccharide, which is referred to as receptor function [5]. The mCD14 is originally described as a myeloid differentiation antigen detected on mature monocytes/macrophages and neutrophils [6] and has been characterized as the most important receptor of these cells that is involved in the process of signal transduction [4].

Soluble CD14 is detectable in several biological fluids like serum, plasma, urine, cord blood, amniotic fluid, cerebrospinal fluid, synovial fluid and most importantly gingival crevicular fluid of human origin [7]. It's source in biological fluid is thought to be due to the spontaneous or stimulated shedding from monocytes/macrophages by the action of proteases or phospholipases [8]. Alternatively, some CD14 molecules may escape the phosphatidylinositol (PI) anchoring mechanism and can be secreted [6]. The sCD14 has been revealed to be responsible for the LPS-mediated activation of cell systems lacking mCD14 (9) Depending on it's concentration sCD14 either functions as a receptor for neutralizing the LPS-LBP (lipopolysaccharide binding protein) complex thereby preventing further stimulation of inflammatory cells or interacts with nonmyeloid cells that do not normally express CD14 enabling their LPS activation [10].

Several studies have demonstrated that the concentration of sCD14 in serum is elevated under many pathological conditions of both bacterial and viral origin [11-14]. It has also been shown that sCD14 levels are increased in sera of periodontitis patients when compared to healthy subjects [15]. Recently, the study of sCD14 in gingival crevicular fluid of untreated adult periodontitis has shown a negative correlation between the severity of the disease and sCD14 levels [16].

Till today no studies have projected the levels of sCD14 in subjects with periodontal disease keeping healthy subjects as controls and also there are no reports correlating the levels of sCD14 before and after treatment of periodontitis.

Keeping the above facts in mind this study is designed to explore further in understanding the role played by sCD14 in the pathogenesis of periodontal disease and also to gain insight into the levels of sCD14 in health, disease and after treatment of periodontitis affected individuals.

Materials and Methods

60 subjects (30 males and 30 females) constituting 20 healthy, 20 gingivitis and 20 chronic periodontitis were selected from group of patients visiting our dental hospital.

Patients with systemic disease, habits of smoking and alcoholism , with gross oral pathology, anomalies of immune system , hematological disorder, liver disorders ,pregnant and lactating mothers, history of bacterial and viral infection and who had taken medication(anti- inflammatory and antibiotics) for at least 6 months prior to sampling procedure, and also patients who had received periodontal therapy in the preceding 6 months were excluded from the study.

Written informed consent was obtained from those who agreed to participate and the ethical clearance was obtained from institutional ethical review board, Government Dental College and Hospital, Rajiv Gandhi University of Health Sciences, Karnataka, India and were recruited for the study conducted in January to February 2006.

Subjects were categorized into three groups based on clinical attachment level ,gingival index scores and radiographic evidence of bone loss. After full mouth periodontal probing, bone loss was recorded dichotomously (presence or absence) to differentiate chronic periodontitis patients from other groups without any delineation in the extent of alveolar bone loss. Group I (Healthy) consisted of 20 subjects with clinically healthy periodontium and gingival index <1 ,pocket probing depth (PPD) of $\leq$ 1mm and no attachment loss. Group II (Gingivitis) consisted of 20 subjects who showed clinical signs of gingival inflammation (GI$>$1) and PPD of $\leq$3mm, without any attachment loss. Group III (chronic periodontitis) consisted of 20 subjects who showed clinical signs of inflammation (gingival index $>$1), attachment loss of $>$1mm and PPD of $\geq$ 4 mm.

Site Selection and Fluid Collection

Subjects selected for sampling were made to sit comfortably in an upright position on the dental chair with proper illumination. After drying the area with a blast of air, supragingival plaque was removed without touching the marginal gingiva and GCF was collected. From each test site, a standardized volume of 1 μL was collected using the calibration on white color-coded 1-5 μL calibrated volumetric microcapillary pipettes[1] with an extracrevicular approach .Each sample collection was allotted a maximum of 20 minutes and some test sites in healthy group, which did not express any volume of GCF, were excluded from the study. Further, micropipettes, which were suspected to be contaminated with blood and saliva, were excluded from the study. Periodontal treatment which included scaling and root planing (SRP) was performed for both gingivitis and periodontitis patients at the same appointment after GCF collection. After 8 weeks GCF was collected from the same sites of the subjects of group III. For this 8 week period subjects were called at one week interval and plaque control measures were performed. The GCF collected was immediately transferred to airtight plastic vial and stored at -70^0 C till the time of assay.

Soluble CD14 Assay

The samples were assayed for soluble CD 14 levels by using soluble CD14 ELISA kit using solid phase sandwich ELISA.[2] This method makes use of a monoclonal antibody specific for sCD114 precoated onto a microplate . Standards containing known volumes of s CD14 and samples to be estimated are pipetted into the wells and any sCD14 present is bound by immobilized antibody. After washing away any unbound substances, an enzyme linked polyclonal antibody specific for sCD14 is added to the wells. Following a wash to remove any unbound antibody –enzyme reagent, a substrate solution is added to the wells and color develops in proportion to the amount of sCD14 bound in initial step. The color development is stopped and the intensity of color is measured. The levels of soluble CD14 in tested samples were calculated using the standard curve plotted using the standard curve plotted using optical density values with standards.

Statistical Analysis

All data were analyzed using a software program[3]. Kruskal-Wallis test was used to compare the mean values of levels of sCD14 between groups. Duncan test was used to compare sCD14 in GCF among study groups. The Spearman's rank correlation was used to correlate the soluble CD14 levels to GI scores and CAL in group III and Group IV.

Results

The GI score,PPD and CAL obtained in all the four groups are listed in the Table 1. Marked clinical improvement was found in group III patients after non surgical periodontal therapy as shown in Table 1.

All the samples in the group tested positive for sCD14 assay. The mean concentration of sCD14 along with standard deviations, are shown in Table 2 and Graph 1. The highest mean

---

[1] Sigma-Aldrich, St. Louis, MO.

[2] *Quantikine*® human sCD14 Immunoassay kit, RandD systems ,Minneapolis USA (catalog no. DC140)

[3] Systat, version 11, and SigmaStat, Systat Software, Point Richmond, CA.

concentration of sCD14 was obtained for group I i.e (1652.50 pg/μl) and least mean concentration was obtained for group III (828.70 pg/μl).

Table 1. Mean clinical paramters for all the groups

Group	*GI*	*PPD*	*CAL*
I	*0.33*	*1*	*0*
II	*1.99*	*2.1*	*0*
III	*2.43*	*6.7*	*4.55*
IV	*1.21*	*3.9*	*2.8*

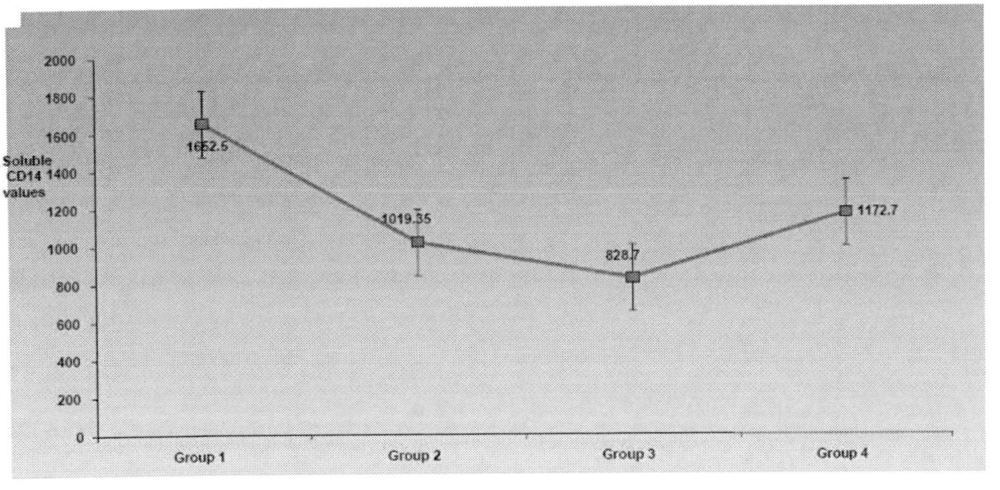

Graph 1. Mean values of levels of soluble CD14 among Study Group.

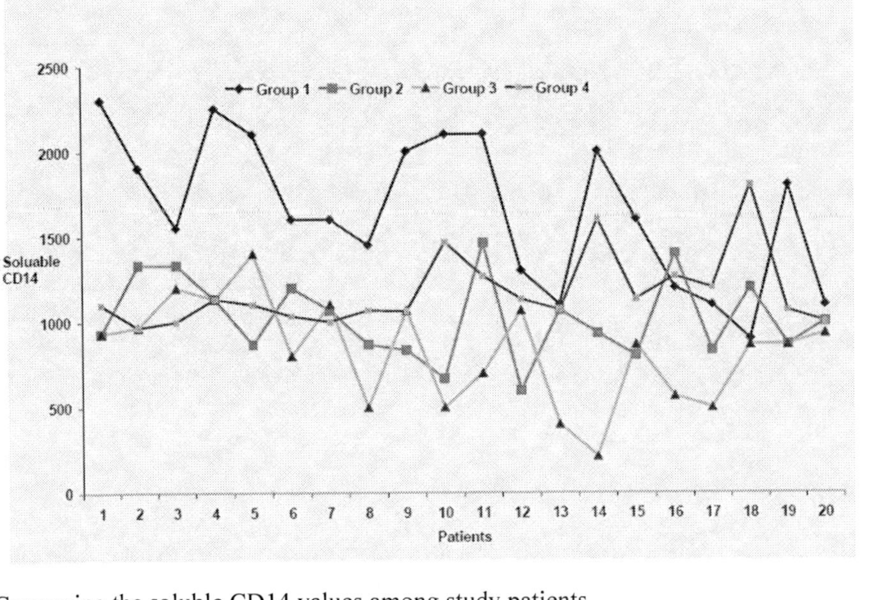

Graph 2. Comparing the soluble CD14 values among study patients.

The mean concentration of the group II i.e (1019.35 pg/µl) and group IV (1172.7 pg/µl ± 216.93) fell between group I and group III. Multiple comparisons between groups were done to explore which pair or pairs differ significantly. The results showed that differences were statistically significant between groups I and II , group I and III , group I and IV and group III and IV. ($p<0.05$). (table 3 and graph 2).

However, comparison of group II and III , group II and IV showed no statistical difference. Significant negative correlation were found between the GCF and clinical variables (viz GI and CAL) in group III which suggests that there is an increase in periodontal inflammation with decreased levels of sCD14. In group IV also, negative correlation were found between concentrations of sCD14 and GI scores and CAL. (Table 4 and 5).

Table 2. Comparison of mean values of levels of soluble CD14 between groups

Group	N	Mean	Median	Std Dev.	Minimum	Maximum
1	20	1652.50	1600	433.61	900.00	2300.00
2	20	1019.35	966.50	243.06	600.00	1460.00
3	20	828.70	866.00	304.46	213.00	1400.00
4	20	1172.70	1100.00	216.93	966.00	1800.00

Table 3. Multiple comparison test (Duncan test) results of sCD14 in GCF amongst the study groups

Comparison	P-value
Group I vs Group II	P<0.05*
Group I vs Group III	P<0.05*

Table 3. (Continued)

Comparison	P-value
Group I vs Group IV	P<0.05*
Group II vs Group III	P<0.05*
Group II vs Group IV	P<0.05*
Group III vs Group IV	P<0.05*

*P<0.05-Significant.

Table 4. Spearman's Correlation between soluble CD14 levels to GI scores and CAL in Group III and Group IV

Correlation	Group III	Group IV
sCD14 vs GI	-0.93*	-0.30
sCD14 vs CAL	-0.90*	-0.33

*indicates there is significant correlation between pairs of variables.

Table 5 .Comparison of mean values of sCD14 levels with respect to CAL in Group III

CAL	N	Mean	Median	Std Dev.	Min.	Max.	F value	P value
3	5	1179.80	1133.00	132.67	1066.00	1400.00	17.93	<0.0001
4	6	927.33	933.00	90.29	800.00	1066.00		
5	3	688.67	700.00	183.26	500.00	866.00		
6	5	566.40	500.00	177.67	400.00	866.00		
7	1	213.00	213.00		213.00	213.00		

This table shows significant difference between the levels of sCD14 and CAL (P<0.0001).

Discussion

The CD14 molecule , 55kDa glycoprotein , exist in a membrane bound (m CD14) and a circulating soluble (s CD14) state [4]. Both can function as receptors for the lipopolysaccharides of gram negative bacteria and for various cell wall products of Gram positive bacteria [17]. Binding of LPS to mCD14 enhances signaling by Toll-like receptor -2 , resulting in activation of the cell and release of proinflammatory mediators like TNF-alpha, IL-1 alpha , IL-6 and IF –gamma [18,19] oxygen free radicals and prostaglandins , (20) all of which are known to play an important role in pathogenesis of periodontitis.

LPS- sCD14 complexes can bind to cells that do not normally express mCD14 , resulting in cellular activation [9]. Moreover, circulating levels of sCD14 have been correlated with LPS exposure experimentally.

Previous study has shown that systemic level of sCD14 receptor significantly increased in patients with periodontal disease [15]. The expression of cell adhesion molecules such as E-selectin [20] and ICAM-1 [21] in human gingival fibroblasts are all in response to host cells to CD14 complexed with microbial LPS. On the contrary, previous data have also shown that the expression of CD14 within periodontal tissues is negatively correlated with amount of attachment loss [16]. Altogether, these observations emphasize the strong relevance of CD14 receptor activity in the clinical manifestations and development of peridontitis.

However currently, no data is available correlating the GCF levels of sCD14 in subjects with periodontal disease keeping healthy subjects as controls and also there are no reports correlating the levels of sCD14 before and after the treatment of the periodontitis. The present study is thus the first case control study to investigate concentrations of sCD14 in GCF of subjects with periodontal health, disease and after treatment of periodontitis.

The origin of s CD14 is from multiple sources. It could be due to local production [16] or may be released spontaneously by monocytes, macrophages and gingival fibroblasts in response to microbial LPS [6,8]. Since sCD14 is constantly present in serum of healthy individuals and fluid component of GCF may also be derived from serum it could be a possible source [22].

In the present study, confounding factors influencing the levels of sCD14 like age and sex were nullified by selecting subjects with equal number of males and females who fell under the narrow age range of 29-39 years, for all the study groups. Extracrevicular (unstimulated) method of GCF collection using microcapillary pipettes was employed to ensure the atraumatism , to obtain an undiluted sample of native GCF whose volume can be accurately assessed and also to avoid non-specific attachment of the analyte to filter paper fibers [23].

Results of our study showed highest concentrations of sCD14 in the healthy group with mean concentrations of 1652.50 ±433.61 pg/µl. However, as there are no previous studies in GCF evaluating the levels of sCD14 in healthy subjects, values couldn't be compared. Further, the mean GCF sCD14 concentrations in periodontitis group was lowest , value being 828.70± 304.46 pg/ µl. concentrations of gingivitis group (1019.35± 243.06pg/ µl.) and after the treatment of periodontitis (1172.7± 216.93pg/ µl.) group fell between the highest and lowest values. This pattern shows a negative correlation between concentrations of sCD14 and periodontal disease progression which is statistically significant. The correlation between clinical parameters like GI scores and CAL has shown a negative correlation with levels of s CD14. When concentrations of s CD14 between different CAL values was compared using Duncan test analysis, significantly lower levels of sCD14 were observed at sites with advanced attachment loss, which were significant lower levels of sCD14 were observed at sites with advanced attachment loss , which were significant among the different values of CAL. This observed trend is in accordance with that of Jin and Darveau's study, [16] who also reported negative correlation between sCD14 levels and periodontal probing depth in untreated adult periodontits patients. However, the mean concentrations of sCD14 obtained for Group III (chronic periodontitis) from our study (828+30.46pg/ µl) were significantly lower than that of Jin and Darveau's study who reported higher concentration of sCD14 (14.04 ± 4.15 µg/ml). The differences in values between two studies may be explained in different ways; the differences in study population may have led the differences in the data, different methods used to collect GCF and failure to control adequately for potential confounding factors in the previous study may have role in the inconsistencies between the results. Finally the complexities of the local bacteria host interactions in periodontitis patients may also have added to the difference.

Nonetheless, this study differs from the Jin and Darveau's s study [16], where in our study consists of four groups (healthy, gingivitis, periodontitis and after treatment of periodontitis), former study has compared values among the subjects of untreated adult peridontitis only. Having additional groups of healthy as controls, gingivitis and after treatment group assisted us better in evaluating the role played by sCD14 in different stages of periodontal disease , during conversion from health to severe disease also after treatment of the disease.

The observation that concentrations of sCD14 in the GCF was higher in healthy subjects and lower in patients with periodontal disease, suggests it's protective role. This could be explained, as sCD14 is responsible for the initial inflammatory response to keep in check the invading pathogens until a more specific response is mounted [24]. Apart from its role as a cell activating receptor, sCD14 may also serve as an opsonin, thereby promoting bacterial pathogens until a more specific response is mounted. It has also been shown that sCD14 functions as a shuttle in the neutralization of LPS by facilitating the movement of LPS to HDL which effectively neutralizes its biological potency both in vitro and in vivo [25]. A new protective functions has also been suggested for CD14 which involves scavenging LPS and apoptotic cells with a charged surface and presenting them to other components of innate host defense system for clearance [26]. Although the exact pathophysiological role of sCD14 is not understood, LPS binding proteins like sCD14 play a pivotal role in physiology as well as pathophysiology of gram negative infections [24] like periodontitis.

However, as the periodontal disease progresses , protective effect of sCD14 on gingiva is lot owing to decline in sCD14 concentration . The mechanism underlying it's decline is attributed to the action of bacterial proteinases (gingipains) which cleave CD14 , resulting in attenuation of the cellular recognition of bacteria and as a consequence sustain chronic inflammation [27]. Since deep periodontal pockets are colonized by multiple gram negative bacteria producing proteinases , levels of sCD14 could be decreased owing to their action.

The chronic periodontitis subjects were treated by non surgical periodontal therapy (SRP) and strict oral hygiene measures were instituted. Again rise in the concentrations of sCD14 in this group with decrease in disease component supports the protective role of sCD14 in this group with decrease in disease component supports the protective role of sCD14 . However, it is surprising outcome of the study that, the observed negative relation after treatment is not statistically significant. This may be attributed to the different stages of inflammatory resolution after the treatment.

The variability of GCF sCD14 concentrations observed in each group could be ascribed to the different stages of the disease process at the time of collection of GCF samples. Since expansion of sCD14 is determined by several factors like LPS, cytokines and also other stimuli and activity of the periodontopathogens present, local host response at the time of collection may influence the levels of sCD14 and explains for the great unevenness of observed values among different subjects in the same group. A few of the samples of group I showed values nearing that of group II which could be due to presence of subclinical inflammation in the healthy group. A few samples of gingivitis group also showed values similar to the healthy group which could again be either due to partial resolution of the inflammation or inactive lesion. Overlapping of values between group II and group III may be due to near conversion of gingivitis lesion to periodontitis lesion that is not detectable clinically, or due to the partial resolution of inflammation in periodontitis group. Further, there was a considerable overlap values between gingivitis group and after treatment (of chronic periodontitis) group which can be attributed to the individual variations in the resolution of periodontitis after the treatment of the same.

Currently, as our data shows inverse relationship between the levels of sCD14 and the clinical parameters like CAL and GI scores, which indicate the inflammatory conditions of periodontal tissue, we speculate thatsCD14 could be used as an inflammatory biomarker. However, carefully controlled longitudinal, population based studies are needed to verify this possibility.

List of Names and Addresses to Send Complimentary Review Copies

[1] Prof. De Stefano Dorigo Elettra - Ospedale Maggiore via Stuparich,1- 34125 Trieste (ITALIA).

[2] Prof. Matteo D'Angelo – Policlinico "P. Giaccone" via del Vespro, 129 -90127 Palermo (ITALIA).

[3] Prof. Giovanni Dolci - Università degli Studi di Roma "La Sapienza" - Clinica Odontoiatrica - Viale Regina Elena, 287/a - 00161 Roma (ITALIA).
[4] Prof. Antonella Polimeri - Università degli Studi di Roma "La Sapienza" - Clinica Odontoiatrica - Viale Regina Elena, 287/a - 00161 Roma (ITALIA).
[5] Prof. Livia Ottolenghi - Università degli Studi di Roma "La Sapienza" - Clinica Odontoiatrica - Viale Regina Elena, 287/a - 00161 Roma (ITALIA).
[6] Prof. Pierluigi Sapelli – P.le Spedali Civili, 1 – 25123 Brescia (ITALIA).
[7] Prof. Giuseppe Gallina - Policlinico "P. Giaccone" via del Vespro, 129 -90127 Palermo (ITALIA).
[8] Prof. Ersilia Barbato - Università degli Studi di Roma "La Sapienza" - Clinica Odontoiatrica - Viale Regina Elena, 287/a - 00161 Roma (ITALIA)
[9] Prof. Mario Capogreco – Clinica Odontoiatrica: Ed. Delta 6 località Coppito, 67100 L'Aquila (ITALIA).
[10] Prof. Paolo Pera – DI.S.T.BI.M.O. Pad. 4 Ospedale san Martino – Largo Rosanna Benzi 10 – 16132 Genova (ITALIA)
[11] Prof. Egidio Bertelli – Via della quercia,10 Monteresi 53035 Monteriggioni – Siena (ITALIA)
[12] Prof. Leonardo Trombelli – Corso Giovecca 203 -44100 –Ferrara (ITALIA)
[13] Prof. Mario Caltabiano – Az. Policlinico, Sezione Odontostomatologia 2 – Via S. Sofia,78 – 95125 Catania (ITALIA)
[14] Prof. Domenico Cicciù - via G. Moranti, 14 -95027 –San Gregorio di Catania
[15] Prof. Ugo Consolo – Vicolo Botta, 3 – 37126 –Verona (ITALIA)
[16] Prof. Potito D'Errico – Dipartimento Scienze Chirurgiche Radiologiche e Odontostomatologiche – Sez. odontoiatria – Policlinico Monteluce – via Brunamonti 0600 Perugia (ITALIA)
[17] Prof. Pier Luigi Foglio Bonda - Ospedale Maggiore della carità di Novara – Viale piazza d'armi,1 – 28100 Novara (ITALIA)
[18] Prof. Mario Giudice - corso di laurea specialistica in medicina e chirurgia –corso di malattie odontostomatologiche - viale Europa -campus universitario di Germaneto – 88100 Catanzaro (ITALIA)
[19] Prof. Enrico Gherlone – Via Olgettina, 48 – 20132 Milano (ITALIA)
[20] Prof. Gregorio Laino - Corso di Laurea in odontoiatria e Protesi Dentaria –Università degli Studi di Napoli –II Facoltà - Via Sant'Andrea delle Dame,6 -80139 Napoli (ITALIA)
[21] Prof. Lorenzo Lo Muzio – Corso Cairoli,62 -71100 Foggia (ITALIA)
[22] Prof. Antonio Carrassi – Dipartimento di Chirurgia ed Odontoiatria Milano –Via di Udinì, 8 – 20142 Milano (ITALIA)
[23] Prof. Roberto Scotti - Via Segantini, 54/2 – 10024 Moncalieri Torino (ITALIA)
[24] Prof. Giuseppe Sfondrini – Dip. Di discipline odontostomatologiche "Silvio Palazzi" – Policlinico San Matteo – P.le Golgi,2 -27100 Pavia (ITALIA)
[25] Prof. Antonio Pittau – Dipartimento Scienze Stomatologiche Università degli studi di Cagliari-via San Giorgio, 12 - 09124 Cagliari (ITALIA)
[26] Prof. Cordasco Giancarlo via Centone, 211 – 98100 Messina (ITALIA)
[27] Prof. Coltella Giuseppe Dipartimento di Discipline Odontostomatologiche, Ortodontiche e Chirurgiche Via S. Andrea delle Dame, 6 – 80138 Napoli (ITALIA).

In: Clinical Dentistry
Editor: Scardina Giuseppe Alessandro

ISBN: 978-1-61122-354-5
© 2011 Nova Science Publishers, Inc.

Chapter 16

ORAL CAVITY OVERINFECTION DURING NON SURGICAL CANCER THERAPIES: REVIEW OF THE LITERATURE[#]

***Daniela Alterio**[*1], **Barbara A. Jereczek-Fossa**[1,3], **Gaia Piperno** [1], **Antonio Laudati**[1], **Anna Maria Ferrari**[1] **Gioacchino Giugliano**[2] and **Roberto Orecchia**[1,3]*

[1]Division of Radiotherapy
[2]Division of Head and Neck Surgery of European Institute of Oncology
[3]University of Milan, Milan Italy

ABSTRACT

Introduction. Oral mucositis represents one of the most frequent acute side effects during cancer therapies (chemotherapy and/or radiotherapy). It has been hypothesized that microbial (bacteria, fungi) overinfection of oral mucosa may enhance intensity and duration of mucositis. For this reason, a lot of studies have been performed in order to evaluate the efficacy of oral cavity bacterial decontamination and/or prevention and treatment of oral candidiasis.

Patients and methods. A comprehensive search of MEDLINE up to December 2007 (with no language restriction) was performed. "Mucositis", "Chemotherapy" and "Radiotherapy" were the key words used.

Results. Sixty clinical studies matched the key words listed above. Most papers were focused on oral cavity bacterial decontamination and prevention and/or treatment of oral

---

[#] A version of this book was also published as a chapter in *International Journal of Clinical Dentistry, Volume 1, Issue 3*, published by Nova Science Publishers, Inc. It was submitted for appropriate modifications in an effort to encourage wider dissemination of research.

[*] Author to whom correspondence should be sent: Alterio Daniela MD, Division of Radiation Oncology, European Institute of Oncology, Via Ripamonti 435. 20141 Milan. Italy. e-mail: daniela.alterio@ieo.it. Tel. +39.02.57489037. Fax.+39.02.94379227

candidiasis. Recent international guidelines and critical reviews of literature were also considered.

Conclusion. Available literature data do not support the use of preventive bacterial decontamination of oral cavity by antimicrobial agents. On the contrary, some evidences exist that prophylaxis of oral candidiasis with antimicotic agents (like fluconazole) could to be efficacious to reduce the impact of oral mucositis but further larger randomized trials are needed.

INTRODUCTION

Oral cavity mucositis represents one of the most frequent acute side effect during non surgical cancer therapies and represents one of the main dose-limiting toxicity in these patients. Intensity of oral mucositis may be related to different factors: patients-related factors (age, concomitant disease), technical characteristics of radiotherapy (extention of radiation fields, total dose, dose fractionaction, treatment plan dosimetry), toxicity profile and schedule of agents used for chemotherapy.

Damage of oral mucosa during cancer treatments leads to pathologic colonisation of bacteria, fungi and viruses. In addition, the reduction of saliva production, which contains immunoglobulins (IgA) and washes away intraoral debris and bacteria, may modify the normal bacterial flora lying in upper aerodigestive tract. These events were described by Sonis (Sonis 1998, Sonis 2007) who highlighted that damaged mucosa could be colonised by aerobic Gram-negative bacteria during last phases of inflammation process. The subsequent release of endotoxins and the stimulation of cytokine release leads to further amplification of mucositis. Based on these observations, clinical studies have been advocated aimed to evaluate if reduction of oral aerobic Gram-negative colonies may reduce intensity and duration of oral mucositis (Epstein 1990, Donnelly 2003, Martin 1992, Brown 1989).

Oral candidiasis also represents a frequent event during cytotoxic therapies: prevention and treatment of this condition have been evaluated by different authors.

The aim of our study was to performed an updated review of the literature on oral cavity overinfection during non surgical cancer therapies. Prevention and treatment strategies for bacterial, fungi and viruses infections were analysed. A comprehensive review of the other diagnostic and therapeutic aspects of treatment-induced oral mucositis in cancer patients has been published elsewhere (Alterio 2007).

METHODS

A comprehensive search of MEDLINE up to December 2007 (with no language restriction) was performed using "Mucositis", "Radiotherapy" and "Chemotherapy" as main key words. Review of oral mucositis pathobiology and recent international guidelines for prevention and treatment of oral mucositis were evaluated. Both phase III randomized and not randomized trial were considered.

Table 1. Modified and updated from Alterio 2007.

Agent	Treat.	Therapy (T) Prophylaxis (P)	Favourable		Not Favourable		Study design
			Author	N.of pts	Author	N.of pts	
Antibiotic agents	RT	P	Symonds 1996	275	Stokman 2003	65	R
			Okuno	54	Wijers	77	
			Matthews	59	El Sayed 2002	137	
		P	Spijkervet 1990	15			NR
			El Sayed 2002	17			
			Oguki	52			
	HDCT	P			Ferra	37	NR
					Yuen	70	R
Chlorhexidine	CT	T			Dodd 2003	23	R
		P	Cheng 2004	34	Dodd 1996	222	R
					Pitten	47	
					Wahlin	28	
		P	Luglie	66			NR
			Cheng 2001	42			
			Cheng 2003	40			
	RT	P	Ferretti 1990	30			R
			Cheng 2006	14			
			Spijkervert 1990	45			NR
					Spijkervet 1989	30	R
					Foote	52	
					Samaranayake		
	HDCT	P	McGaw	16	Epstein 1992	86	R
			Ferretti 1988	51	Weisdorf	100	
			Ferretti 1987	40	Raether	47	
			Ratkaukas				
Iseganan	RT	P			Trotti	545	R
	CT	P			Giles	323	R
Nystatin	CT	P			Barret	33	NR
	RT	T	Rotwell				NR

Table 1. (Continued)

Agent	Treat.	Therapy (T) Prophylaxis (P)	Favourable		Not Favourable		Study design
			Author	N.of pts	Author	N.of pts	
	HDCT				Epstein 1992	86	R
	RT/CT	PT	Hasenau				NR
Amphotericin B	CT	T			Lefebvre	123	R
					Hejna	31	
	RT	P	Spijkervert 1991	15			NR
Miconazole	CT	P	Brinker	30			R
		T	Jordan	37			NR
	RT	T	Oguchi	25			NR
Clotrimazole	CT	P	Yeo	202			R
		T	Shechtman	13			R
	RT	P	Yeo	202	El-Sayed2002	137	R
		P	Matthews	59			NR
		T	Yap	52			R
			Schechtman	13			
	RT/CT	P	Yeo	202			R
		T	Yap	52			R
			Shechtman	13			
Itraconazole	RT	P	Belazi	39			NR
Fluconazole	CT	T	Epstein 2002	19			NR
		PT	Allison	40			NR
		T	Finlay	73			
			Lefebvre	123			R
	RT	P	Mucke	50			NR
			Belazi	39			
			Nicolatou-G	63			R
		T	Epstein	19			NR
		PT	Allison	40			NR
		T	Lefebvre	123			R

Table 1. (Continued)

Agent	Treat.	Therapy (T) Prophylaxis (P)	Favourable		Not Favourable		Study design
			Author	N.of pts	Author	N.of pts	
	HDCT	T	Epstein	19			NR
		P	Gava	80			R
			Koc	80			
	RT/CT	P	Samonis				R
			Bodey	112			
Antiviral agents	CT	T	Kubesova	34			NR
	RT	P			Bubley	57	R
	HDCT	P	Epstein 1996	83			NR

Legend: Treat.= treatment; n.of pts= number of patients; RT= radiotherapy; CT= chemotherapy; HDCT= high dose chemotherapy; RT/CT= concomitant radiochemotherapy; R= randomized trials; NR = not randomized trial.

RESULTS

In Table 1 all analysed studies were summarized. This table represents a revised and updated table of an already published paper on oral mucositis (Alterio 2007). All studies were divided according to cancer therapy (radiotherapy, chemotherapy, chemoradiotherapy, high dose chemotherapy), purpose of the study (prevention or treatment of mucositis) and the study design (phase III randomized or not randomized trial). The number of enrolled patients was also specified for most studies.

Guidelines of Multinational Association of Supportive Care in Cancer (MASCC)/International Society of Oral Oncology (ISOO) for prevention and treatment of oral mucositis were considered (Barash 2006). Recent reviews and meta-analyses were also evalutated (Stokman 2006, Keefe 2007)

Basic Oral Care

Oral cavity hygiene has been shown to be of great importance in preventing oral mucositis during anticancer treatments. A lot of studies demonstrated that poor oral care with concomitant dental and periodontal pathology (such as dental caries, periodontal and pulpal disease, third molar pathology, defective dental restoration, dental absesses, ill-fitting prosthesis, orthodontic appliances and other potential sources of mucosal or gingival irritation) may lead to a greater risk for oral or systemic complications (Karthaus 1999, Raber-Durlacher 1999, Shih 2002, Greenberg 1982, Symonds 1998). Careful inspection of the oral cavity allows for the differentiation of oral mucositis from preexisting changes (pemphigoid, lichen planus, leukoplakia). Meticoulous pretreatment assessment with periodontal, dental and radiographic evaluation and, when necessary, restorative dental procedures performed at least three weeks before the beginning of mucosatoxic therapy have all been shown to reduce incidence and duration of mucositis (Borowski 1994, Sonis 1990, Shieh 1997). During mucosatoxic therapy, patients should avoid to wear removable prostheses (except while eating), to eat meals which may cause irritation (hot, spicy and coarse foods), fruits and beverages with high acid content and alcohol while a soft bland diet is advised. In addition, patients should perform frequent and effective mechanical plaque removal, using a soft toothbrush and dental floss or foam brushes and rinsing solution in order to avoid microtruama. To maintain oral moistness and to decrease cariogenic flora, patients should rinse with 0,9% saline or bicarbonate solution at least 10-12 time a day, use lip lubricants and employ sugarfree products (Jansma 1992, Dose 1995, Shubert 1999, Feber 1995). Patients should refrain from smoking because duration of mucositis has been demonstrated to be longer in patients who smoke compared with patients who do not (Rugg 1990, Dodd 1999).

A standardized protocol of oral care is not yet been validated. Different protocols of oral hygiene have been studied but no consensus has been obtained since today (Jasma 1992, Borowski 1994, Shiesh 1997, Ezzone 1993, Armstrong 1994, Hatton-Smith 1994, Borowski 1994). Daily review of symptoms by a radiation therapy nurse, combined with a well–defined strategy for mouth care and analgesics administration resulted in improved management of radiation-related mucositis compared with sporadic nursing intervention and absence of analgesic protocol (Janjan 1992). The use of oral assessment guide ensures that all patients receive the same high–quality care (Feber 1995).

A survey of prevention and treatment regimens for oral sequelae resulting from head and neck radiotherapy used in Dutch radiotherapy Institutes showed a great diversity in the preventive approach of head and neck cancer patients. The most comprehensive counselling was performed by those centers in which a dental team was active, particularly when an oral hygienist was a member of such a team (Jansma 1992). In 1995 Federation of the French Cancer Center (FNCLCC) decided to formulate the "Standard, Option and Recommendation (SOR) for good practices in dentistry for head and neck cancer patients". Risk factors for treatment-related late effects, safety and quality of life, efficacy of dental preventive measures and treatments were main and points considered (Maire 1999).

Xerostomia should also be avoided during and after cancer therapies. Xerostomia may be ameliorated by treatment of hunderlying preexisting autoimmune disease, avoiding drugs that decrease salivary flow and by mechanical cleaning of the dorsum of the tongue. In addition, stimulation of salivary flow may be achieved by the use of nonirritanting, cinnamon-free, mint-free and sugar-free drops or shewing gum, alkaline or saline solutions, by low dose of pilocarpine or using substitutes containing methylcellulose or mucopoly-saccharides (Wolfgang 2001).

In spite of these accordance, some studies did not found any differences in incidence, severity and time to onset of mucositis between patients with presence of dental appliances, history of oral lesions, history of smoking and practice of dental hygiene and care and patients without these characteristics (Dodd 1999, Peters 1993).

In conclusion, most literature data showed a reduction in mucositis incidence and duration when accurate pre-treatment assessment of oral cavity hygiene was performed and when a frequent review of symptoms combined with a well-defined protocol for palliative treatment was applied to all treated patients.

Antibiotic Agents

First clinical studies showed that elimination of Gram-negative bacilli resulted in a lower incidence of oral mucositis therefore selective decontamination of oral cavity has been emphasised by many authors (Matthews 1996, Spijkervert 1990, Symonds 1996). Five clinical randomised trials were performed in order to test a mixed antibiotic-antimycotic lozenge (polimixine E, tobracyn, amphotericin B) called APT lozenge (Symonds 1996, Spijkervert 1991, Okuno 1997). Three of these trials found a reduction of oral mucositis (Symonds 1996, Spijkervert 1991, Okuno 1997) whereas two trials failed to show any clinical benefit (Stokman 2005, Wijers 2001).

Because of high estimated cost of APT lozenge, El-Sayed at al. performed a pilot study followed by a randomised trial in order to evaluate a less costly lozenge containing bacitracin, clotrimazole and gentamicine (BCoG lozenge). Results showed that BCoG lozenge was safe, tolerable and microbiologically effective (El Sayed 2002) but randomised trial failed to obtain a statistically significant clinical impact on severity of oral mucositis (El Sayed 2002) and quality of life between patients treated with BCoG lozenge and control group (Duncan 2005).

Ferra et al evaluated efficacy in reducing oral mucositis of ciprofloxacine, associated with pentoxifilline and steroids. Unfortunately, none relevant result was obtained (Ferra 1997).

Only one study showed that systemic administration of clarithromycin was found to reduce oral mucositis in patients submitted to bone marrow transplant (Yuen 2001).

Based on literature data, MASCC/ISOO guidelines recommend against use of antibiotic lozenges for the prevention of radiation-induced oral mucositis (Barash 2006, Keefe 2007). In a recent meta-analyses, Stockman et al found that PTA resulted to have a significant preventive effect on the development of ulceration with an OR of 0.61 (CI 0.39 – 0.96) with no effect on the prevention of mucositis in patients treated with radiotherapy.

In conclusion, these controversial results suggests that bacterial infections are probably not primarily involved in the pathogenesis of oral mucositis but could make worse the course of a pre-existent oral inflammation. Up to now no clear evidence exists that antibiotic prophylaxis may reduce oral mucositis during cancer treatments.

Only patients therefore suspected to carry a well-known high pathogenic flora due to underlying oral pathology could probably benefit from prophylactic use of antibacterial agents but well designed clinical trial are required to confirm this hypothesis.

In presence of a clinical diagnosis of bacterial oral cavity over infection an antibiotic regimen must be administrated; an aminopenicillin with a beta-lactamase inhibitor or a penicillin in combination with metronidazole should be preferred for outpatients treatments (Epstein 2007).

a) Iseganan

Iseganan is a synthetic protegrin (IB-367), analog to Protegrin-1 a naturally occurring peptide with broad-spectrum microbicidal activity. Iseganan is a well-tolerated agent probably because of lack of systemic absorption when topical oral administration was performed. In spite of preliminary promising results on hamster, two phase III randomised clinical trials did not show an impact of this agent on mucositis (Giles 2003, Trotti 2004).

b) Clorhexidine

Chlorhexidine is a broad-spectrum antiseptic agent (gram-positive and gram-negative bacilli and yeast). Chlorhexidine mouthwashes were found to be efficacious in reducing oral mucositis in several clinical trials (Symonds 1996, McGaw 1985, Ferretti 1987, Ferretti 1988, Ratkauskas 1993, Luglie 2002, Cheng 2001) but these results were in contrast with other studies in which a clinically demonstrable additional therapeutic advantage was not obtained (Dodd 1996, Spijkervert 1989, Weisdorf 1989, Raether 1989, Worthington 2004, Wahlin 1989, Foote 1994, Pitten 2003). Chlorhexidine was also studied in combination with nystatin but, because of a low solubility of the chlorhexidine-nystatin complex, a not soluble salt was formed. This combined drugs complex was therefore not useful in clinical practice (Barkvoll 1989).

Chlorhexidine efficacy was also compared with different agents like salt and soda, a mixed mouthwash (lidocaine, benadryll and maalox) (Dodd 2003), benzydamine (Samaranayake 1988, Cheng 2003, Cheng 2004), nystatine and salin solution (Epstein 1992) and a mixed antibiotic lozenge (Polymyxin E, tobramycin and amphotericin B) (Spijkervert 1991). Results of these clinical trials were controversial.

Based on literature data also MASCC/ISOO continued to recommend against the use of chlorhexidine for treatment of chemotherapy induced oral mucositis (Barash 2006).

Antifungal Agents

Between the opportunistic fungi, candida albicans represents the commonest species found in oral cavity but also other species may be found. Martin et al pointed out that all yeast isolated during radiation therapy were found to be sensitive to miconazole, ketoconazole, amphotericin B and nystatin (Marin 1981).

Clinical importance of Candida prophylaxis was evaluated in a meta-analysis published in 1994 in which a strong beneficial effect of antifungal prophylaxis in reducing incidence of oropharyngeal candidiasis was found (Meunier 1994).

a) Polyene Antifungal Agents

Nystatin, when administrated as a single agent or in association with other products, was not found to be efficacious in preventing oral mucositis in most clincal trials (Epstein 1992, Poland 1989, Barrett 1984). Only mixed solutions composed with nystatin associated with H2O2, povidone iodine, and dexpanthenol (Hasenau 1988) or hydrocortisone, tetracycline and diphenhydramine solution (Rothwell 1990) were found to obtain clinical benefit in reducing oral mucositis. *Amphotericin B* was found to be less efficacious compared with fluconazole (Lefebvre 2002) and GM-CSF topical application (Hejna 2001) while tolerance was found to be worst compared with nystatin (Epstein 2004). Only when combined with polymyxin and tobramycin, amphotericin B seems to be efficacious in reduction of oral mucositis (Spijkervert 1991).

b) Imidazole Antibiotics and Triazolic Antimycotic Agents

Many not randomised and randomised trials provided that prophylactic and therapeutic systemic and topical application of imidazole antibiotics like *miconazole* (Brincker 1978, Oguki 1998, Jordan 1979), *clotrimazole* (Yeo 1985, Yap 1979, Aviles 1987, Shechtman 1984, Spijkervert 1990) and *ketoconazole (*Poland 1989, Moody 1980), and triazolic antimycotic agents like *fluconazole* (Mucke 1997, Mucke 1998, Epstein 2002, Gava 1996, Koc 2003, Samonis 1990, Bodey 1990, Belazi 2004, Redding 1999, Nicolatou-Galitis O 2005,) and *itraconazole* (Belazi 2004) significantly reduces incidence and duration of oropharyngeal candidiasis and oral mucositis. Compared to amphotericin B, fluconazole was found to be more efficacious in reducing oral mucositis (Finlay 1996, Lefebvre 2002). Association of fluconazole with Sucralfate had been also demonstrated to be efficacious both in preventing and in treating cancer treatment-related mucositis (Allison 1995). In contrast to these studies, in a double-blind phase III randomised controlled study, a lozenge containing bacitracin, clotrimazole and gentamycin was not found to significantly impact on severity of mucositis (El Sayed 2002). A recent review published by Clarkson JE et al showed that only ketoconzole and clotrimazole were found to be effective for eradication of oral candidias (Clarkson 2002).

In conclusion, literature data seems to suggest that prevention of oral candidiasis may reduce the impact of oral mucositis but further randomized trial are needed.

Antiviral Agents

Oral cavity virus overinfection represents a rare event during non surgical cancer therapies except for patients submitted to high dose chemotherapy and bone marrow transplant (BMT) (Montgomery 1986, Woo 1990). The presence of a virus overinfection seems to be a negative prognostic factor in particular for patients submitted to BMT (Gomez 2001). For this reason some authors advocated a prophylaxis regimen in these high risk group of patients (Redding 1990). Herpes simplex virus type I (HSVI), varicella zoster virus and less frequently cytomegalovisur may make worse a pre-existent oral mucositis but literature data are not conclusive.

In case of a clinically diagnosed virus overinfection, treatment was mainly performed by acyclovir and valacyclovir (Bubley 1989, Wpstein 1996, Eisen 2003, Kubesova 1998, Spijkervert 1990, Woo 1990).

Conclusion

Literature data are not sufficient to justify prophylaxis of oral cavity bacterial overinfection in clinical practice during non surgical cancer therapies. On the contrary prevention of oral candidiasis seems to be effective in reducing oral mucositis but further studies are required. Prophylaxis of viruses infection seems to have a role mainly in patients submitted to high dose chemotherapy and bone marrow transplant but not conclusive data are available.

References

Allison RR, Vongtama V, Vaughan J, et al: Symptomatic acute mucositis can be minimized or prophylaxed by the combination of sucralfate and fluconazole. *Cancer Invest.* 1995;13(1):16-22.

Alterio D, Jereczek-Fossa BA, Fiore MR et al: Cancer treatment-induced oral mucositis *Anticancer Res.* 2007 Mar-Apr;27(2):1105-25.

Armstrong TS: Stomatitis in the bone marrow transplant patient. An overview and proposed oral care protocol. *Cancer Nurs*. 1994 Oct;17(5):403-10.

Aviles A: Clotrimazole treatment for prevention of oral candidiasis in patients with acute leukemia undergoing chemotherapy. *Am. J. Med.* 1987 Apr;82(4):867-8.

Barasch A, Elad S, Altman A et al: Antimicrobials, mucosal coating agents, anesthetics, analgesics, and nutritional supplements for alimentary tract mucositis. *Supp. Care Cancer* 2006 14:528-532.

Barkvoll P, Attramadal A: Effect of nystatin and chlorhexidine digluconate on Candida albicans. *Oral Surg. Oral Med. Oral Pathol.* 1989 Mar;67(3):279-81.

Barrett AP: Evaluation of nystatin in prevention and elimination of oropharyngeal Candida in immunosuppressed patients. *Oral Surg. Oral Med. Oral Pathol.* 1984 Aug;58(2):148-51.

Belazi M, Velegraki A, Koussidou-Eremondi T, et al: Oral Candida isolates in patients undergoing radiotherapy for head and neck cancer: prevalence, azole susceptibility profiles and response to antifungal treatment. *Oral Microbiol. Immunol.* 2004 Dec;19(6):347-51.

Bodey GP, Samonis G, Rolston K: Prophylaxis of candidiasis in cancer patients: *Semin Oncol.* 1990 Jun;17(3 Suppl 6):24-8.

Borowski B, Benhamou E, Pico JL, et al: Prevention of oral mucositis in patients treated with high-dose chemotherapy and bone marrow transplantation: a randomised controlled trial comparing two protocols of dental care. *Eur. J. Cancer B Oral Oncol.* 1994;30B(2):93-7.

Brincker H: Prophylactic treatment with miconazole in patients highly predisposed to fungal infection. A placebo-controlled double-blind study. *Acta Med. Scand.* 1978;204(1-2):123-8.

Brown AT, Sims RE, Raybould TP, et al: Oral gram-negative bacilli in bone marrow transplant patients given chlorhexidine rinses. *J. Dent Res.* 1989 Jul;68(7):1199-204.

Bubley GJ, Chapman B, Chapman SK, et al: Effect of acyclovir on radiation- and chemotherapy-induced muouth lesion. *Antimicrob Agents Chemother.* 1989 Jun; 33 (6): 862-65.

Cheng KK, Yuen Ka Tsui J: A pilot study of Chlorhexidine and Benzydamine oral rinses for the prevention and treatment of irradiation mucositis in patients with head and neck cancer. *Cancer Nursing* 2006 29(5): 423-430.

Cheng KK, Chang AM, Yuen MP: Prevention of oral mucositis in paediatric patients treated with chemotherapy; a randomised crossover trial comparing two protocols of oral care. *Eur. J. Cancer.* 2004 May;40(8):1208-16.

Cheng KK, Chang AM: Palliation of oral mucositis symptoms in pediatric patients treated with cancer chemotherapy. *Cancer Nurs.* 2003 Dec;26(6):476-84.

Cheng KK, Molassiotis A, Chang AM, et al: Evaluation of an oral care protocol intervention in the prevention of chemotherapy-induced oral mucositis in paediatric cancer patients. *Eur. J. Cancer.* 2001 Nov;37(16):2056-63.

Clarkson JE, Worthington HV, Eden OB: Interventions for treating oral candidiasis for patients with cancer receiving treatment. *Cochrane Database Syst. Rev.* 2002;(1):CD001972.

Dodd MJ, Larson PJ, Dibble SL, et al: Randomized clinical trial of chlorhexidine versus placebo for prevention of oral mucositis in patients receiving chemotherapy. *Oncol. Nurs. Forum.* 1996 Jul;23(6):921-7.

Dodd MJ, Miaskowski C, Greenspan D, et al: Radiation-induced mucositis: a randomized clinical trial of micronized sucralfate versus salt and soda mouthwashes. *Cancer Invest.* 2003;21(1):21-33.

Dodd MJ, Miaskowski C, Shiba GH, et al: Risk factors for chemotherapy-induced oral mucositis: dental appliances, oral hygiene, previous oral lesions, and history of smoking. *Cancer Invest.* 1999;17(4):278-84.

Donnelly JP, Bellm LA, Epstein JB, et al: Antimicrobial therapy to prevent or treat oral mucositis *Lancet Infect. Dis.* 2003 Jul;3(7):405-12.

Dose AM: The symptom experience of mucositis, stomatitis, and xerostomia. *Semin. Oncol. Nurs.* 1995 Nov;11(4):248-55.

Eisen D, Essell J, Broun ER, Sigmund D, et al:. Clinical utility of oral valacyclovir compared with oral acyclovir for the prevention of herpes simplex virus mucositis following autologous bone marrow transplantation or stem cell rescue therapy. *Bone Marrow Transplant.* 2003 Jan;31(1):51-5.

El-Sayed S, Epstein J, Minish E, et al: A pilot study evaluating the safety and microbiologic efficacy of an economically viable antimicrobial lozenge in patients with head and neck cancer receiving radiation therapy. *Head Neck*. 2002 Jan;24(1):6-15.

El-Sayed S, Nabid A, Shelley W, et al: Prophylaxis of radiation-associated mucositis in conventionally treated patients with head and neck cancer: a double-blind, phase III, randomized, controlled trial evaluating the clinical efficacy of an antimicrobial lozenge using a validated mucositis scoring system. J Clin Oncol. 2002 Oct 1;20(19):3956-63.

Epstein JB: Infection prevention in bone marrow transplantation and radiation patients. *NCI Monogr*. 1990;(9):73-85.

Epstein JB, Gorsky M, Caldwell J: Fluconazole mouthrinses for oral candidiasis in postirradiation, transplant, and other patients. *Oral Surg. Oral Med. Oral Pathol. Oral Radiol. Endod*. 2002 Jun;93(6):6.

Epstein JB, Vickars L, Spinelli J, et al: Efficacy of chlorhexidine and nystatin rinses in prevention of oral complications in leukemia and bone marrow transplantation. *Oral Surg. Oral Med. Oral Pathol.* 1992 Jun;73(6):682-9.

Epstein JB, Truelove EL, Hanson-Huggins K, et al: Topical polyene antifungals in hematopoietic cell transplant patients: tolerability and efficacy. *Support Care Cancer*. 2004 Jul;12(7):517-25. Epub 2004 Apr 24.

Epstein JB, Ransier A, Sherlock CH, et al: Acyclovir prophylaxis of oral herpes virus during bone marrow transplantation. *Eur. J. Cancer B Oral Oncol*. 1996 May; 32 B (3): 158-162.

Ezzone S, Jolly D, Replogle K, et al: Survey of oral hygiene regimens among bone marrow transplant centers. *Oncol. Nurs. Forum*. 1993 Oct;20(9):1375-81.

Feber T. Mouth care for patients receiving oral irradiation. *Prof. Nurse*. 1995 Jul;10(10):666-70.

Ferra C, de Sanjose S, Lastra CF, et al: Pentoxifylline, ciprofloxacin and prednisone failed to prevent transplant-related toxicities in bone marrow transplant recipients and were associated with an increased incidence of infectious complications. *Bone Marrow Transplant*. 1997 Dec;20(12):1075-80.

Ferretti GA, Ash RC, Brown AT, et al: Control of oral mucositis and candidiasis in marrow transplantation: a prospective, double-blind trial of chlorhexidine digluconate oral rinse. *Bone Marrow Transplant*. 1988 Sep;3(5):483-93.

Ferretti GA, Hansen IA, Whittenburg K, et al: Therapeutic use of chlorhexidine in bone marrow transplant patients: case studies. *Oral Surg. Oral Med. Oral Pathol.* 1987 Jun;63(6):683

Ferretti GA, Raybould TP, Brown AT, et al: Chlorhexidine prophylaxis for chemotherapy- and radiotherapy-induced stomatitis: a randomized double-blind trial. *Oral Surg. Oral. Med. Oral Pathol.* 1990 Mar;69(3):331-8.

Finlay PM, Richardson MD, Robertson AG: A comparative study of the efficacy of fluconazole and amphotericin B in the treatment of oropharyngeal candidosis in patients undergoing radiotherapy for head and neck tumours. *Br. J. Oral Maxillofac Surg.* 1996 Feb;34(1):23-5.

Foote RL, Loprinzi CL, Frank AR, et al: Randomized trial of a chlorhexidine mouthwash for alleviation of radiation-induced mucositis. *J. Clin. Oncol.* 1994 Dec;12(12):2630-3.

Gava A, Ferrarese F, Tonetto V, et al: [Can the prophylactic treatment of mycotic mucositis improve the time of performing radiotherapy in head and neck tumors?] *Radiol. Med.* (Torino). 1996 Apr;91(4):452-5.

Giles FJ, Miller CB, Hurd DD, et al : A phase III, randomized, double-blind, placebo-controlled, multinational trial of iseganan for the prevention of oral mucositis in patients receiving stomatotoxic chemotherapy (PROMPT-CT trial). *Leuk Lymphoma.* 2003 Jul;44(7):1165-72.

Gomez RS, Carneiro MA, Souza LN, et al: Oral recurrent human herpes virus infection and bone marrow transplantation survival. *Oral Surg. Oral Med. Oral Pathol. Oral Radiol. Endod.* 2001 May;91(5):552-6.

Hasenau C, Clasen BP, Roettger D: [Use of standardized oral hygiene in the prevention and therapy of mucositis in patients treated with radiochemotherapy of head and neck neoplasms] *Laryngol. Rhinol. Otol. (Stuttg).* 1988 Nov;67(11):576-9.

Hatton-Smith CK: A last bastion of ritualised practice? A review of nurses' knowledge of oral healthcare. *Prof. Nurse.* 1994 Feb;9(5):304, 306-8.

Hejna M, Kostler WJ, Raderer M, et al: Decrease of duration and symptoms in chemotherapy-induced oral mucositis by topical GM-CSF: results of a prospective randomised trial. *Eur. J. Cancer.* 2001 Nov;37(16):1994-2002.

Janjan NA, Weissman DE, Pahule A: Improved pain management with daily nursing intervention during radiation therapy for head and neck carcinoma. *Int. J. Radiat. Oncol. Biol. Phys.* 1992;23(3):647-52.

Jansma J, Vissink A, Spijkervet FK, et al: Protocol for the prevention and treatment of oral sequelae resulting from head and neck radiation therapy. *Cancer.* 1992 Oct 15;70(8):2171-80.

Jordan WM, Bodey GP, Rodriguez V, et al: Miconazole therapy for treatment of fungal infections in cancer patients. *Antimicrob Agents Chemother.* 1979 Dec;16(6):792-7.

Karthaus M, Rosenthal C, Ganser: A Prophylaxis and treatment of chemo- and radiotherapy-induced oral mucositis - are there new strategies? *Bone Marrow Transplant.* 1999 Nov;24(10):1095-108.

Keefe DM, Schubert MM, Elting LS et al: Updated clinical practice guidelines for the prevention and treatment of mucositis. *Cancer* 2007 109(5); 820-831.

Koc M, Aktas E: Prophylactic treatment of mycotic mucositis in radiotherapy of patients with head and neck cancers. *Jpn. J. Clin. Oncol.* 2003 Feb;33(2):57-60.

Kubesova H, Penka M, Kral Z, et al: Herpes simplex infection as possible etiology for febrile neutropenia and mucositis in patients treated for hematological malignancies. *Acta Med Austriaca.* 1998;25(2):57-60.

Lefebvre JL, Domenge C: Study Group of Mucositis. A comparative study of the efficacy and safety of fluconazole oral suspension and amphotericin B oral suspension in cancer patients with mucositis. *Oral Oncol.* 2002 Jun;38(4):337-42.

Luglie PF, Mura G, Mura A, et al: Prevention of periodontopathy and oral mucositis during antineoplastic chemotherapy. *Clinical study Minerva Stomatol.* 2002 Jun;51(6):231-9.

Maire F, Borowski B, Collangettes D, et al: [Standards, Options and Recommendations (SOR) for good practices in dentistry for head and neck cancer patients. Federation of the French Cancer Centres (FNCLCC)] *Bull Cancer.* 1999 Jul-Aug;86(7-8):640-65.

Martin MV, van Saene HK. The role of oral microorganisms in cancer therapy. *Curr. Opin. Dent.* 1992 Sep;2:81-4.

Martin MV, Al-Tikriti U, Bramley PA. Yeast flora of the mouth and skin during and after irradiation for oral and laryngeal cancer. J Med Microbiol. 1981 Nov;14(4):457-67.

Matthews RH, Ercal N: Prevention of mucositis in irradiated head and neck cancer patients. *J. Exp. Ther Oncol.* 1996 Mar;1(2):135-8.

McGaw WT, Belch A: Oral complications of acute leukemia: prophylactic impact of a chlorhexidine mouth rinse regimen. *Oral Surg. Oral Med. Oral Pathol.* 1985 Sep;60(3):275-80.

Meunier F, Paesmans M, Autier P: Value of antifungal prophylaxis with antinfungal drugs against oropharygeal candidiasis in cancer patients. *Eur. J. Cancer B Oral Oncol.* 1994 May; 30 B (3): 196-9.

Montgomery MT, Redding SW, LeMaistre CF: The incidence of oral herpes virus infection in patients undergoing cancer chemotherapy. *Oral Surg. Oral Med. Oral Pathol.* 1986 Mar 61 (3):238-42.

Moody MR, Young VM, Morris MJ, et al: In vitro activities of miconazole, miconazole nitrate, and ketoconazole alone and combined with rifampin against Candida spp. and Torulopsis glabrata recovered from cancer patients *Antimicrob Agents Chemother.* 1980 May;17(5):871-5.

Mucke R, Kaben U, Libera T, Knauerhase H, et al: Use of fluconazole as antimycotic prophylaxis in radiotherapy of patients with head and neck tumors] *Mycoses.* 1997;40 Suppl 1:53-5.

Mucke R, Kaben U, Libera T, et al: Fluconazole prophylaxis in patients with head and neck tumours undergoing radiation and radiochemotherapy. *Mycoses.* 1998 Nov;41(9-10):421-3.

Nicolatou-G. O, Velegraki A, Sotiropoulou-Lontou A et al: Effect of fluconazole antifungal prophylaxis on oral mucositis in head and neck cancer patients receiving radiotherapy. *Support Care Cancer* 2006 14: 44-51.

Oguchi M, Shikama N, Sasaki S, et al: Mucosa-adhesive water-soluble polymer film for treatment of acute radiation-induced oral mucositis. *Int. J. Radiat. Oncol. Biol Phys.* 1998 Mar 15;40(5):1033-7.

Okuno SH, Foote RL, Loprinzi CL et al: A randomized trial of a nonabsorbable antibiotic lozenge given to alleviate radiation-induced mucositis. *Cancer* 1997 Jun 1;79(11):2193-9.

Pitten FA, Kiefer T, Buth C, et al: Do cancer patients with chemotherapy-induced leukopenia benefit from an antiseptic chlorhexidine-based oral rinse? A double-blind, block-randomized, controlled study. *J. Hosp. Infect.* 2003 Apr;53(4):283.

Poland JM: The role of Candida infections as an adverse effect upon head and neck cancer patients undergoing therapeutic radiation and the effect of antimycotic treatment. *Mycoses.* 1989;32 Suppl 2:39-41.

Raber-Durlacher JE: Current practices for management of oral mucositis in cancer patients. *Support Care Cancer.* 1999 Mar;7(2):71-4.

Ratkauskas JS, Davis JW: Effects of chlorhexidine during immunosuppressive chemotherapy. A preliminary report. *Oral Surg. Oral Med. Oral Pathol.* 1993 Oct;76(4):441-8.

Raether D, Walker PO, Bostrum B, et al: Effectiveness of oral chlorhexidine for reducing stomatitis in a pediatric bone marrow transplant population. *Pediatr. Dent.* 1989 Mar;11(1):37-42.

Redding SW, Haveman CW: Treating the discomfort of oral ulceration resulting from cancer chemotherapy .*Compend. Contin. Educ. Dent.* 1999 Apr;20(4):389-92, 394, 396.

Redding SW: Role of herpes simplex virus reactivation in chemotherapy-induced oral mucositis. *NCI Monogr*. 1990;(9):103-5.

Rothwell BR, Spektor WS: Palliation of radiation-related mucositis. *Spec. Care Dentist*. 1990 Jan-Feb;10(1):21-5.

Rugg T, Saunders MI, Dische S: Smoking and mucosal reactions to radiotherapy. *Br. J. Radiol*. 1990 Jul;63(751):554-6.

Samaranayake LP, Robertson AG, MacFarlane TW et al: The effect of chlorhexidine and benzydamine mouthwashes on mucositis induced by therapeutic irradiation. *Clin. Radiol.* 1988 May;1939(3):291-4.

Samonis G, Rolston K, Karl C, Miller P, Bodey GP: Prophylaxis of oropharyngeal candidiasis with fluconazole. *Rev. Infect. Dis*. 1990 Mar-Apr;12 Suppl 3:S369-73.

Shechtman LB, Funaro L, Robin T, et al: Clotrimazole treatment of oral candidiasis in patients with neoplastic disease. *Am. J. Med.* 1984 Jan;76(1):91-4.

Shieh SH, Wang ST, Tsai ST, et al: Mouth care for nasopharyngeal cancer patients undergoing radiotherapy. *Oral Oncol*. 1997 Jan;33(1):36-41.

Shih A, Miaskowski C, Dodd MJ, et al: A research review of the current treatments for radiation-induced oral mucositis in patients with head and neck cancer. *Oncol. Nurs Forum*. 2002 Aug;29(7):1063-80.

Shubert MM: Oral complication. Hematopoietic cell transplantaion. 2nd ed. Malden Mass: Blackwell. *Science* Inc. 1999 pp 751-763.

Sonis ST: Pathobiology of Oral mucositis: novel insights and opportunities. Supportive *Oncologoy* 5(9)Supp 4;3-11,2007.

Sonis ST, Woods PD, White BA: Oral complications of cancer therapies. Pretreatment oral assessment. *NCI Monogr*. 1990;(9):29-32.

Sonis ST, Mucositis as a biological process: a new hypothesis for the development of chemotherapy-induced stomatotoxicity. Oral Oncol 1998 Jan;34(1):39-43.

Spijkervet FK, van Saene HK, Panders AK, et al: Effect of chlorhexidine rinsing on the oropharyngeal ecology in patients with head and neck cancer who have irradiation mucositis. *Oral Surg. Oral Med. Oral Pathol.* 1989 Feb;67(2):154-61.

Spijkervet FK, van Saene HK, van Saene JJ, et al: Mucositis prevention by selective elimination of oral flora in irradiated head and neck cancer patients. *J. Oral Pathol. Med.* 1990 Nov;19(10):486-9.

Spijkervet FK, Van Saene HK, Van Saene JJ, et al: Effect of selective elimination of the oral flora on mucositis in irradiated head and neck cancer patients. *J. Surg. Oncol*. 1991 Mar;46(3):167-73.

Stokman MA, Spijkervet FK, Burlage FR et al: Oral mucositis and selective elimination of oral flora in head and neck cancer patients receiving radiotherapy: a double-blind randomized clinical traial. *Br. J. Cancer* 2003 Apr 7;88(7):1012-6.

Stokman MA, Spijkervet FKL, Boezen HM et al: Preventive intervention possibilities in radiotherapy and chemotherapy-induced oral mucositis: results of meta-analyses. *J. Dent Res*. 85(8) 2006; 690-700.

Symonds RP: Treatment-induced mucositis: an old problem with new remedies. *Br. J. Cancer*. 1998 May;77(10):1689-95.

Symonds RP, McIlroy P, Khorrami J, et al : The reduction of radiation mucositis by selective decontamination antibiotic pastilles: a placebo-controlled double-blind trial. *Br. J. Cancer.* 1996 Jul;74(2):312-7.

Trotti A, Garden A, Warde P, et al: A multinational, randomized phase III trial of iseganan HCl oral solution for reducing the severity of oral mucositis in patients receiving radiotherapy for head-and-neck malignancy. *Int. J. Radiat Oncol. Biol. Phys.* 2004 Mar 1;58(3):674-81.

Wahlin YB. Effects of chlorhexidine mouthrinse on oral health in patients with acute leukemia. *Oral Surg. Oral Med. Oral Pathol.* 1989 Sep;68(3):279-87.

Weisdorf DJ, Bostrom B, Raether D, et al: Oropharyngeal mucositis complicating bone marrow transplantation: prognostic factors and the effect of chlorhexidine mouthrinse. *Bone Marrow Transplant.* 1989 Jan;4(1):89-95.

Wijers OB, Levendag PC, Harms ER, et al: Mucositis reduction by selective elimination of oral flora in irradiated cancers of the head and neck: a placebo-controlled double-blind randomized study. *Int. J. Radiat Oncol. Biol. Phys.* 2001 Jun 1;50(2):343-52.

Woo SB, Sonis ST, Sonis AL: The role of herpes simplex in the development of orla mucositis in bone marrow transplant recipients. *Cancer* 1990 Dec 1;66 (11): 2375-9.

Worthington HV, Clarkson JE, Eden OB: Interventions for treating oral mucositis for patients with cancer receiving treatment. *Cochrane Database Syst. Rev.*2004;(2):CD001973.

Yap BS, Bodey GP: Oropharyngeal candidiasis treated with a troche form of clotrimazole. *Arch. Intern. Med.* 1979 Jun;139(6):656-7.

Yeo E, Alvarado T, Fainstein V, et al: Prophylaxis of oropharyngeal candidiasis with clotrimazole. *J. Clin. Oncol.* 1985 Dec;3(12):1668-71.

Yuen KY, Woo PC, Tai JW et al: Effects of clarithromycin on oral mucositis in bone marrow transplant recipients. *Haematologica* 2001 May;86(5):554-5.

In: Clinical Dentistry
Editor: Scardina Giuseppe Alessandro

ISBN: 978-1-61122-354-5
© 2011 Nova Science Publishers, Inc.

Chapter 17

ANTERIOR ESTHETIC RESTORATIONS : THE IMPORTANCE OF TEAMWORK FOR A SUCCESSFUL OUTCOME[#]

***Serge Dibart*[*1] *and Andre Hashem*[2]**

[1]Department of Periodontology and Oral Biology,
Boston University School of Dental Medicine, 100 East Newton street,
Boston MA 02118

[2]Department of Restorative Sciences and Biomaterials,
Boston University School of Dental Medicine, 100 East Newton street,
Boston MA 02118

INTRODUCTION

As the saying goes, "beauty is in the eye of the beholder." Oral esthetics is part art and part science. The enhancement of a person's smile culminates in the individualization of the general rules governing dental esthetics to that person. Every patient is different, and yet a nice smile is the result of several components coming together in an orderly fashion. Knowing the general guidelines that make a smile appealing and tailoring them to the individual patient gives that smile uniqueness.

The esthetic zone has been defined as the area encompassed by the upper and lower lip. It is the harmonious relationship between the dentition (premolar to premolar), the periodontium (gingival line) and the lips that will make or break a smile [1].

[#] A version of this book was also published as a chapter in *International Journal of Clinical Dentistry, Volume 1, Issue 3*, published by Nova Science Publishers, Inc. It was submitted for appropriate modifications in an effort to encourage wider dissemination of research.

[*] Corresponding author: Serge Dibart DMD, Department of Periodontology and Oral Biology, Boston University School of Dental Medicine, 100 East Newton street, Boston MA 02118, sdibart@bu.edu, telephone: 617-638-4762, facsimile: 617-638-4765.

In 1984, Tjan and Miller [2], after observing several hundred dental and hygiene students, defined a standard of normalcy in an esthetic smile. From their findings, a pleasant smile line revealed 75 to 100% of the maxillary anterior teeth and the Interproximal gingiva only; the maxillary incisal curve is parallel with the lower lip and the gingival margins of the central incisors and canines are located horizontally at the same level, whereas the gingival margins of the Laterals are 2 mm below (Figure 1). Rufenacht [3] in 2000 and Snow [4] in 1999 added the following dental guidelines: the position of the anterior contact point progresses from incisal to cervical, the gingival zenith is distal to the long axis of the teeth for centrals and canines but coincides with it for the laterals. Finally, the suggested ideal width ratio between the anterior teeth (canine to canine) is 1.6:1.0 between central and lateral incisor and 1.0:0.6 between lateral and canine (Figure 2).

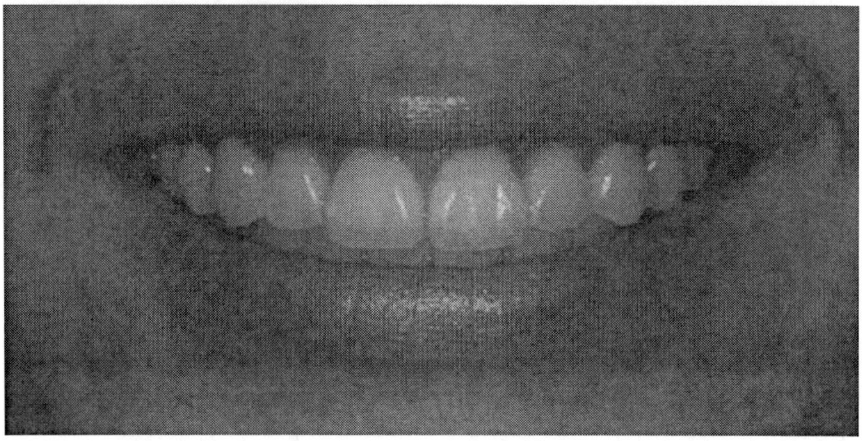

Figure 1. A pleasant smile line revealing 75 to 100% of the maxillary anterior teeth and the interproximal gingiva only; the maxillary incisal curve is parallel with the lower lip and the gingival margins of the central incisors and canines are located horizontally at the same level, whereas the gingival margins of the laterals are 2 mm below.

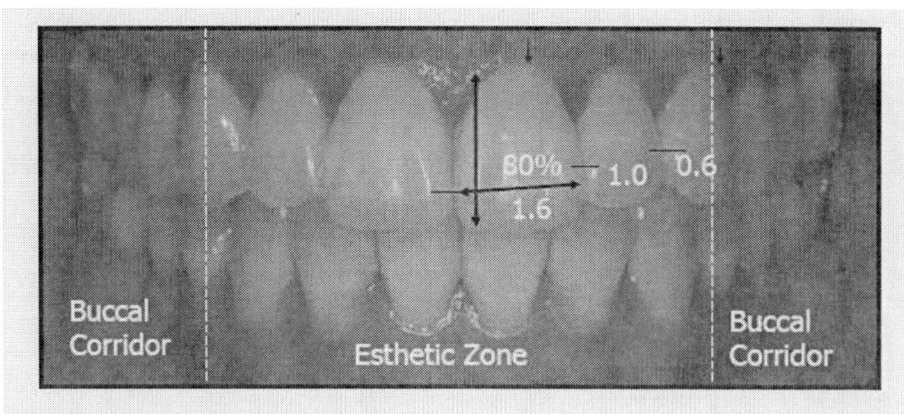

Figure 2. Intraoral picture showing the position of the anterior contact points (progressing from incisal to cervical), the gingival zenith (distal to the long axis of the teeth for centrals and canines) and the suggested ideal width ratio between the anterior teeth (canine to canine): 1.6:1.0 between central and lateral incisor and 1.0:0.6 between lateral and canine.

The Importance of Teamwork

There are 3 components when rebuilding a smile: the gingival margins, the prosthetic restorations and the patients desire. The good working relationship between the first two is critical to the successful outcome of the case. Consistent and effective communication between the periodontist and the restorative dentist is the key factor for smooth case management and treatment progression. The dental specialists need to appraise each other of the slightest changes in the treatment plan as it may affect the order of procedure scheduling. Finally the patients desire for a beautiful smile can not be underestimated; more often then not patients will come with older pictures of themselves or from a magazine and will ask the dental practitioners to duplicate them. It is the team's responsibility to inform the patient's of the feasibility of such request and guide them toward a solution that is both acceptable and pleasing.

The Surgical Phase

The most common surgical procedure used to recreate a pleasant smile, around natural teeth, is the crown lengthening procedure. This procedure can be done macrosurgically or microsurgically depending on the case, the quality of the soft tissues and the extent of the surgery.

There are two aspects to the crown lengthening procedure: esthetic and functional. In both cases the surgical procedure is aimed at re-establishing the biological width apically, while exposing more tooth structure. The biological width is defined as the sum of the junctional epithelium and supracrestal connective tissue attachment [5].

Gargiulo [6] in 1961 measured the dentogingival junction in humans. He found that the average space occupied by the sum of the junctional epithelium and the supracrestal connective tissue fibers was 2.04 mm. Violation of that space by restorations impinging on the biological width has been associated with gingival inflammation, discomfort, gingival recession, alveolar bone loss, pocket formation, etc [7,8,9].

To have a harmonious and successful long-term restoration, Ingber [10] advocated a 3 mm distance of sound supracrestal tooth structure between bone and prosthetic margins. This would allow for the reformation of the biological width plus sulcus depth. This can be achieved surgically (crown lengthening) or orthodontically (forced eruption) or a combination of both [11,12,13].

General indications for crown lengthening:

- To improve esthetics and treat a gummy smile in a patient with a high smile line.
- To rehabilitate a dentition that is compromised by the presence of extensive caries, short clinical crowns, traumatic injuries, or severe parafunctional habits.
- To restore gingival health when the biological width has been violated by a prosthetic restoration that is too close to the alveolar bone crest.

Crown lengthening can be limited to the soft tissues, when there is enough gingiva coronal to the alveolar bone allowing for surgical modification of the gingival margins without the need for osseous recontouring (i.e., pseudo pockets in cases of gingival hyperplasia). An external or internal bevel gingivectomy (gingivoplasty) is the procedure of choice for these cases. The biological width has not been compromised, and, as a result, the soft tissue pocket is eliminated and the teeth exposed without the need for osseous resection. Unfortunately, the majority of cases will involve bone re-contouring as well as gingival resection to accommodate esthetics and function. This is a more delicate procedure that will require exposing root surface, positioning gingival margins at the desired height, and apically re-establishing the biological width.

The crown lengthening procedure will enable the restorative dentist to develop an adequate zone for crown retention without extending the crown margins deep into periodontal tissues. Once the procedure is performed it is customary to wait six to eight weeks before taking the final impression. In the esthetic zone, a waiting period of at least six months is recommended before final impression [14]. This will reduce the chances of gingival recession following prosthetic crown insertion, specifically if there is a thin biotype.

Special Cases: The Microsurgical Crown Lengthening Surgery

In the areas of high esthetic demand, where papilla and soft tissue conservation is of paramount importance, the use of a microsurgical technique is recommended. There will be smaller incisions and they will not involve the papillae.

Flap reflection will be minimal, and the sutures will allow a very close adaptation of the flaps. This, in turn, will result in minimal inflammation, scarring, and patient discomfort. Because of the minimally invasive nature of the procedures and the superior wound adaptation, quick healing and enhanced esthetics are to be expected. Proficiency in periodontal microsurgery requires additional training and daily practice in order to keep and perfect these newly developed neuro-motor skills.

Case Number 1

A 42 year old female came for consultation to her restorative dentist, stating that she was unhappy with her smile. Upon analysis the clinical crowns were deemed to be too short and square, giving her a feeling of embarrassment when she smiled (figure 3). After the diagnostic wax up was completed, a surgical guide was made by the restorative dentist and given to the periodontist prior to the surgical appointment. The surgical guide delineated the proposed new location of the gingival margins, aiming to accomplish an ideal tooth proportion for each anterior tooth and a proper tooth to tooth ratio from teeth number 6 to 11. Correcting the "gummy smile" by reducing the excessive gingival display via crown lengthening surgery without compromising the proportions of the anterior teeth was also deemed to be critical.

Effective verbal communication, with the models on hand, between the restorative dentist and the periodontist at this stage is critical. This is when the restorative dentist tells the periodontist what the "final picture" will look like. It is when he or she tells the surgical operator where he/she would like the margins to be, based on the esthetic work up that has taken place earlier. The role of the periodontist is to "make it happen" by helping the restorative dentist achieve his/her goal. This will imply using the techniques and armamentarium that are best suited to the individual case, be it purely macrosurgical, microsurgical or a combination of both. At the surgical appointment after giving the patient proper local anesthesia the surgical guide was inserted on the maxilla and the new gingival margins were outlined. Again, using such a guide is critical, since it allows the surgeon to place the gingival margins in the desired position. The periodontist will use this critical tool to position the gingival margins appropriately (Figure 4). After 6 months of healing final impressions are taken and the case is sent to the dental laboratory for ceramic veneers and crowns (Figure 5).

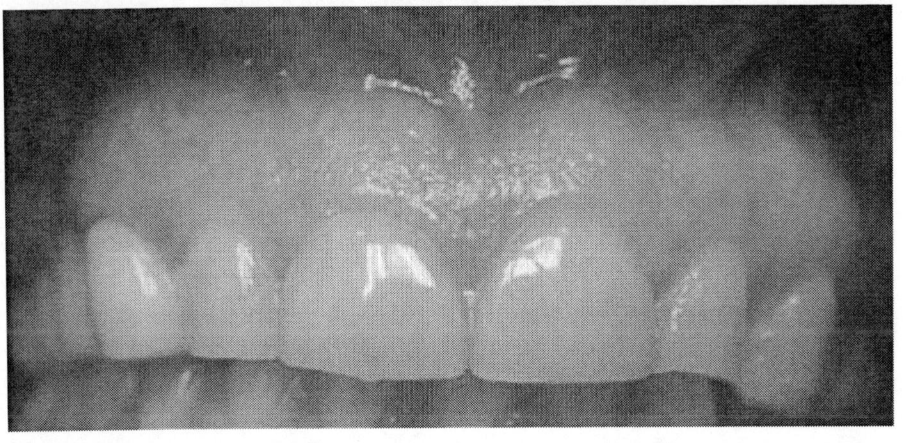

Figure 3. Intraoral photograph of case #1.

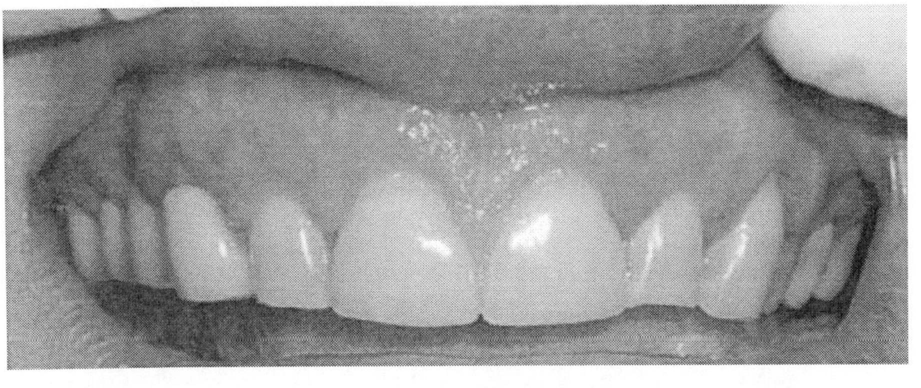

Figure 4. Intra oral photograph of case #1 after crown lengthening surgery teeth # 6-11.

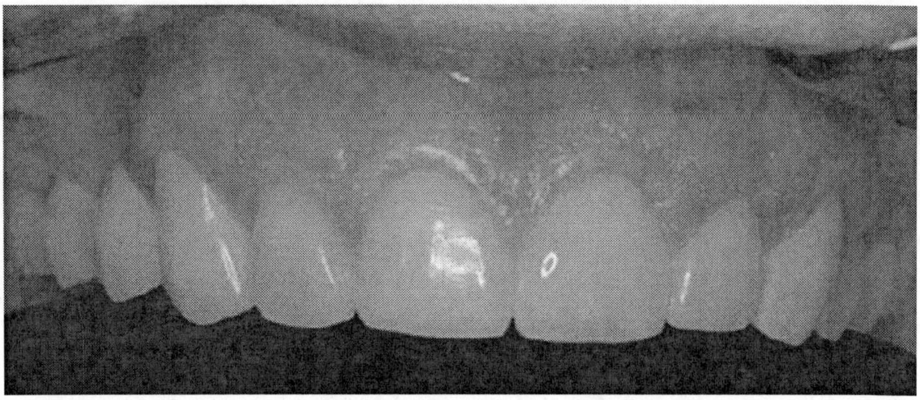

Figure 5. Intra oral photograph of case #1 after prosthetic restoration.

Case Number 2

31 year old male presenting with the complaint of uneven gingival margins affecting teeth #8 and 9 (Figure 6). The patient will be getting married in a few months and is eager to have tooth #8 restored appropriately. He emphasized the fact that he did not want to have repeated surgical procedures or a new implant fixture replacing the existing one.

The challenge in this situation is the presence of a dental implant replacing tooth # 9 next to tooth # 8 which is a natural tooth (Figure 7). A conventional surgical design aimed at lengthening crown #8 that would extend to include the papilla of # 9 could be detrimental to the final esthetic outcome.

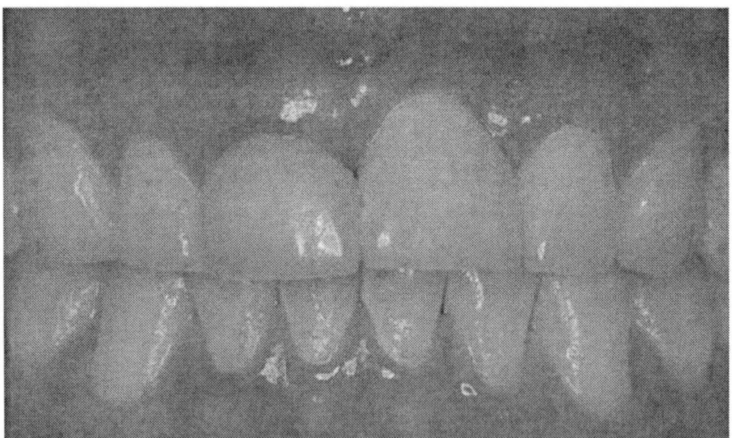

Figure 6. Intra oral photograph of case #2. Notice the uneven gingival margins (#8 and 9).

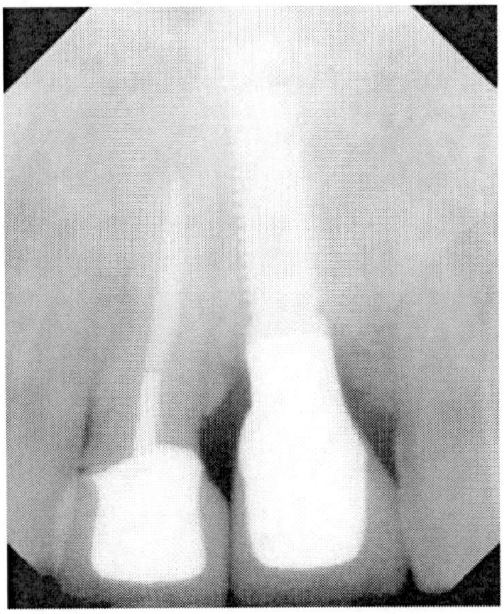

Figure 7. Periapical radiograph of teeth # 8 and 9 (dental implant)

Peri-implant tissues differ from peri-dental gingiva, and it is important to acknowledge this difference when handling peri-implant soft tissues. The mucosa that encircles the fixture presents with more collagen and fewer fibroblasts, with a 2:1 ratio, when compared to the periodontal gingival tissue [15,16].

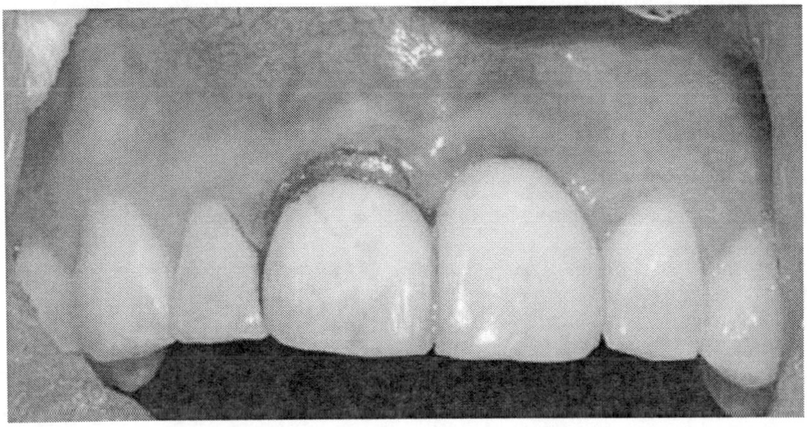

Figure 8. Flap design of the microsurgical crown lengthening procedure using a micro-blade. Notice how the incision respects the adjacent papillae.

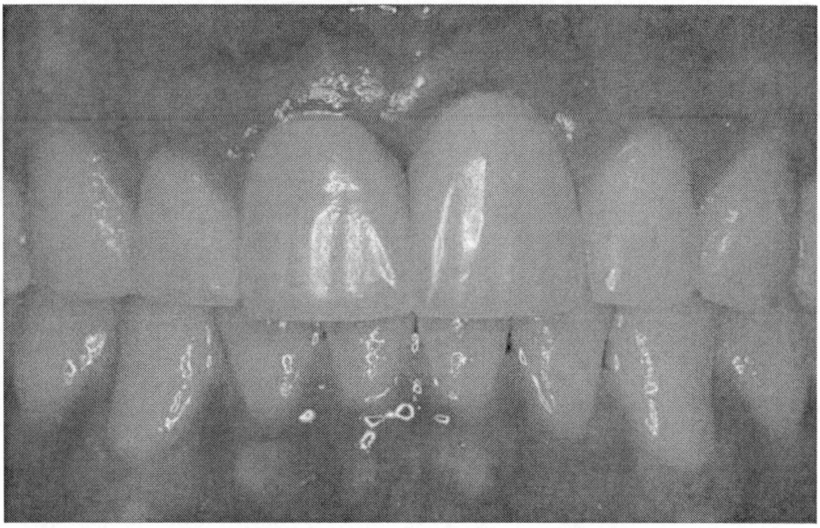

Figure 9. Intra oral photograph that shows the final restoration. Although greatly improved, the case was somewhat compromised by the patients desires for limited treatment and time constraints.

When compared to the supracrestal vessels of a natural dental element, the supracrestal vascular topography surrounding the fixture is reduced and diversely arranged [17,18].

The tissue that encompasses the fixture, with its lower cellularity and reduced vascularity, resembles cicatritial tissue, and requires special care when surgically challenged. In the basic periodontal wound healing processes, after flap elevation, one of the most dynamic tissues involved is the periodontal ligament [19]. The lack of this ligament, with its vessels and cells, must be kept in consideration by the surgeon that is approaching the peri-implant mucosa. This is one of the areas where microsurgical technique can be of interest. Because of the minute instrumentation and the minimally invasive nature of the surgery, the engendered surgical trauma is minimal, which in turns translate to negligible discomfort and maximal patient acceptance. Also the close adaptation of the flaps, due to the high quality of the suturing, will lead to rapid revascularization and faster healing [20].

Conclusion

Communication is a process that allows people to exchange information by using verbal or non verbal methods such as classical writing or emailing. Between the treating dentists and the patient, communication includes acts that confer knowledge and experiences, give advice and ask questions. Such an exchange requires feedback and it is our opinion that feed back given verbally is the most effective way of communicate in a clear and timely fashion. We are all working toward a common goal, which is restoring a patients oral health and esthetics. The success of this mission can only be achieved by the clear understanding of the treatment plan and the expectations of the patient.

REFERENCES

[1] Saadoun, A.P. and LeGall, M.G. (1998) Periodontal implications in implant treatment planning for esthetic results. *Practical Periodontics and Esthetic Dentistry.* 10(5), 655-664.

[2] Tjan, A.H., Miller, G.D., and The JG. (1984) Some esthetic factors in a smile. *The Journal of Prosthetic Dentistry* 51(1), 24-28.

[3] Rufenacht, C.R. (2000) Principles of esthetic integration. Chapter I. Quintessence: London, United Kingdom 13-36.

[4] Snow, S.R. (1999) Esthetic smile analysis of maxillary anterior tooth width: the golden percentage. *The Journal of Esthetic Dentistry* 11(4), 177-184.

[5] Cohen, D.W. (1962) Periodontal preparation of the mouth for restorative dentistry. Presented at the Walter Reed Army Medical Center, Washington, D.C. June 3, 1962.

[6] Gargiulo, A.W., Wentz, F.M., and Orban, B. (1961) Dimensions and relations of the dentogingival junction in humans. *Journal of Periodontology* 32, 261-267.

[7] Tarnow, D. et al.. (1986) Human gingival attachment responses to subgingival crown placement–marginal remodeling. *Journal of Clinical Periodontology* 13, 563-569.

[8] Parma-Benfenati, S, Fugazzotto, P.A., and Ruben, M.P. (1985) The effect of restorative margins on the post surgical development and nature of the periodontium. Part I. *The International Journal of Periodontics and Restorative Dentistry* 5(6), 30-51.

[9] Tal, H. et al.. (1989) Periodontal response to long-term abuse of the gingival attachment by supracrestal amalgam restorations. *Journal of Clinical Periodontology* 16, 654-689.

[10] Ingber, F.J.S., Rose, L.F., and Coslet, J.G. (1977) The biologic width. A concept in periodontics and restorative dentistry. *Alpha Omegan* 10, 62-65.

[11] Ingber, J.S. (1976) Forced eruption II. A method of treating non-restorable teeth-periodontal and restorative considerations. *Journal of Periodontol*ogy 47, 203-213.

[12] Pontoriero, R. et al. (1987) Rapid extrusion with fiber resection: A combined orthodontic-periodontic treatment modality. *The International Journal of Periodontics and Restorative Dentistry* 5, 30-43.

[13] De Waal, H. and Castellucci, G. (1994) The importance of restorative margin placement to the biologic width and periodontal health. Part II. *The International Journal of Periodontics and Restorative Dentistry* 14(1), 70-83.

[14] Pontoriero, R. and Carnevale, G. (2001) Surgical crown lengthening: A 12-month clinical wound healing study. *Journal of Periodontology* 72, 841-848.

[15] Berglundh, T. et al.. (1991) The soft tissue barrier at implants and teeth. *Clinical Oral Implants Research* 2(2), 81-90.

[16] Abrahamsson, I. et al.. (2002) The mucosal attachment to titanium implants with different surface characteristics: An experimental study in dogs. *Journal of Clinical Periodontology* 29(5), 448-455.

[17] Berglundh, T.et al.. (1994) The topography of the vascular systems in the periodontal and peri-implant tissues in the dog. *Journal of Clinical Periodontology* 21(3), 189-193.

[18] Moon, I.S. et al.. (1999) The barrier between the keratinized mucosa and the dental implant: An experimental study in the dog. *Journal of Clinical Periodontology* 26(10), 658-663.

[19] Goldman, H.M. and Cohen, D.W. (1980) *Periodontal Therapy*. Sixth edn. The C.V. Mosby Company: St. Louis, 670-677.

[20] Burkhardt R and Lang NP. Coverage of localized gingival recessions: comparison of micro- and macrosurgical techniques.J Clin Periodontol. 2005 Mar;32(3):287-93.

In: Clinical Dentistry
Editor: Scardina Giuseppe Alessandro

ISBN: 978-1-61122-354-5
© 2011 Nova Science Publishers, Inc.

Chapter 18

FOUR-YEAR CLINICAL EVALUATION OF A SELF-ETCH ADHESIVE IN CLASS V CARIOUS LESIONS[#]

Ali I. Abdalla[*]
Department of Restorative Dentistry
Faculty of Dentistry, University of Tanta, Tanta, Egypt

ABSTRACT

Purpose: To evaluate the clinical performance of a self-etching adhesive in Class V carious lesions with and without acid etching procedures.

Methods: A total of 183 Class V carious cavities with incisal margins in enamel and gingival margins in cementum were selected and restored with Futurabond NR self-etch adhesive and resin composite Grandio. Restorations were made using three different techniques; after etching of the enamel, after etching the whole cavity for 20 seconds and without acid etching (control). The restorations were evaluated at baseline, and every year up to 4 years using USPHS criteria.

Results: No loss of restorations was recorded after four year for all the three restorative techniques. There was no significant difference between the baseline and 4-year results for any of the tested technique. However, restorations made after acid etching showed less marginal discoloration at the enamel margins.

[#] A version of this book was also published as a chapter in *International Journal of Clinical Dentistry, Volume 1, Issue 4*, published by Nova Science Publishers, Inc. It was submitted for appropriate modifications in an effort to encourage wider dissemination of research.

[*] Correspondence: Dr. Ali I. Abdalla, Department of Restorative Dentistry, Faculty of Dentistry, University of Tanta, Tanta, Egypt. E-mail address: ali_abdalla79@yahoo.com .Tel: 00- 2-040 3336654. Fax: 00- 2-040-331800.

Clinical Significance

Futurabond NR demonstrated a good clinical effectiveness in the restoration carious cervical lesions for 4 years. Acid etching of the enamel margin or the whole cavity did not improve the overall quality of the restorations, but displayed less marginal discoloration.

Introduction

Today's adhesives are applied following either total-etch or self-etch technique.

Several clinical studies have shown that reliable and long lasting adhesive restorations can be obtained following the total-etch technique [1-6]. In contrast, scarce information is available on the clinical performance of self-etch adhesives [7-9]. When using the total-etch technique, the quality of resin-dentin adhesion can be greatly influenced by the duration of the acid etching process and the amount of surface wetness left prior to adhesive application [3,10]. By using this strategy, some problems could occur, such as the collapse of the collagen networks following the application of etching agent, the necessity of rinsing or the correct interpretation of the wet or dry bonding [8].

Self-etching primers use non-rinsed acidic monomers that simultaneously dissolve the smear layer, demineralize the dentin surface beyond the smear layer and prime dentin as well as the enamel [11] The adhesive in two-step self-etching adhesives agent is often a solvent-free component. Newer self-etching systems combine the etchant, primer and adhesive in one container [12]. As they etch, they also infiltrate the exposed collagen with hydrophilic monomers, where they copolymerize with the placed adhesive resin to the same depth in the dentin [13]. The result is the formation of a hybridized complex; a hybridized smear layer and hybrid layer which thickness is related to the aggressiveness of the self-etching agent [13]. With these systems the smear layer is a bonding substrate. Moreover, these systems are used under dry bonding conditions.

Laboratory studies evaluating self-etch materials showed different findings. Some studies [14-17] have reported that self-etch adhesives bond less effectively to enamel than total etch systems. Others, [18-20] however, have noted that both self-etch and total-etch adhesive systems perform equally well on ground enamel. Self-etch adhesives have also been reported to interact less effectively with dentin compared to total-etch ones [21-23]. In particular, with regard to bond durability, a bond produced by self-etch adhesives appears more vulnerable to degradation due to areas of increased permeability present at the hybridized adhesive dentin interface [24]. Water was suggested to be incompletely removed and resulted in regions of incomplete polymerization making the interface permeable and more degradation sensitive.

Though *in vitro* testing methodology tends to predict clinical performance, clinical trials remain necessary to ultimately evaluate the clinical efficacy of adhesives. To date two clinical trials [25, 26] are available on the influence of prior acid etching of enamel on the clinical performance of self-etch adhesives. They reported no differences in clinical performance of the tested adhesive when applied with and without prior etching of enamel.

The objective of this study was to evaluate the effect of prior acid etching of enamel only or etching enamel and dentin on the clinical performance of a self-etch adhesive in Class V carious lesions.

MATERIALS AND METHODS

Two experimental and one control groups were tested. In the experimental groups Futurabond NR[1] (Table 1) was applied on phosphoric acid etched enamel or enamel and dentin. In the control group it was applied according to the manufacture's instructions on non-etched enamel and dentin.

Fifty four subjects with age ranging between 18-44 years participated in this study. A total of 183 Class V carious lesions were restored after randomization. Only carious lesions were selected in maxillary and mandibular premolars and maxillary anterior (incisors and cuspid) teeth (Table 1).

Table 1. Composition of the adhesive system used in the study

Adhesive system	Component	Composition	Manufacturer
Futurabond NR	Liquid A	Water, ethanol, silicium dioxide	Voco, Cuxhaven Germany
	Liquid B	Acid modified methacrylate (methacrylate ester), HEMA, camphorquinone.	
Vococid		36% Phosphoric acid	

Patients were selected so that each one must had at least three class V carious lesions. Patients having only one or two lesions were not included. So the three tested adhesive techniques were placed under the same condition.

Subjects with a compromised medical history, severe or chronic periodontitis, extreme caries, and abnormal occlusion were excluded from the study. All procedures were explained to the patients and their written informed consents were obtained.

Table 2. Distribution of restorative techniques and tooth location

Adhesive techniques	Max anterior	Maxillary premolar	Mandibular premolar	Total
Enamel etching	20	18	16	54
All etch	25	20	19	64
No etch	27	23	15	65
total	72	61	50	183

[1] Voco, cuxhaven, Germany.

Restorative Procedures

Operative procedures were carried out by the author. Local anaesthesia was obtained with 2% Lidocaine solution (Mepacaine)[2]. All restorative procedures were done under rubber dam isolation using gingival retraction clamps. The teeth to be restored were first cleaned with a non-fluoridated prophylaxis paste[3] on a rubber cup and subsequently rinsed with water. A Class V cavity was prepared on the buccal surface of each tooth using a # 56 bur[4] at high speed with water coolant. An attempt was made to prepare cavities of comparable size; 3-4 mm occlusogingivally, 2-3 mm mesiodistally and 1 mm deep in dentin. Cavities that exceeded these dimension or those that were difficult to be isolated properly were excluded from the study. A 1-2 mm short bevel was placed on the enamel margin to increase surface area for bonding and to enhance aesthetics. Deep caries, if found, was removed with # 4 round bur at low speed and a thin layer of calcium hydroxide Dycal[5] was placed on the deep portion of the cavity.

The materials were used according to the manufacturers' instructions as follows: One drop of liquid A and one drop of liquid B of Futurabond NR[1] was mixed in the mixing palette for 5 seconds. The material was then applied to the whole cavity, massaged for 20 seconds, air-dried for 5 seconds and light-cured for 20 seconds using light curing unit (Heliolux DLX)[6] The output of the light curing unit was regularly checked with a curing radiometer[7] to be at least 600 mW/mm^2.

Three restorative techniques were used:

- The enamel margins were etched with 36% phosphoric acid (Vococid, Voco) for 15 seconds, rinsed with water spray for 20 seconds and dried with mild air for 3-5 seconds.
- The entire cavity was etched with phosphoric acid for 15 seconds, rinsed with water spray and air dried for 20 seconds.
- The material was applied without acid etching (control).

All cavities were restored with resin composite Grandio[1] (Voco) using an incremental technique. Each increment (thickness < 2 mm) was light cured for 40 seconds.

Finishing was accomplished using contouring diamond at high speed and polishing was done with flexible discs[8] (Sof-Lex Pop-on set) and finishing strips at low speed hand piece with water cooling.

---

[2] El Ameria Co. Alexandria, Egypt.

[3] Prophy jet, Septodont, St-Maur, France.

[4] Komet, Lemgo, Germany.

[5] Dentsply Caulk, Milford, DE, USA.

[6] Ivoclar Vivadent, Schaan, Liechtenstein.

[7] Kerr Demetron, Danbury, CT, USA.

[8] 3 M ESPE, AG, Seefeld, Germany

Evaluation Procedures

Each restoration was clinically evaluated after finishing and polishing and every year up to 4 years in accordance with the US Public Health Service (USPHS) criteria [27]. The variables evaluated were: color match, anatomic form, marginal adaptation, marginal discoloration, postoperative sensitivity and recurrent caries. Two independent examiners familiar with USPHS criteria were chosen for evaluation of the restorations. The evaluators were blinded to the adhesive technique used in any given restoration. When disagreement occurred during evaluation, consensus evaluations were obtained between evaluators. An initial agreement of at least 85% between evaluators was considered statistically significant.

Only the data on each variable evaluated at the 4-year time point was used for a statistical analysis. The analysis was based on comparing the adhesive techniques at base line and 4-year results.

The obtained data were tabulated and statistically analyzed with a McNemar Chi-square test at a level of significance of 5% ($p < 0.05$).

RESULTS

The data for color match, anatomic form, marginal adaptation and cavosurface marginal discoloration for the tested techniques are presented in Table 3a.

Table 3a. Clinical evaluation of Futurabond NR restorations after 4- year

Adhesive technique	Color match A B C	Anatomic form A B C	Marginal adaptation A B C	Marginal discoloration A B C	Retention rate (%)
Enamel etching					
Baseline (54)	54 0 0	54 0 0	54 0 0	54 0 0	100%
4-year (44)	41 3 0	40 4 0	42 2 0	41 2 1	100%
Total etching					
Baseline (64)	64 0 0	64 0 0	64 0 0	64 0 0	100%
4-year (50)	50 0 0	48 2 0	47 3 0	46 4 0	100%
No etching					
Baseline (65)	65 0 0	65 0 0	65 0 0	65 0 0	100%
4-year (53)	49 4 0	47 3 3	48 3 2	47 5 1	100%

( ) indicate the number of restorations evaluated.

Table 3b. Sites of marginal discoloration for various restorative groups

Adhesive techniques	Enamel margin only	Dentin margin only	Both enamel and dentin margins
Enamel etching	0	3/44	0
Total etching	0/50	4/50	0
No etching (control)	0/53	0/53	6/53

After 4 year, 166 restorations were available for evaluation (recall rate 91 %). No loss of restoration was recorded (retention rate 100%).

Restorations made after *enamel etching* showed three restorations with Bravo rating for colour match. For anatomic form, four restorations were rated Bravo. For marginal adaptation, two restorations were rated Bravo. These marginal defects were localised mainly at the gingival margins. For cavosurface marginal discoloration, two restorations showed minor localized area of discoloration (Bravo score) and one restoration showed extensive discoloration (Charlie). This discoloration was located at the gingival margins of the restorations.

For *the total-etch group*, all restorations showed Alfa rating regarding all color match. For anatomic form, two restorations showed bravo rating. As regarding marginal adaptation, three restorations showed Bravo rating. For marginal discoloration, four restorations showed Bravo score. These stains were mainly located at the gingival margins of the restorations.

For *control group (no etch),* four restorations showed Bravo score for colour match. For anatomic form, three restorations showed bravo score and two restorations were rated Charlie. For marginal adaptation three restorations showed Bravo score and two other restorations showed Charlie rating. For cavosurface marginal discoloration five restorations (9.4%) were rated Bravo and one restoration (1.9 %) showed Charlie score. In these restorations stains were located both at enamel and dentin margins.

Statistical analysis revealed no significant differences (P>0.05) between the 4-year and baseline evaluation for the three tested methods regarding colour match, anatomic from and marginal adaptation and marginal discolorations. Restorations made without acid etching (control) showed increase in marginal discolorations than that of base line evaluation. The sites of marginal discoloration for various restorative groups are shown in Table 3b.

None of the restorations showed secondary caries and no teeth became non vital due to the placed restorations.

Postoperative sensitivity (Table 3c): After four year, mild postoperative sensitivity was reported with two and three restorations for enamel etch and no etch groups respectively.

Table 3c. Results of postoperative sensitivity of Futurabond NR restorations after 4-years

Adhesive techniques	Postoperative sensitivity		
	A	B	C
Enamel etching			

Table 3c – Continued

Baseline (54) 4-year (44)	54 42	0 2	0 0
Total etching Baseline (64) 4-year (50)	 64 50	 0 0	 0 0
No etching Baseline (65) 4-year (53)	 65 50	 0 3	 0 0

( ) indicate the number of restorations evaluated.
A: No sensitivity.
B: Mild sensitivity.
C: Sever sensitivity.

Discussion

In the present study, the effect of acid etching on the quality of restorations made with a self-etch adhesive and resin composite was evaluated after 4 years.

This clinical trial was randomized and the examiners were blinded for the adhesive technique applied for any restoration. The rationale for this study design was that laboratory studies, [19,20,28] on bond strength reported high bond strength of self etch adhesives to enamel after acid etching compared to those produced without etching.

This study revealed that both enamel etching and total-etch procedures had no improvement in the quality of Class V resin composite restorations after 4 years compared to the baseline values. However, restorations made after enamel etching procedures showed less deterioration in regards to marginal adaptation and marginal staining. This difference in clinical performance although not significant may raise some concern about the etching capability of self-etch adhesives on enamel. In contrast, restorations made after total etching showed more deterioration at the dentin margins compared to other groups. These findings are in agreement with those from other clinical investigations. Van Meerbeek et al., [25] reported no differences in clinical performance when a mild two-step self etch was applied following either with and without enamel etching. However, they reported more marginal defects at the enamel side when enamel was not beforehand etched. In a similar study, Peumans et al., [26] showed a significant difference only in the number of small marginal defects at the enamel side in non-etch group. They also reported slightly increased in marginal discoloration in the non-etch group that was related to the higher frequency of small incisal marginal defects.

The favorable clinical effectiveness of Futurabond NR in this study may have resulted from the strong and reliable bond obtained when the material was applied to dental tissues [29]. Futurabond NR contains polyfunctional adhesive monomers (phosphoric acid modified methacrylate esters). These acid esters when mixed with water produced a pH value of 1.4.

Accordingly, the smear layer was mobilized and the hydroxyl apatite was solublized (demineralized). The resulting collagen network and the open dentin tubules are then penetrated by the hydrophilic bonding agent [26]. Chemical bonding also take place in the surface of tooth structure due to complexation of the calcium by the adhesive monomers [30]. In addition; Futurabond is a nano-filled adhesive which forms a thicker adhesive layer and a more flexible interface [31]. Again, such a flexible intermediate resin layer may help to counteract stress resulting from polymerization shrinkage of resin composite [32].

Another contributing factor to such favorable performance is that the adhesion stage is a part of etching the tooth structure. When using total-etch systems, excessive etching of the dentin could result in the deminerlized collagen layer becoming too thick, thus inhibiting the bonding agent from properly penetrating it. This results in nano-leakage and reduced adhesion [33]. In case of over drying of the dentin after etching, the collagen network may collapse, inhibiting the hybrid layer being penetrated properly. The bond strength is reduced and, therefore, the dentin bond becoming hypersensitive. Such technique sensitivity can be ruled out with Futurabond NR as etching and bonding procedures can happen together.

Restorations made without acid-etching (control) showed localized area of marginal discrepancies and stains at the enamel margins. This marginal enamel discrepancies and stains may raise a concern about the etching capability of self-etch adhesives. The etching pattern resulting from self-etch adhesive is less defined when compared to that resulting from phosphoric acid etching [34]. This shallower etching pattern and subsequent reduced micromechanical retention might reduce bond strength [35].

Restorations made after total-etch technique showed less marginal defects at the enamel margins. However, there was increased tendency toward marginal discrepancies and stains at the gingival margins. Several studies [36-39] have shown increased bond strength of self etch adhesive when applied to etched enamel. The increased in bond strength may have been attributed to the increased surface roughness and irregularities associated with acid etching. In a study on bond strength, Van Landuyt *et al* [40] failed to find any detectable resin tag formation on enamel treated only with the self-etching adhesive. In contrast, distinct infiltration of the self-etching resin into enamel tags was evident after prior acid etching.

The reported deterioration at the gingival margin seems to come from the reverse effect of etching on dentin-bond produced by self-etch adhesives. This was attributed to the incomplete infiltration of the bonding resin to the demineralized collagen [41]. As Futurabond NR-etch group was applied following the "dry bond" technique, collapse and shrinkage of collagen networks could have occurred. This may prevent efficient resin infiltration leading to porous zone at the bottom of hybrid layer.

In conclusion, enamel etching prior application of Futurabond NR had no improving effect on the qualities of composite resin restorations. However, more marginal defects at the enamel side were noticed when enamel was not etched. These defects were small and of clinical negligible relevance. Etching the whole cavity, however, resulted in more deterioration at the gingival walls of the restorations.

REFERENCES

[1] Browning WD, Brackett WW, Gilpatrick RO. Two-year clinical comparison of a microfilled and a hybrid resin-based composite in non-carious Class V lesions. *Oper. Dent.* 2000; 25: 46-50.

[2] van Dijken JW. Clinical evaluation of three adhesive systems in class V non-carious lesions. *Dent. mater.* 2000; 16: 285-291.

[3] Van Meerbeek B, De Munck J, Yoshida Y, Inoue S, Vargas M, Vijay P, Van Landuyt K, Lambrechts P, Vanherle G. Buonocore memorial lecture. Adhesion to enamel and dentin: current status and future challenges. *Oper. Dent.* 2003; 28: 215-235.

[4] Van Meerbeek B, Perdigão J, Lambrechts P, Vanherle G. The clinical performance of adhesives. *Dent. mater.* 1998; 26: 1-20.

[5] Van Meerbeek B, Peumans M, Gladys S, Braem M, Lambrechts P, Vanherle G. Three-year clinical effectiveness of four total-etch dentinal adhesive systems in cervical lesions. *Quintessence Intl.* 1996; 27: 775-784.

[6] Van Meerbeek B, Peumans M, Verschueren M, Gladys S, Braem M, Lambrechts P, Vanherle G. Clinical status of ten dentin adhesive systems. *J. Dent. Res.* 1994; 73: 1690-1702.

[7] Brackett WW, Covey DA, St Germain HA, Jr. One-year clinical performance of a self-etching adhesive in class V resin composites cured by two methods. *Oper. Dent.* 2002; 27: 218-222.

[8] Swift EJ, Jr. Dentin/enamel adhesives: review of the literature. *Pediatric Dentistry* 2002; 24: 456-461.

[9] Turkun SL. Clinical evaluation of a self-etching and a one-bottle adhesive system at two years. *Dent. mater.* 2003; 31: 527-534.

[10] Tay FR, Gwinnett AJ, Wei SH. The overwet phenomenon: a transmission electron microscopic study of surface moisture in the acid-conditioned, resin-dentin interface. *Am. J. Dent.* 1996; 9: 161-166.

[11] De Munck J, Van Meerbeek B, Yoshida Y, Inoue S, Vargas M, Suzuki K, Lambrechts P, Vanherle G. Four-year water degradation of total-etch adhesives bonded to dentin. *J. Dent. Res.* 2003; 82: 136-140.

[12] Tay FR, Pashley DH. Dental adhesives of the future. *J. Adhes Dent.* 2002; 4: 91-103.

[13] Perdigão J. Dentin bonding as a function of dentin structure. *Dent. Clinic North Am.* 2002; 46: 277-301

[14] Hara AT, Amaral CM, Pimenta LA, Sinhoreti MA. Shear bond strength of hydrophilic adhesive systems to enamel. *Am. J. Dent.* 1999; 12: 181-184.

[15] Kanemura N, Sano H, Tagami J. Tensile bond strength to and SEM evaluation of ground and intact enamel surfaces. *Dent. mater* 1999; 27: 523-530.

[16] Tay FR, Pashley DH, Suh BI, Carvalho RM, Itthagarun A. Single-step adhesives are permeable membranes. *Dent. mater.* 2002; 30: 371-382.

[17] Torii Y, Itou K, Nishitani Y, Yoshiyama M, Ishikawa K, Suzuki K. Effect of self-etching primer containing N-acryloyl aspartic acid on enamel adhesion. *Dent. mater* 2003; 19: 253-258.

[18] Hannig M, Reinhardt KJ, Bott B. Self-etching primer vs phosphoric acid: an alternative concept for composite-to-enamel bonding. *Oper. dent.* 1999; 24: 172-180.

[19] Ibarra G, Vargas MA, Armstrong SR, Cobb DS. Microtensile bond strength of self-etching adhesives to ground and unground enamel. *J. Adhes dent.* 2002; 4: 115-124.

[20] Pashley DH, Tay FR. Aggressiveness of contemporary self-etching adhesives. Part II: etching effects on unground enamel. *Dent. mater.* 2001; 17: 430-344.

[21] Inoue H, Inoue S, Uno S, Takahashi A, Koase K, Sano H. Microtensile bond strength of two single-step adhesive systems to bur-prepared dentin. *J. Adhes. Dent.* 2001; 3: 129-136.

[22] Oliveira SS, Pugach MK, Hilton JF, Watanabe LG, Marshall SJ, Marshall GW, Jr. The influence of the dentin smear layer on adhesion: a self-etching primer vs. a total-etch system. *Dent. mater.* 2003; 19: 758-767.

[23] Tay FR, Pashley DH. Aggressiveness of contemporary self-etching systems. I: Depth of penetration beyond dentin smears layers. *Dent. mater.* 2001; 17: 296-308.

[24] Tay FR, King NM, Chan KM, Pashley DH. How can nanoleakage occur in self-etching adhesive systems that demineralize and infiltrate simultaneously? *J. Adhes. Dent.* 2002; 4: 255-269.

[25] Van Meerbeek B, Kanumilli P, De Munck J, Van Landuyt K, Lambrechts P, Peumans M. A randomized controlled study evaluating the effectiveness of a two-step self-etch adhesive with and without selective phosphoric-acid etching of enamel. *Dent. mater* 2005; 21:375-383

[26] Peumans M, Munck J, Van Landuyt K, Lambrechts P, Van Meerbeek B Three-year clinical effectiveness of a two-step self-etch adhesive in cervical lesions. *Eur. J. Oral Sci*. 2005:113:512-518.

[27] Cvar JF, Ryge G. Reprint of criteria for the clinical evaluation of dental restorative materials. 1971. *Clinical Oral Investigation 2005*; 9: 215-232.

[28] Van Landuyt KL, Peumans M, De Munck J, Lambrechts P, Van Meerbeek B. Extension of a one-step self-etch adhesive into a multi-step adhesive. *Dent. mater*. 2006; 22:533-544.

[29] Abdalla AI, Garcia-Godoy F. Effect of hydrostatic pulpal water pressure on microtensile bond strength of self-etch adhesives to dentin. *In press*. *Am. J. Den*. 2008

[30] German Cecilia C, Garcia Ballesta C, Cortes Lillo O, Perez Lajarin L. Shear bond strength of a self-etching adhesive in primary and permanent dentition. *Am. J. Dent.* 2005; 18: 331-334.

[31] Can Say E, Nakajima M, Senawongse P, Soyman M, Ozer F, Ogata M, Tagami J. Microtensile bond strength of a filled vs unfilled adhesive to dentin using self-etch and total-etch technique. *Dent. mater*. 2006; 34:283-291.

[32] Perdigão J, Geraldeli S. Bonding characteristics of self-etching adhesives to intact versus prepared enamel. *J. Esth. Rest. Dent.* 2003; 15: 32-41; discussion 42.

[33] Ajlouni R, Bishara SE, Soliman MM, Oonsombat C, Laffoon JF, Warren J. The use of Ormocer as an alternative material for bonding orthodontic brackets. *Angle Ortho*. 2005; 75:106-108.

[34] Van Meerbeek B, Yoshida Y, De Munck J, Inoue S, Vargas M, Lambrechts P, Vanherle G. Correlative morphologic and clinical characterization of tooth biomaterial interaction In: Self-etching primer: current status and its evolution. *Proceedings of the international symposium '01*, Tokyo 2001; P. 41-55.

[35] Yoshida Y, Nagakane K, Fukuda R, Nakayama Y, Okazaki M, Shintani H, Inoue S, Tagawa Y, Suzuki K, De Munck J, Van Meerbeek B. Comparative study on adhesive performance of functional monomers. *J. Dent. Res.* 2004; 83: 454-458.

[36] Misra DN. Adsorption from solutions on synthetic hydroxyapatite: nonaqueous vs. aqueous solvents. *J. Biomed. Mater. Res.* 1999; 48: 848-855.

[37] Van Landuyt KL, Peumans M, De Munck J, Lambrechts P, Van Meerbeek B. Extension of a one-step self-etch adhesive into a multi-step adhesive. *Dent. mater.* 2006; 22:533-544.

[38] Frankenberger R, Tay FR. Self-etch vs etch-and-rinse adhesives: effect of thermo-mechanical fatigue loading on marginal quality of bonded resin composite restorations. *Dent. mater.* 2005; 21: 397-312.

[39] Blunck U, Roulet JF. Effect of one year water storage on the effectiveness of dentin adhesive in class V composite resin restorations. *J. Dent. Res.* 2002; 81: A-39 (Abstract 946).

[40] Van Landuyt KL, Kanumilli P, De Munck J, Peumans M, Lambrechts P, Van Meerbeek B. Bond strength of a mild self-etch adhesive with and without prior acid-etching. *Dent. mater* 2006; 34:77-85.

[41] Moll K, Park HJ, Haller B. Effect of simulated pulpal pressure on dentin bond strength of self-etching bonding systems. *Am. J. Dent.* 2005; 18: 335-339.

In: Clinical Dentistry
Editor: Scardina Giuseppe Alessandro

ISBN: 978-1-61122-354-5
© 2011 Nova Science Publishers, Inc.

Chapter 19

NUMB CHIN SYNDROME: A SYMPTOM OF MALIGNACY PROGRESSION (NUMB CHIN AND CARCINOMATOUS MENINGITIS)*

***Silvia Chiandussi*[1], *Matteo Biasotto*[1], *Giorgio Mustacchi*[2], *Giancarlo Tirelli*[3], *Michela Faraon*[1] and *Roberto Di Lenarda*[1]**

[1]School of Dental Sciences, University of Trieste
[2]Università di Trieste, Centro Oncologico ASS1 triestina, Italy
[3]Department of Otorhinolaryngology, Head and Neck Surgery, Cattinara Hospital, University of Trieste, Italy

ABSTRACT

Purpose The numb chin syndrome is a mental nerve neuropathy that origins in the absence of a mandibular lesion or a dental cause. In most occasions it can be the first symptom of a malignancy. *Methods* We present a series of four oncologic patients that were complaining of oral and facial numbness associated with neuralgia. All subjects underwent neurological and dental examinations. Computed tomography, magnetic resonance imaging and bone scan were also carried out. Neoplastic neurological involvement was suspected and the analysis of the cerebrospinal fluid was performed.

Results The neurological examination, combined with the radiological features and the cerebrospinal fluid analysis confirmed the diagnoses of numb chin syndrome associated with carcinomatous meningitis.

* A version of this book was also published as a chapter in *International Journal of Clinical Dentistry, Volume 1, Issue 4*, published by Nova Science Publishers, Inc. It was submitted for appropriate modifications in an effort to encourage wider dissemination of research.

Clinical Significance

The numb chin syndrome is an underappreciated though well documented manifestation of neurological metastases. The medical and dental professions should be able to recognise it at an early stage as a possible presenting symptom of underlying, or progressing malignancy.

Introduction

The numb chin syndrome is a rare neurological condition which is most often associated with malignancy. Patients develop oro-facial paraesthesia which is typically localized to the chin and lower lip. We present a series of four cases of carcinomatous meningitis that were diagnosed following the development of mental numbness.

Case Series

Four female oncologic patients that had been diagnosed with breast cancer were followed-up at the Dental Institute, University of Trieste. Three of them had received intravenous bisphosphonates (zoledronic acid) as treatment for their bone metastases and they regularly attended our Department as they were at risk of developing bisphosphonates associated osteonecrosis of the jaws. The fourth subject had been treated with taxolo for twelve weeks and, subsequently, with fulvestrant obtaining a good control of the progression of her disease.

Their mean age was 66.2 years. In two subjects liver metastases were evident, while in the other two cases there was lymph nodes involvement.

All patients developed oral and facial numbness with associated neuralgia involving the chin and the lower lip. In one case there was associated paralysis of the facial nerve. At the onset of the condition, in all subjects the symptoms were monolateral. In one case, as the disease was progressing, the numbness involved the controlateral mental region. Examination revealed an area of spontaneous paraesthesia in the distribution of the mental nerve and the intraoral examination showed no dental or periodontal lesions that could have been associated with the described symptoms. No bone exposure was evident as a possible clinical sign of osteonecrosis. In all patients a digital panoramic radiograph was taken (Kodac 8000C Digital Panoramic and Cephalometric System) and it allowed to exclude a dental problem or a mandibular lesion as the origin of the numbness. A computed tomography scan (CT scan) was carried out (Toshiba Aquilion 16) and it did not show the presence of mandibular metastases or osteonecrosis. Our patients were all having regular technetium-99m-methylene diphosphonate ($^{99}Tc^{m}$ –MDP) three-phase bone scans in planar and SPECT technique (Infinia-Hawkeye) to monitor the neoplastic bone involvement. In all cases the Nuclear Medicine imaging was judged negative for the presence of mandibular bone lesions as it did not show abnormal localized metabolic activity.

The symptoms and the clinical examination arouse the suspicion of neoplastic neurological involvement. In all subjects, the gadolinium-enhanced magnetic resonance imaging (Philips Gyroscan Intera) showed thickening of meninges, which was not evident at the computed tomography (Figures 1 and 2). The magnetic resonance imaging (MRI) of the brain was normal.

For three subjects a neurological examination was carried out. The cerebrospinal fluid (CSF) analysis was performed and it revealed the presence of carcinomatous cells in two patients, while in the third one it showed evident increase in proteins level and decrease in glucose concentration. The neurological examination, combined with the radiological features and the CSF analysis confirmed the diagnoses of carcinomatous meningitis.

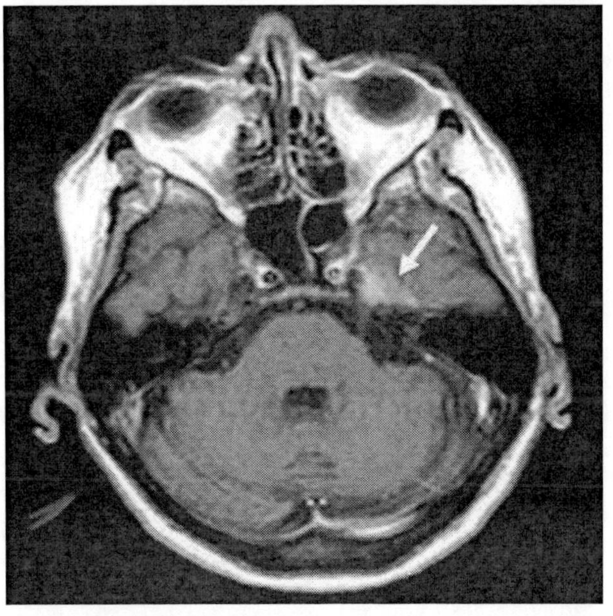

Figure 1. MRI of a patient with NCS showing a meningeal involvement (white arrow).

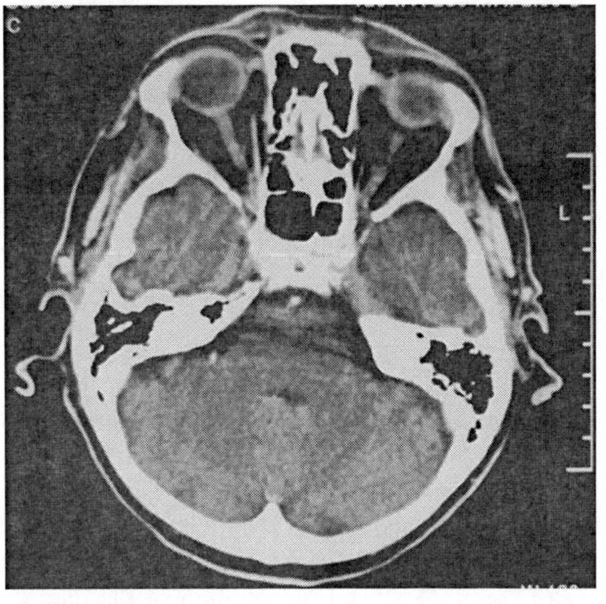

Figure 2. CT scan of the same patient showed on figure 1.

In all patients the oro-facial numbness was the first sign that led to the diagnosis of meningeal metastases. In three subjects partial remission of the numbness was obtained with systemic chemotherapy but disease progression led rapidly to death. The third patient was treated with systemic therapy and carbamazepine for the neuralgia, obtaining symptomatic relieve. Table 1 summarises the clinical features of our series of patients (Table 1).

Table 1. Clinical features of our series of patients

Patients	1	2	3	4
Primary tumor	Breast cancer	Breast cancer	Breast cancer	Breast cancer
Onset of the tumor	1989	1993	1991	1993
Onset of NCS	2006	2005	2004	2007
Presence of neuralgia	Yes	Yes	Yes	Yes
Associated paralysis of VII nerve	Yes	No	No	No
Leptomeningeal involvement at MRI	Yes	Yes	Yes	Yes
CSF examination	↑ proteins and ↓glucose	Carcinomatous cells	Carcinomatous cells	Not performed
Treatment	Systemic therapy and carbamazepine	Systemic therapy and carbamazepine	Systemic therapy and gapapentin	Systemic therapy and carbamazepine
Follow up	No remission	Partial remission but death occured in 2006	Partial remission but death occured in 2005	Partial remission but death occured in 2007

Discussion

The numb chin syndrome (NCS) is characterised by oral and facial numbness restricted to the distribution area of the mental nerve. NCS has been well documented in the literature as a symptom of malignancy that usually occurs in a late stage of the disease [1-16].

The symptom is typically characterised by oro-facial hypoesthesia, paresthesia or pain over the chin.

As suggested by Burt et al. [5] a frequent aetiology is malignant infiltration of the inferior alveolar nerve sheath or compression of mental or inferior alveolar nerves by jaw metastases or local tumour. The literature review by Laurencet et al. suggests that lymphoma and adenocarcinoma of the breast are the primary tumours most likely to metastatise to the mandible [17]. Numb chin syndrome may also be caused, in up to 14% of cases, by metastases to the base of the skull [2; 10]. Penetration of the dura and involvement of the leptomeninges is an uncommon feature, though estimation of its prevalence may be low due to underdiagnosis [18].

There are other possible systemic factors, not related to malignancy, that can cause NCS: diabetes, sarcoidosis, amyloidosis, multiple sclerosis, HIV, sickle cell anaemia and Sjögren's syndrome [19].

In three of our patients, bisphosphonates-associated osteonecrosis of the jaws was considered in the differential diagnosis of the numbness. Bisphosphonates are regarded as the standard therapy for treatment of metastatic osteolytic lesions, but an increasing number of osteonecrosis of the jaws in patients treated with these drugs has been reported in the literature [20].

In patients with suggestive symptoms, CT scan and scintigraphy are of crucial value to exclude both metastases and osteonecrosis of the jaws. Where no lytic lesions of the mandible are evident at the CT scan and where no abnormal uptake is detected through a bone scan, either penetration of the dura and involvement of the leptomeninges or cerebral malignancy should be suspected. The clinical examination must therefore always be accompanied by diagnostic imaging (CT, MRI and scintigraphy) in order to carry out a proper diagnosis. In the case of carcinomatous meningitis, lesions may be visualized by gadolinium-enhanced MRI, which has been shown to be superior to CT scan for diagnosing nerve involvement [21].

Treatment consists of systemic chemotherapy. In accordance to Lossos and Siegal [2], these patients have a better prognosis if the Numb Chin Syndrome depends on leptomeningeal involvement compared to mandibular metastases. This is why it is important not only the recognition of the syndrome, but also its attribution to a causal factor. Though rare, the NCS may be the first symptom and manifestation in the presentation of an underlying malignancy. As an early diagnosis can have a significant improvement of treatment course and prognosis, we emphasise that dentists and physician should consider metastatic cancer in patients presenting with NCS in the absence of other local causes.

Conclusions

Although the numb chin syndrome has frequently been described in the literature, it remains often unrecognized by most primary care physician as a possible symptom of progressing malignancy. It is essential that the medical and dental professions are able to recognise the numb chin syndrome at an early stage as a possible presenting symptom of underlying or progressing malignancy, where no other obvious cause for this complaint is found.

References

[1] Massey EW, Moore J, Schold SC. Mental neuropathy from systemic cancer. *Neurology* 1981; 31:1277-1281.

[2] Lossos A, Siegal T. Numb chin syndrome in cancer patients: etiology, response to treatment, and prognostic significance. *Neurology* 1992; 42:1181-1184.

[3] Newman NJ. Multiple cranial neuropathies: presenting signs of systemic lymphoma. *Surv. Ophthalmol.* 1992; 37:125-129.

[4] Kuroda Y, Fujiyama F, Ohyama T et al. Numb chin syndrome secondary to Burkitt's cell acute leukemia. *Neurology* 1991; 41: 453-454.

[5] Burt RK, Sharfman WH, Karp BI, Wilson WH. Mental neuropathy (numb chin syndrome). A harbinger of tumor progression or relapse. *Cancer* 1992; 70:877-881.

[6] Hashimoto N, Kurihara K, Yamasaki H et al. Pathological characteristics of metastatic carcinoma in the human mandible. *J. Oral Pathol.* 1987; 16:362-367.

[7] Eppley BL, Snyders RV. Mental neuropathy as a sign of distant malignancy: report of cases. *J. Oral Maxillofac. Surg.* 1992; 50:1117-1119.

[8] Vincent SD, Lilly GE, Hupp JR. Paresthesia of the mandibular division, trigeminal nerve. *J. Oral Maxillofac Surg.* 1993; 51:565-569.

[9] Penarrocha Diago M, Bagan Sebastian JV, Alfaro Giner A, Escrig Orenga V. Mental nerve neuropathy in systemic cancer. Report of three cases. *Oral Surg. Oral Med. Oral Pathol.* 1990; 69:48-51.

[10] Bar-Ziv J, Slasky BS. CT imaging of dental nerve neuropathy: the numb chin syndrome. AJR *Am. J. Roentgenol.* 1997; 168: 371-376.

[11] Bruyn RP, Boogerd W. The numb chin. *Clin. Neurol. Neurosurg* 1991; 93:187-193.

[12] Turner-Iannacci A, Mozaffari E, Stoopler ET. Mental nerve neuropathy: case report and review. *Can. J. Emerg. Med.* 2003; 5: 259-262.

[13] Halachmi S, Madeb R, Madjar S et al. Numb chin syndrome as the presenting symptom of metastatic prostate carcinoma [abstract]. *Urology* 2000; 55: 286.

[14] Glaser C, Lang S, Pruckmayer M et al. Clinical manifestations and diagnostic approach to metastatic cancer of the mandible. *Int. J. Oral Maxillofac. Surg.* 1997; 26: 365-368.

[15] Silverstein LH, Szikman M, Melkonian R, Dubovsky D. Mental neuropathy associated with malignant disease: a case report. *J. Oral Implantol.* 1994; 20: 63-64.

[16] Baskaran RK, Krishnamoorthy, Smith M. Numb chin syndrome – a reflection of systemic malignancy. *World J. Surg. Oncol.* 2006; 4: 52.

[17] Laurencet FM, Anchisi S, Tullen E, Dietrich PY. Mental neuropathy: report of five cases and review of the literature. *Crit. Rev. Oncol. Hematol.* 2000; 34: 71-79.

[18] Dispenzieri A, Kyle RA. Neurological aspects of multiple myeloma and related disorders. *Best Pract. Res. Clin. Haematol.* 2005;18: 673-688.

[19] Sève P, Gachon E, Petiot P et al. Successful treatment with rituximab in a patient with mental nerve neuropathy in primary Sjögren's syndrome. *Rheumatol. Int.* 2007; 28:175-177.

[20] Poznak C, Estilo C. Osteonecrosis of the jaw in cancer patients receiving IV bisphosphonates. *Oncology* 2006; 20:1053-1062.

[21] Marsot-Dupuch K, Matozza F, Firat MM et al. Mandibular nerve: MR versus CT about 10 proved unusual tumors. *Neuroradiology* 1990; 32:492-496.

In: Clinical Dentistry
Editor: Scardina Giuseppe Alessandro

ISBN: 978-1-61122-354-5
© 2011 Nova Science Publishers, Inc.

Chapter 20

ESTHETIC MANAGEMENT OF GINGIVAL FENESTRATION USING PLASTIC SURGICAL PROCEDURE[#]

A. R. Pradeep*[*]*, Swati Pradeep Patel and Shikha Chowdhry
Department of Periodontics,
Government Dental College and Hospital,
Bangalore, India

ABSTRACT

Purpose: Gingival fenestration is a rare pathological entity, scarcely described in the literature. The purpose of this paper is to report a case of a tooth with a gingival fenestration which was successfully treated by the periodontal plastic surgical procedure with excellent aesthetic results.

Methods: A 27 year old male patient reported with a "Gingival fenestration" which persisted after a periapical surgery and apicectomy. The lesion was successfully treated using a modified free gingival graft with successful aesthetic and functional outcome. The hypothesis for the formation of such isolated gingival defect have been proposed.

Results: The aesthetic result obtained by the surgical procedure was successfully maintained during the one year follow up period.

[#] A version of this book was also published as a chapter in *International Journal of Clinical Dentistry, Volume 1, Issue 4*, published by Nova Science Publishers, Inc. It was submitted for appropriate modifications in an effort to encourage wider dissemination of research.

[*] Corresponding author: Dr. A.R. Pradeep, Professor and Head, Department of Periodontics, Government Dental College and Research Institute, Bangalore-2. India. Email: periodontics_gdc@yahoo.co.in; Ph. 91-98450-81190.

Clinical Significance

This in this report we highlight the need of identifying gingival fenestration as distinct pathological entity and suggest a variation from traditional techniques in treating such lesions. Furthermore, the importance of preserving the marginal gingiva to maintain the aesthetics is highlighted.

Fenestration is the term derived from the Latin word "Fenestra" meaning window. It is used frequently in the periodontal literature to describe areas in the alveolar bone devoid of bone, creating the window exposing the root surface. The term "gingival fenestration" has been discussed decades ago [1], but till now fails to be identified as a distinct pathological entity. It is an opening through oral mucosa, usually unattached keratinized gingiva and is usually seen associated with heavy subgingival deposits on the root surfaces in suprabony pockets. The lesion is infrequent in clinical practice and usually presents with lack of acute symptoms. The lesion is considered the transitory stage in the development of gingival cleft and surgical correction is usually not required except prophylaxis and brushing [1]. There are very few reports in the literature concerning this lesion and no definitive aetiology or treatment plan has been discussed.

The purpose of this presentation is to report a case of a tooth with a gingival fenestration which was successfully treated by the free gingival graft with excellent aesthetic results.

Case Report

A 27 year old male patient was referred to the department of Periodontics, Government Dental College and Research Institute, Bangalore, for an unusual complaint of food lodgement in the maxillary anterior region. The food lodgement was associated with halitosis and patient reported no associated acute symptoms such as pain or bleeding.

Patient reported having been hit by a cricket ball in the region of maxillary left central incisor seven years previously. The accident resulted in a laceration of the upper lip and increased mobility of the tooth, which subsided a few months after the trauma. The tooth remained asymptomatic for about four years, after which patient developed pain and swelling in the labial vestibule apparently related to the same tooth.

Following dental consultation, endodontic therapy was performed. Five months after the endodontic therapy, periapical surgery with apicectomy was done due to recurrent infection and persistent sinus tract. Eight months following the surgery, although, there was no recurrence of pain or pus discharge, but the periapical sinus persisted as an inflammation free gingival fenestration and patient complained of food lodgement in the same region. Patient was referred to the Department of Periodontics. Governement Dental College and Research Institute. Bangalore for futher management.

On clinical examination, a gingival fenestration exposing the apical third of the root was seen in relation to maxillary left incisor. The fenestration was located at the junction of attached gingiva and alveolar mucosa and was about 2.5 mm in diameter (Figure 1) The tooth was found to be restored with a complete crown. On Intraoral periapical radiograph endodontically treated maxillary left central incisor with completely healed periapical area was noted. (Figure 2).

Patient was a non smoker and his medical and family history was unremarkable.

Surgical Procedure

Under local anaesthesia, recipient site was prepared leaving 3 mm of marginal gingiva coronally. Laterally the recipient bed preparation extended up to the line angles of the adjacent teeth, avoiding the prominences of these teeth. (figure 3) Apical extent was 4 mm from the margin of the fenestration. The template was prepared using a sterile tin foil. (Figure 4).The template was then used to harvest a soft tissue graft from the premolar region of the left side of the palate.(Figure 5).

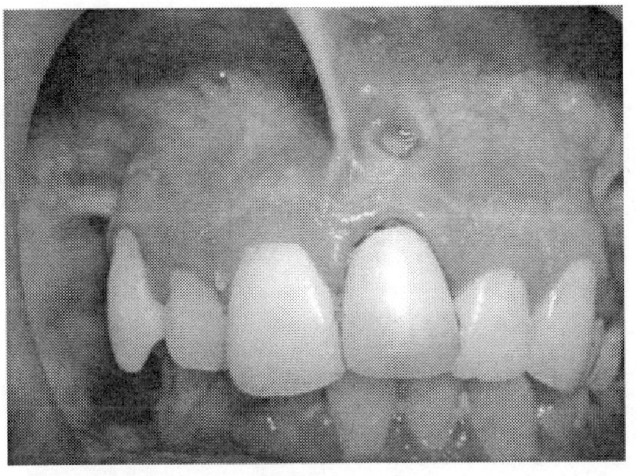

Figure 1. Gingival fenestration exposing the apical third of the root in relation to maxillary left central incisor.

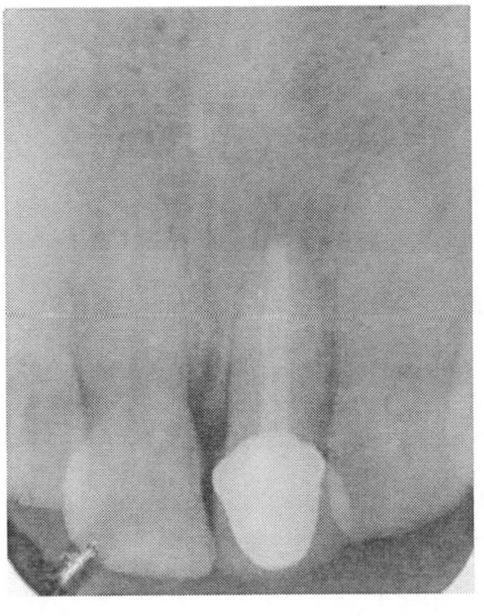

Figure 2. Radiograph of the same region.

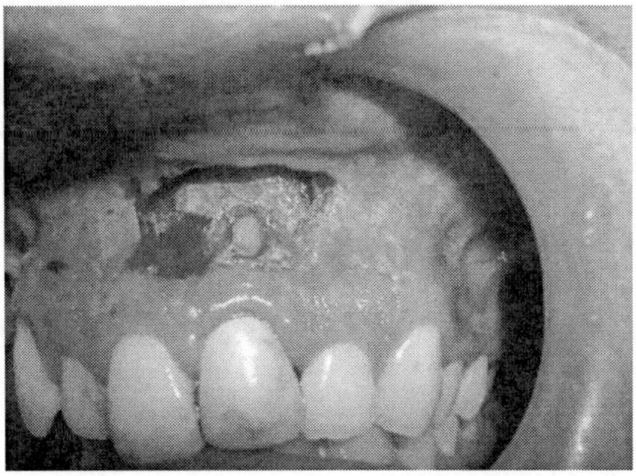

Figure 3. Recipient bed preparation to receive the free gingival graft.

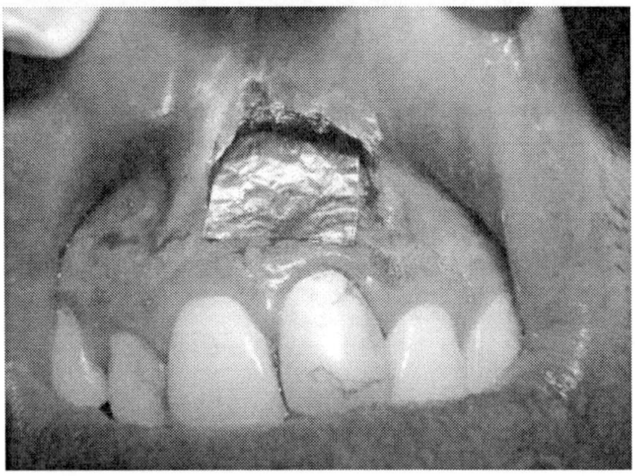

Figure 4. Preparation of the surgical template to harvest the graft using sterile tin foil.

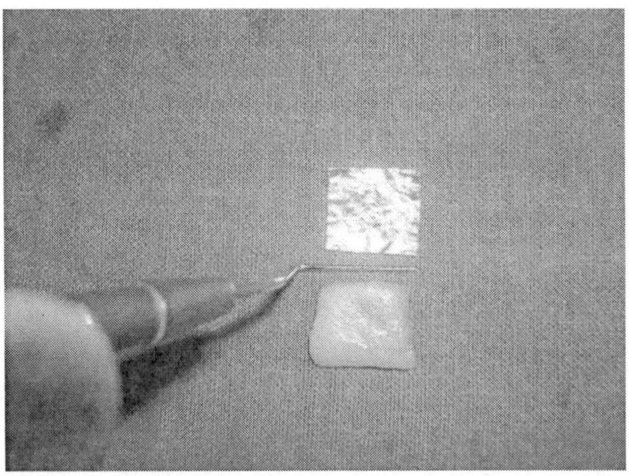

Figure 5. Graft harvested from the palate.

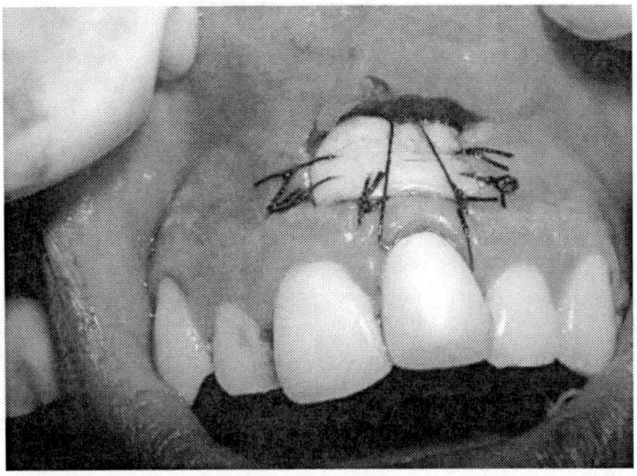

Figure 6. Free gingival graft secured at the recipient bed with sutures.

After appropriate thinning, the graft was sutured at the recipient site using 4-0 black braided silk suture material (Mersilk ®) with interrupted sutures and additional adaptation was achieved by a sling suture around the maxillary left central incisor (concavity suture). Non-eugenol periodontal dressing was placed over the surgical area.(Figure 6)

At the donor site, the haemostasis was achieved and the non eugenol periodontal dressing (COE PAK ™ ,GC AMERICA INC. USA) was given which was retained using an acrylic stent.

Post Operative Instructions

Patient was prescribed ibuprofen (400 mg, three times a day while necessary) for pain relief and 0.2 % chlorhexodine rinse (diluted 1:1 with water, 10 ml for 2 minutes, two times for 21 days).

RESULT

Ten Days Post Operative (Figure 7)

Ten days post operatively periodontal dressing and sutures were removed. Successful graft uptake with adequate vascularization was noticed. Patient was given instructions for home care and recalled after a month. Healing of the donor site was adequate and patient reported minimum pain and discomfort.

In the surgical area, mechanical oral hygiene in the form of toothbrushing and flossing was initiated at the end of second week.

One month post-operative (Figure-8) complete healing of the area with successful coverage of the fenestration was achieved and patient was satisfied with the results.

One year post operative (Figure-9) Coverage of the fenestration defect was maintained and no recurrence was seen.

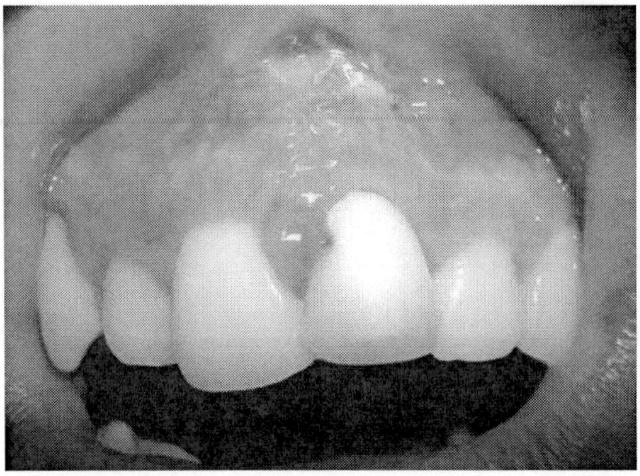

Figure 7. Successful graft uptake 10 days post-operatively.

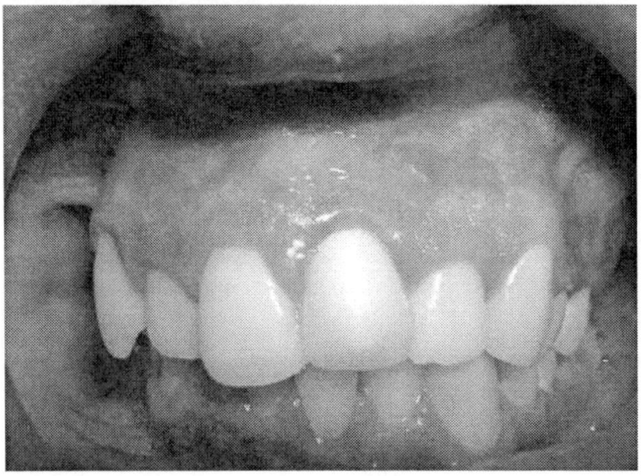

Figure 8. Adequate healing 1 month post operative.

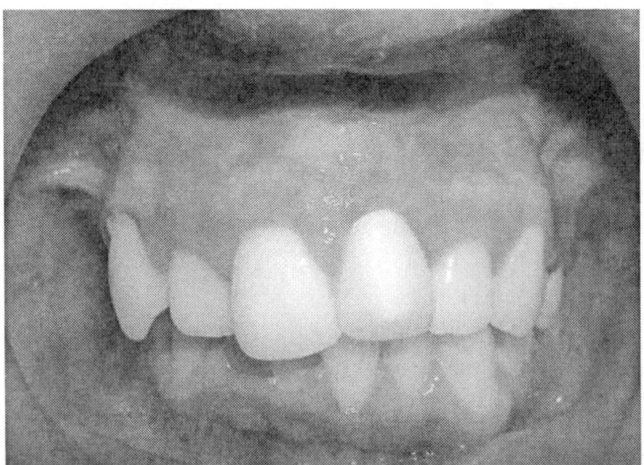

Figure 9. No recurrence 6 months post operatively.

DISCUSSION

This paper describes an unusual case of gingival fenestration which persisted following the incomplete healing of a periapical sinus. Gingival fenestration is a rare pathologic entity reported scarcely in the literature. Such lesions are most commonly reported to involve the primary maxillary incisors in children below six years of age [2,3,4]. The suggested eitiology in such cases is disturbed root resorption, loss of vitality of the resorbing teeth, or possible pressure from the erupting permanent teeth.

Gingival fenestration defect in permanent incisors have been reported in a few reports, primarily presenting in the region of attached gingiva in teeth with heavy band of subgingival calculus [5]. These lesions are considered as transitory stage in the formation of gingival cleft. According to a proposed hypothesis [1], the cause for the formation of gingival cleft is some form of marginal irritation such as marginal plaque or improper brushing, leading to inflammation of marginal tissue with a resultant downgrowth of long epithelial ridges. These ridges fuse with the surface epithelium producing an isolated area of connective tissue ischaemia causing degradation of overlying epithelium resulting in fenestration.

But to our knowledge, persistence of periapical sinus as a symptom free gingival fenestration has never been reported in the literature. Thus, the presented case is the first report of such pathology. The formation of isolated gingival defect in our case could be explained similarly. The periapical infection would have resulted in isolated ischaemia of overlying epithelium with subsequent degeneration. Alternatively, the lesion presented here could be a considered as an epithelialised sinus tract with resolution of the underlying infection.

Most of these fenestration lesions are asymptomatic which might be the reason for lack of reports. In most of the reports the defects have been followed by no treatment other than prophylaxis and oral hygiene with a final outcome of apical positioning of the gingival margin. Lane et al [1] suggested that such defects should be treated as gingival recessions extending up to the apical border of the recession.

In our case, we deviated from the conventionally suggested treatment plan by preserving the uninvolved, marginal gingiva coronal to the fenestration. The recipient bed to receive the soft tissue graft was prepared sparing 3 mm of the marginal gingiva coronally. The purpose of preserving the marginal gingiva was two fold:

1. Avoiding the patch like appearance of the free gingival graft in the aesthetic area of the patients gingiva.
2. Avoiding undue morbidity to the patient by harvesting bigger graft for the recipient bed involving the marginal gingiva.

The collar of the gingiva which was devoid of the apical blood supply, survived successfully with no signs of congestion or necrosis. This could be attributed to the lateral blood supply to the marginal gingiva as suggest Tarnow in 1986 [6].

Thus we report an unusual case of gingival fenestration treated successfully using soft tissue graft in the unconventional way. This in this report we highlight the need of identifying gingival fenestration as distinct pathological entity and suggest a variation from traditional techniques in treating such lesions. Furthermore, the importance of preserving the marginal gingiva to maintain the aesthetics is highlighted.

REFERENCES

[1] Lane JJ.Gingival fenestration. *J. Periodontol.* 1977; 48:225-7.

[2] Menendez OR. Bone fenestration by roots of deciduous teeth. *Oral Surg. Oral Med. Oral Pathol.* 1967;24: 654-658.

[3] Serrano J. Gingivo-osseous pathologic fenestration. *Oral Surg. Oral Med. Oral Pathol.* 1971;32: 697-700.

[4] Kelly JR, Keeton JM, Barr ES. Apical fenestration. *ASDC J. Dent. Child* 1976;43 :96-98.

[5] Aguilo LJ, Bagan JV. Pyogenic granuloma subsequent to apical fenestration of a primary tooth. *JADA* 2002, 133; 559- 602.

[6] Tarnow DP. Semilunar coronally positioned flap. *J. Clin. Periodontol.*. 1986, 13; 182-185.

In: Clinical Dentistry
Editor: Scardina Giuseppe Alessandro

ISBN: 978-1-61122-354-5
© 2011 Nova Science Publishers, Inc.

Chapter 21

KNOWLEDGE AND PRACTICAL ATTITUDES TOWARDS GLOVES USE IN DENTAL PRACTICE[#]

***Fethi Maatouk**[*1] **and Afef Zribi**[2]*

[1]Paediatric Dentistry, Dentistry School of Monastir, Tunisia
[2]Private practice Tunis, Tunisia

ABSTRACT

Nowadays hygiene and asepsis took an important place in all the medical fields and particularly in Dentistry, because the "hand of the dentist" can constitute a important source of infection. So, one basic measure of infection control, supposes a careful hand washing and the use of gloves which form a physical barrier and protect the Health Care Workers from occupational exposure to blood and saliva.

Our study carried out with the University Dental Clinic of Monastir (Tunisia) aims to evaluate knowledge in dental practice and to investigate their attitudes and practices toward the use of the gloves. It consists of a survey by auto-administrated questionnaire managed to a sample of 106 dental practitioners including 16 teachers, 26 trainees and 64 dental students.

Findings revealed that about 78.3% of dentists wore gloves, 21.7% wore masks and 2% wore protective eyeglasses. The students have a minimum necessary knowledge about gloves use but do not have a correct practice while the other practitioners have the good knowledge and the good practical attitudes.

Our study shows an important need to improve the students' behaviour with respect of occupational hygiene and safety conditions in order to reduce occupational blood exposure hazards.

[#] A version of this book was also published as a chapter in *International Journal of Clinical Dentistry, Volume 1, Issue 4*, published by Nova Science Publishers, Inc. It was submitted for appropriate modifications in an effort to encourage wider dissemination of research.

[*] Address: Pr. Fethi Maatouk. Paediatric Dentistry Department. Dentistry School Avicenne Avenue 5019 Monastir. TUNISIA. Tel. + 216 73 460 832 / Fax. + 216 73 461 150 / E-Mail fethi.maatouk@fmdm.rnu.tn Web Site: http://maatouk.tripod.com

Keywords: MeSH, Asepsis, Attitude to health, Dental staff, Dental practice, Nosocomial infection control, Gloves, Protective/utilization.

The hygiene and the asepsis took today an important place in all the medical fields and particularly in Dentistry. The patients are aware for this problem, which becomes the major concern of our society. This concern is not recent because since the sixteenth century Semmelweiss encouraged the fight against the infection and mortality in maternities by a simple washing of the hands. Later in 1867, "The Lancet" published the article of Lister on the concept of the disinfectant surgery [1, 2]. But at the base of the great principles of asepsis and sterilization, we find the famous work of Louis Pasteur (1822-1895) who wrote: "Instead of effort to eliminate the microbes in the wounds, it would be more reasonable not to introduce some".

Today, the strict hygiene and the nosocomial infections control must be an absolute priority for all the health care workers, especially for the dental care staff because it can constitute a very important link in the transmission of the infections from a patient to another and also towards all the dentist entourage, particularly the family [3]. It is a risk of “cross contamination" complicated and increased by the characteristics of the dentistry practice, in particular, the multiplication and the diversity of care acts, the miniaturization of the instruments... So the respect of the asepsis, which is the guarantee of an optimal quality of care and comfort for the patient and a medico-legal protection for the practitioner, remains a true challenge with the dentistry [4, 5, 6].

It is known that the "hand of the dentist" plays, as a source of infection, a role which should not be underestimated. Indeed the hands are the first vector of the contamination, and it is estimated that 70 to 80% of the infections are carried by hands. So, one basic measure of infection control, supposes firstly a careful hand washing and secondly the use of gloves which are a personal protective equipment (PPE). These two factors constitute an essential elements for the nosocomial infection control since the glove forms a physical barrier which protects the dentist from direct exposure to blood and body fluids like saliva (occupational blood exposure hazards: OBE). In dentistry, the circumstances of gloves use are so varied that only one type of glove cannot satisfy the whole of the dentist needs [7].

In 1889, the American physician "William halsted" used the glove for the first time at the surgical operation [8]. Until the discovery of rubber, the gloves were manufactured from animal bladders, leather or cotton.

Since 1985 with the AIDS epidemic the frequency of the gloves use increased. Indeed the appearance of this affection was a real catalyst which modified the behaviour of the Care health professionals and also at the origin of the concepts of universal precautions against contamination risk from blood and biological products. These standard precautions were stated in 1989 by Occupational Safety and Health Administration (OSHA) and Centers for Disease Control (CDC). Their purpose is to avoid or control the cross infection.[9, 10]

The objectives of the present study were to measure knowledge among dental care staff about rational use of gloves in order to prevent nosocomial hazards, to investigate their practice towards the use of the gloves and to look for any relationship between knowledge and practice.

1. Material and Methods

Our investigation carried out with the university dental clinic of Monastir (Tunisia) was conducted between April and May 2006. It consisted of a survey by questionnaire managed to a sample of 106 dental care workers including 16 teachers, 26 trainees, 32 students of last form and 32 students of 5th form.

In fact, the questionnaire was distributed directly to 111 practitioners but despite that anonymity and confidentiality of the answers was guaranteed 5 of them refused to answer it, so the participant rate was about 95.5%.

Study Tool

The self administrated questionnaire with open answers was adapted from the literature that reported on the understanding and attitudes toward the control of nosocomial infection by wearing gloves. The items of the questionnaire were divided in two headings:

- Knowledge with 7 questions.
- Practical attitude towards gloves use with 17 questions.

A pilot study with 20 subjects was used to validate the questionnaire which was found to be consistent, reliable and easy to read.

Sample Presentation

The sample presentation given in table 1 shows that girls constitute 55.6% of studied subjects which age varied from 25 to 50 years with mean of 27.5 ± 4.3 years. Experience duration varied from 0 to 27 years with average of 2.84 ± 5.78 years for all subjects and 15.25 ± 5.71 years for teachers.

Table 1. Sample presentation

Gender	Male		Female		Total	
Variables	N	%	N	%	N	%
Age (years)						
25-29	36	76.6	54	91.5	90	84.9
30-39	4	8.5	3	5	7	6.6
40-50	7	14.9	2	3.4	9	8.5
Level of education						
Student 5th form	15	31.9	17	28.8	32	30.2
Student last form (diploma)	13	27.7	19	32.2	32	30.2
Trainees (University diploma)	8	17	18	30.5	26	24.5
Teacher (Bachelor degree)	11	23.4	5	8.5	16	15.1

Table 1. (Continued)

Gender	Male		Female		Total	
Variables	N	%	N	%	N	%
Years of experience						
0-5	36	76.6	54	91.5	90	84.9
6-10	3	6.4	2	3.4	5	4.7
11-15	3	6.4	1	1.7	4	3.7
>15	5	10.5	2	3.4	7	6.4
Total	47	44.4	59	55.6	106	100

All dental specialties were involved as shown in table 2.

Table 2. Distribution according to specialties

	None	PD	CD	Ortho	Perio	OS	CP	FP	RPP	Total
N	32	12	9	9	9	11	6	9	9	106
%	30,1	11,3	8,5	8,5	8,5	10,4	5,7	8,5	8,5	100

PD: pediatric dentistry CD: conservative dentistry Ortho: orthodontics Perio: periodontology OS: oral surgery CP: complete prosthesis FP: fixed prosthesis RPP: Removable partial prosthesis.

Statistical Analysis

After validation of the forms, the data were collected by computer system and the statistical analysis was performed with the Epi-Info software version 6.04. The Pearson chi-squared test was used at 5% level of significance to compare different percentages [11].

2. Results

2.1. Knowledge

Table 3 summarizes the knowledge of respondents about gloves and gives percentages of correct answers.

- Principal materials of the gloves: 98 subjects (92.4%) knew only latex probably because it is the unique gloves' material used in the university dental clinic. Only two respondents knew also the vinyl and one knew in more the nitril and the neoprene.

- Type of powder used to lubricate the gloves (Starch of corn, talc...): the answers were all for talc and any response for the corn starch. The use of talc is banned since about 15 years for allergic problems and only the modified corn starch is used now.
- Types of gloves used in dental practice (Examination gloves / sterile operating gloves /sterile gloves for surgery): the respondents make the difference between examination gloves and sterile glove of surgery without knowing the sterile glove of care.
- Level of gloves protection.
  Complete protection 2- Partial protection 3- Does not protect at all
  4- Protection from cuts 5- Protection from the punctures)

The greatest number of practitioners (97.2 %) believed in the true protection of the gloves. That explains the important use for the gloves. Only 3 dentists (2.8 %) have false idea on the protection of the gloves.

In fact the wearing of gloves does not reduce the frequency of sharps injuries, but may confer some protection by virtue of their wiping action on the sharp object on penetration [8].

- Risks related to gloves' use for the dentist and the patient: 86% admitted risk from gloves' wear for dentist and only 44% admitted risk for patients. It was thought that the risk is primarily the allergy to latex and that it is higher for the dentist who is with the direct and close contact with this material.
- Possibility to wash the gloves: those which confirmed the washing of the gloves did it when the gloves are soiled by blood, saliva or impression material. This wrong idea more frequent in students (12.7%) is due to a fact that they must buy gloves.
- Evaluation of knowledge: according to answers' of the 7 preceding questions, knowledge was scored with 1 for a correct answer and 0 for an incorrect one. Scores are ranged from 0 to 7, with a median of 3. A cut-off score was calculated based on the median value. Participants scoring at or above the median value of the total knowledge score were classified as having good knowledge, while those having a total knowledge score less than the median value were considered as having poor knowledge.

The mean knowledge score was about 3.40 ± 1.02. According to the function, the best marks are recorded among trainees. Indeed 92.2% of them had good knowledge, but the difference is not statistically significative.

Table 3. Knowledge about rational gloves use

Items		% correct answers				
		Students 5th form	Students last form	Trainees	Teachers	Total n = 106
1	Do you know principal materials of the gloves?	90.6	97	100*	75	92.5
2	What type of powder is used to lubricate the gloves?	59.4	78	80.7*	75	72.6
3	Which are the types of gloves used in dental practice?	43.7	62.5	53.8	43.7	51.9

Table 3. (Continued)

Items		% correct answers				
		Students 5th form	Students last form	Trainees	Teachers	Total n = 106
4	What do you think about the protection of the gloves? (partial protection)	100	84.4	96.1	81.2	97.2
5	Are there risks related to the use of the gloves for dentist?	81.2	84.4	96.1	81.2	85.8
6	Are there risks related to the use of the gloves for patient?	46.9	34.3	46.1	56.2	44.3
7	Can we wash the gloves?	87.5	90.6	92.3	93.7	90.6
8	Evaluation of knowledge (score/7)					
	Get good knowledge ≥ 3	68.6	78	92.2	81.1	79.2
	Mean score	3.16±0.9	3.31 ± 1	3.58±0.8	3.75±1.3	3.4 ± 1

* Statistical significative difference $p \leq 0.05$.

2.2. Practical Attitude

Table 4 shows the percentages of correct practical attitude about rational gloves use.

- Frequency and moment of use of personal protective equipment:

An important and systematic use of the gloves in the University Dental Clinic is noted in 78.3%. About 20% used them irregularly and only 1.9% of the respondents never used the gloves. They thought that the risk misses out in complete prosthesis because the patients are toothless. Some believed that the gloves' wearing is unpleasant in some acts of prosthesis and in those needing a tactile sensation like acts of endodontics.

The students were the large consumers of the gloves with 87.5% of them that always used gloves.

Among the answers given about the moment of gloves' use, 5 choices were noted:

1. Face to a patient at risk
2. When glove is available
3. In bloody act
4. In patient with failing oral hygiene
5. In contact with saliva

The majority of those who wore masks were students of last forms (52.1%) and only 2% wore protective glasses.

- About factors which guide the choice of gloves, the respondents had selected 4 factors:

1. The type of glove
2. The size of glove
3. The act to carry out
4. The medical history of patient.

2.8% of them take in account all these 4 factors in their choice. The majority of the respondents that is 86% chose gloves according to size. In our dental university clinic, except in the oral surgery department, only one type of gloves is available, the examination gloves, therefore the choice according to these parameters remains theoretical.

- Jewels and watches: the majority of the practitioners did not remove their jewels, of which 63.6% were woman. The 7.5% "not specified answers" were to men who did not carry jewels in fact.
- Time of hands washing and gloves wearing:

61.3% of the respondents washed their hands before and after the gloves' wearing.

35.8% of them gave a great importance to the handwashing after the use of the gloves since the hands were soiled by the powder and sweating. It is noted that some were rather interested in the visible stain than in the invisible micro-organisms.

23.6% of the practitioners wore the gloves at one time when it is useless to carry them (with the interrogation) an equivalent number of the practitioners make the clinical examination in mouth naked hands.

- Gloves use factors:

The majority of the respondents (86.8%) used one pair of gloves for each patient.

4.7% of them work without gloves for patients whom they judge without risk.

5.5% of the practitioners wore an overglove (double pair of gloves) when they treated patient at contamination risk but 5.7% of them had the false ideas that it can protected from the punctures...

40% of the respondents never used an overglove; among them 45.2% were students because they have only one pair of gloves.

72.6% of the subjects take off the gloves immediately after the care. But 21.7% of the subjects make gestures apart from the mouth with the soiled gloves (wrote the appointments, the prescriptions, the medical certificates, answered to phone call, take X-ray…). More than half of them were students.

- In case of long care procedure (More than 1 hour): Among the 39 practitioners (37%) who wore the gloves for duration longer than one hour, 66.6% were students. That is explained by the fact that the students brought only one pair of gloves for a clinical session of two hours and half.
- In case of an interruption of care: 92 practitioners (86.8%) take off the gloves with the interruption of care but 25 among them (23.6%), whom were mainly students, re-used them when they continued the cares.
- In case of gloves perforation: 11.3% of respondents keep on perforated gloves; more than half of them were students.

That is explained in the same way by the fact that they have only one pair of gloves.

- Assistant or co-workers: among the 61 subjects (58%) that assistant did not wear gloves almost half (47.5%) were students who always work in binomial. Of course, in oral surgery the assistants of surgeons always wear sterile gloves.
- Gloves elimination: the major part of the respondents removed and threw the gloves just at the end of the care in dustbin.
- Allergy to latex gloves: The majority of the practitioners (89.6%) didn't ask the patient if it is allergic to latex.

As the synthetic gloves are not available at the university dental clinic of Monastir, only the 11 dentists (10.4%) which were allergic to latex used synthetic gloves.

In fact, some complains about reactions of dryness, redness, urticaria or burns are reported but these reactions are rare and it is thought that they are surely due to repeated washings and to the other dental materials used rather than with true allergy to latex [12, 13, 14, 15, 16].

- Evaluation of the practical attitudes: According to answers' of the 18 preceding questions, practical attitudes were scored with 1 for a correct practice and 0 for a wrong one. Then the total score (note/18) was calculated for the evaluation of correct attitudes.

A cut-off score was calculated based on the median value. Participants scoring at or above the median value were classified as having good practical attitudes, while those having a total attitudes score less than the median value were considered as having bad practical attitudes. The average note was about 9.7 ± 2.6; about nearly 68% of the respondents had the average.

According to the function, like as knowledge, the best notes were recorded among trainees. Indeed 88.5% of them had note equal or better than 9. The worst marks are recorded in the students.

Table 4. Practical attitude about rational gloves use

Items		% correct attitudes				
		Students 5th form	Students last form	Trainees	Teachers	Total
1	Do you always use gloves?	87.5*	81.3	76.9	56	78.3
2	Do you use mask?	9.4	37.5*	19.2	18.8	21.7
3	Do you use protective glasses?	0	0	3.8	6.3*	1.9
4	Which factor does guide your choice of gloves? (size)	65.6	59.4*	57.7	50	85.8
5	Do you remove jewels and watches before wearing the gloves?	43.8	40.6	38.5	37.5	40.6
6	When do you wash your hands? (Before wearing and after removing gloves)	56.3	40.6	80.8	81.3*	61.3

Table 4. (Continued)

Items		% correct attitudes				
		Students 5th form	Students last form	Trainees	Teachers	Total
7	At which time do you wear the gloves? Just before examination	53	53	57.7*	18.8	52
8	Do you change gloves in case of long care procedure?	50	65.6	84.6*	62.5	65
9	How long do you keep the gloves? (≤1H)	18.8	84.4	73.1	87.5*	62.3
10	Do you use one pair of gloves for each patient? (Yes)	93.8	90.6	80.8	81.3	86.8
11	When do you remove the gloves? (just after care)	59.4	71.9	77	87.5	72.6
12	Where do you throw the (soiled) removed gloves? (in dustbin)	100	97	96.2	87.5	96.2
13	In case of an interruption of care do you change gloves? (yes)	25	59.4	61.5*	56.3	49
14	Do you change gloves if it is perforated?	75	90.6	96.2*	93.8	87.7
15	Do you sometimes wear an overgloves (double pair)?	40.6	78*	73	37.5	59.4
16	Does your assistant wear gloves?	9.4	28	46.2	56.3*	31
17	Do you ask whether the patient is allergic to latex?	9.4	3	7.7	18.8	8.5
18	What do you make for a patient allergic to latex? (use a synthetic gloves)	87.5	75	53.8	50	69.8
19	Evaluation of the practical attitudes (note/18)					
	Mean note	8.5±2.3	10 ± 2.6	10.6±2.2*	9.7±3.1	9.7 ± 2.6
	Get at least a note ≥ 9	43.7	72	88.5	75	68
20	Do you have any allergy to the material of the gloves?	6.25	6.25	19.2	12.5	10.4

* Statistical significative difference p ≤ 0.05.

3. Analysis and Discussion

The frequency of personal protective equipment (PPE) wearing in our study was about 78.3% for gloves, 21.7% for mask and only 2% for protective glasses. The respondents suppose surely that the glasses of sight are also safety goggles but special protective glasses, or goggles are required to provide sufficient eye protection.

These rates are lower than what was reported by Burke et al 1994 in a 2-year follow-up study of 2000 dentists in England and Wales about glove use in clinical practice, they found that 83% of respondents wore gloves routinely for all patients and all procedures, 15% wore gloves for either selected patients or procedures and 2% never wore gloves [17, 18].

Morris et al.1996 showed that about 90% of dentists in Kuwait wore gloves, 75% wore masks and 52% wore eyeglasses [19].

A study conducted in Canada revealed that in 1994 91.8% of dentists in Ontario always wore gloves, 74.8% always wore masks and 83.6% always wore eye protection [20].

The situation is almost the same in Saudi Arabia where it was found that only 2%–4% of dental professionals never wore gloves when treating patients [21]. Al-Omari MA et al 2005, which reported that among 120 dentists of private practice in Jordan 81.8 % wore and changed gloves during treatment and between patients [22].

Our frequency of gloves wearing is higher than reported by Treasure and Treasure in a New Zealand study, where only 42.0% of dentists wore gloves, 64.8% wore masks and 66.4% wore eye protection [23].

According to gender Motamed N. et al [24] and McCarthy et al. [25] showed in their study on knowledge and practices, that women had a significant higher level of knowledge and practice toward universal precautions than men. Hellgren 1994 reported that dentists never using loves at all were older, male practitioners [26]. This is in agreement with our results where girls usemore gloves than boys with respectively 85% and 66% ($p<10^{-2}$). These percentages decrease significantly with age ($p<10^{-9}$) as also reported by McCarthy et al. 1999 [27].

Regarding function, the students are the large users of the gloves (87.5%). This high rate is in relation with the nature of work in the university dental clinic which imposes to the students the use of gloves, but it does not really reflect a true conscience of the importance of gloves use.

It seems that the use of gloves is more related to a fear of the direct occupational blood exposure (OBE) than to a true comprehension of the interests of its use.

Indeed, in comparison with the residents and the teachers a reduced number of students wash their hands before and after gloves wearing.

53% of the students wear the gloves before the clinical examination and 31.2% carry them even before the medical interrogation of the patient. Often, time before clinical examination includes also the call of the patient from the waiting room, the installation of the patient on dental chair, the recovery of the material of work... in fact gestures which do not require gloves wearing.

All the students wear one pair of gloves for each patient, perhaps because the students often treat only one patient by clinical training session. This is in agreement with the results of a study conducted in a province of northern Italy where 99% of the dentists changed gloves after each patient [28].

60% of the students of our study take off their gloves immediately after the end of care. It was supposed that students whose remain keeping on the gloves until patient leaving write the prescriptions, the appointments, the medical certificates... with the soiled gloves.

It is noted that a significant number of students (66.6% $p<10^{-4}$) wear longer than one hour the same gloves. Indeed the gloves are provided to all the practitioners of the university dental clinic except for the students who must bring them themselves and they buy only one pair of glove for a working session of two hours and half.

21.8% of students don't change gloves with the interruption of care.

According to dental specialities the best "practical attitudes scores" are recorded with the departments of periodontology and "oral surgery" which are the departments where the contact with blood and saliva is almost constant with each care. The lowest scores are noted with the prosthesis departments; in the latter the care and the interventions are much less bloody. Also, in these departments the nature of certain acts is incompatible with the gloves wearing like the dental impression, the handling of the wax... The papers of Burke FJ et al 1992 and Epstein JB et al 1995 lead to the same conclusions [29, 30, 31].

In brief, the glove wearing patterns were found to be related to gender, age and function. The reasons given for not wearing gloves routinely included problems of comfort, loss of tactile sensation, cost and the risk of cross-infection, which was perceived to be small. Burke FJ et al. 1994, Gordon BL et al 2001 and Christensen GJ 2001 reported the same reasons in their study [29,32,33].

4. Recommendations with Use of the Gloves: [34, 35]

- Use a glove for each patient and a glove for each care:
- The gloves must be preserved in their box in a dry place safe from heat, light and x-rays.
- The gloves must be used as supplementary measure of nosocomial infection control, they do not replace hands washing.
- The hand washing both prior to placement and following removal of gloves is necessary.
- The gloves must be used before the clinical examination in the new patient and right before the act to carry out at a second appointment.
- The jewels and the watch must be removed before wearing the gloves.
- An order of care must be respected: from cleanest care to more contaminated one.
- The maximum time of wearing of gloves is between 30 minutes and 2 hours. This time decreases more especially as the act has a high risk of contamination.
- In the event of interruption of care, it is necessary to change the gloves as well as the resumption of the whole procedure of antisepsy of the hands.
- The washing of the gloves is to be proscribed owing to the fact that it affects the integrity of the glove and thus its effectiveness.
- The worn gloves are not reusable.
- The elimination of the gloves must be done immediately at the end of the care, in the nearest adapted dustbin.
- Gloves must be eliminated just at the end of the care and more close possible of the place of care in the adapted die of waste. We must take off a first glove and lock up it in the other hand than take off the second glove. The hands should never return in contact with the external soiled face of the glove to eliminate. The removal of the glove is followed of a simple or disinfectant washing of the hands according to the level of contamination of the care which has been just carried out.

Conclusion

As in all the specialities of medicine, the medical gloves are largely used in dentistry. They form an effective physical barrier and constitute the best protection to our hands and to our patients. A few years ago, the wearing of gloves was badly perceived with the dentist and the patient doesn't perceive his utility. However, nowadays, with the evolution of the medical culture of the patients, it is the opposite phenomenon which occurs and the gloves wearing now is perceived very favourably and even regarded as an element of great professionalism which improves the public image of the dentist. The use of the gloves is of course useful, but it is necessary to know to correctly use them according to the predetermined rules and recommendations. Because misused, the gloves become a vector of the infection. There are various materials of the gloves, but the latex remains more used considering its performance and its qualities.

However the use of the gloves is not completely without risk since certain reactions of allergies especially related to natural latex are reported.

- Our study shows that there is a need to improve the dental health team behaviour with respect of occupational hygiene and safety conditions in order to reduce OBE hazards.
- To lead to the correct practice we must start first of all by offering the gloves to all the practitioners without exception including the students.
- There is also a great need to provide infection control courses and guidelines for the students and cycles of continuous training for other practitioners, in addition to distribution of standard infection control manuals that incorporate current infection control recommendations.

Acknowledgments

The authors would like to express their gratitude to all those who helped them in this study especially the students.

References

[1] Chin JE. Control of communicable disease manual, 17th ed. Washington, American Public Health Association, 2000:1–9.

[2] Thomas O, Maiza L. Transmission of infectious diseases. *Encycl. Med. Chir*. (Elsevier Paris) odontologie, 23-841-B-10, 1998,10p.

[3] Hudson-Davies SC, Jones JH, Sarll DW. Cross-infection control in general dental practice: dentists' behaviour compared with their knowledge and opinions. *Br. Dent J.* 1995 May 20;178(10):365-9.

[4] Nash KD. How infection control procedures are affecting dental practice today. *J. Am. Dent. Assoc*. 1992 Mar;123(3):67-73.

[5] CDC. Updated USPHS guidelines for managing occupational exposures to HBV, HCV, and HIV and considerations for dentistry. Journal of the American Dental Association, 2002, 133(12):1627–9.

[6] Stoopler ET. Oral herpetic infections (HSV1-8). *Dent. Clin. N Am*. 2005; 49:15-29.

[7] Aubier M, Kleinfinger S. *Protection des mains au cabinet dentaire*. Paris: CdP, 2001 :80p.

[8] Upton LG, Barber HD. Double-gloving and the incidence of perforations during specific oral and maxillofacial surgical procedures. *J. Oral Maxillofac Surg*. 1993;51:261–3.

[9] CDC. Recommended infection-control practices for dentistry. *MMWR* 1993;35:237-42.

[10] Bolyard EA, Tablan OC, Williams WW et al. Guideline for infection control in health care personnel. *American Journal of Infection Control* (1998;26:289-354)

[11] Abramson JH, Abramson ZH. Making Sense of Data: A Self-Instruction Manual on the Interpretation of Epidemiological Data. Oxford University Press US, 2001.

[12] Ahmed DD, Sobczak SC, Yunginger JW. Occupational allergies caused by latex. *Immunology Allergy Clin. North Am.* 2003;23:205-19.

[13] Chardin H. Hypersensibilités en pratique odontostomatologique : cas particuliers de l'allergie au latex et de l'allergie aux métaux. *Encycl. Med. Chir.* (Elsevier Paris) *odontologie,* 23-841-C-15, 1997,4p.

[14] Yip E, Cacioli P. The manufacture of gloves from natural rubber latex. *J. Allergy Clin. Immuno*l. 2002;110(2 Suppl):S3-14.

[15] Barbara J, Santais MC, Levy DA, et al. Immunoadjuvant properties of glove cornstarch powder in latex-induced hypersensitivity. *Clin. Exp. Allergy* 2003;33:106-112.

[16] Huber MA, Terezhalmy GT. Adverse Reactions to Latex Products: Preventive and Therapeutic Strategies. *J. Contemp. Dent. Pract.* 2006 February;(7)1:097-106.

[17] Burke FJ, Wilson NH, Cheung SW. Glove use by dentists in England and Wales: results of a 2-year follow-up survey. *Br. Dent. J.* 1994 May 7;176(9):337-41.

[18] Burke FJ, Wilson NH, Cheung SW. Trends in glove use by dentists in England and Wales: 1989-1992. Int Dent J. 1994 Jun;44(3):195-201.

[19] Morris E et al. Infection control knowledge and practices in Kuwait: a survey on oral health care workers. Saudi dental journal, 1996, 8:19–26.

[20] McCarthy GM, MacDonald JK. The infection control practices of general dental practitioners. Infection control and hospital epidemiology, 1997;18(10):699–703.

[21] Al-Rabeah A, Mohamed AG. Infection control in the private dental sector in Riyadh. *Annals of Saudi medicine*, 2002, 22(1–2):13–7.

[22] Al-Omari MA, Al-Dwairi ZN. Compliance with infection control programs in private dental clinics in Jordan. *J. Dent. Educ*. 2005 Jun;69(6):693-8.

[23] Treasure P, Treasure ET. Survey of infection control procedures in New Zealand dental practices. International dental journal, 1994, 44(4):342–8.

[24] Motamed N, BabaMahmoodi F, Khalilian A, Peykanheirati M and Nozari M Knowledge and practices of health care workers and medical students towards universal precautions in hospitals in Mazandaran Province. EMHJ,2006;12, 5.

[25] McCarthy GM, MacDonald JK. Gender differences in characteristics, infection control practices, knowledge and attitudes related to HIV among Ontario dentists. *Community Dent. Oral Epidemiol*. 1996 Dec;24(6):412-5.

[26] Hellgren K. Use of gloves among dentists in Sweden--a 3-year follow-up study. *Swed. Dent. J.* 1994;18(1-2):9-14.

[27] McCarthy GM, Koval JJ, MacDonald JK, John MA. The role of age- and population-based differences in the attitudes, knowledge and infection control practices of Canadian dentists. *Community Dent. Oral Epidemiol.* 1999;27:298–304.

[28] Veronesi L, Bonanini M, Dall'Aglio P, Pizzi S, Manfredi M, Tanzi ML, Health hazard evaluation in private dental practices: a survey in a province of northen Italy. *Acta Bio Medica Ateneo Parmense* 2004; 75; 50-55.

[29] Burke FJ, Wilson NH, Shaw WC, Cheung SW. Glove use by orthodontists: results of a survey in England and Wales. *Eur. J. Orthod.* 1992 Jun;14(3):246-51.

[30] Burke FJ, Wilson NH, Cheung SW, Shaw WC. Glove use by orthodontists in England and Wales: changes since 1989 and comparisons with general dental practitioners. *Eur. J. Orthod.* 1994 Jun;16(3):241-4.

[31] Epstein JB, Mathias RG, Bridger DV. Survey of knowledge of infectious disease and infection control practices of dental specialists. *J. Can. Dent. Assoc.* 1995 Jan;61(1):35-7, 40-4.

[32] Gordon Bl, Burke FJT, Bagg J, Marlborough HS, McHugh ES. Systematic review of adherence to infection control. Guidelines in dentistry. *J. Dent.* 2001; 29: 509-16.

[33] Christensen G.J : Operating gloves : The good and the bad. *J. Am. Dent. Assoc*, 2001; 132, 10: 1455-57.

[34] Harte JA, Charlton DG. Characteristics of infection control programs in U.S. Air Force dental clinics. A survey. *J. Am. Dent. Assoc*, 2005; 136, 7: 885-892.

[35] Kohn WG, Collins AS, Cleveland JL, Harte JA, Eklund KJ, Malvitz DM; Centers for Disease Control and Prevention. Guidelines for infection control in dental health-care settings—2003. *MMWR Recomm. Rep.* 2003;52(RR-17):1–61.

In: Clinical Dentistry
Editor: Scardina Giuseppe Alessandro

ISBN: 978-1-61122-354-5
© 2011 Nova Science Publishers, Inc.

Chapter 22

THE GROWING NEED FOR FURTHER COLLABORATION BETWEEN DENTISTRY AND MEDICINE: INTERDISCIPLINARY MANAGEMENT FOR IMMUNOCOMPROMISED PATIENTS*

Nermin Yamalik[1] and Tolga F. Tözüm[2]
[1]Department of Periodontology, Faculty of Dentistry,
University of Hacettepe, Ankara, Turkey
[2]Department of Periodontology, Faculty of Dentistry,
University of Hacettepe, Ankara, Turkey

ABSTRACT

There is a bilateral relationship between oral health and general health and, without doubt, interdisciplinary management increases the efficiency of diagnosis and treatment, reduces complications and unnecessary treatment, and improves the quality of care and quality of life. Dental and medical professionals have always been in close cooperation particularly for the provision of comprehensive care for patients with specific needs; however, there seems to be a need for further improvement of the collaboration between the two health disciplines. Immunocompromised patients may well serve as a good example of the growing need for such an improved treatment alliance between the two health disciplines for provision of efficient care for special in-need groups, because of the increasing number of immunocompromised patients, particularly the bone marrow or solid organ transplant candidates and recipients, and due to the many areas of interface between dentistry and medicine regarding these patients, Recent advances in both disciplines are also likely to provide new opportunities for dental and medical professionals to provide comprehensive care for many of the immunocompromised patients. Further, an active team approach may enable both health professionals to

---

* A version of this book was also published as a chapter in *International Journal of Clinical Dentistry, Volume 1, Issue 3*, published by Nova Science Publishers, Inc. It was submitted for appropriate modifications in an effort to encourage wider dissemination of research.

significantly increase their part of contribution to the improvement of general health, oral health, well being, and quality of life of this specific patient category.

Keywords: immunocompromised patients, transplantation, interdisciplinary care.

Clinical significance: Due to the development of more advanced and innovative models for diagnosis and care arising from clear scientific and technical advances that is experienced in both disciplines, it is likely that many categories of patients with specific needs benefit from a further improved collaboration between dentistry and medicine.

Dentistry and medicine interface at many levels and comprehensive care, most often, requires the integration of the knowledge, skills, and experience of both disciplines [1]. Currently, further improvement of the collaboration between dental and medical professionals is likely to be needed as:

- The concept of 'health' and 'oral health' is broadened. New definitions are not confined solely to the biomedical status [2,3].
- Peoples' perception of oral health changes [8] and quality of life becomes an important measure of health [2,4,5].
- The functional and bilateral relationship between oral and systemic health/diseases is better clarified [1,2,4,5,6,7].
- Advances in medical and dental sciences provide new circumstances and opportunities for more active teamwork [3].
- Interdisciplinary care can provide better treatment outcomes, reduce unnecessary or ineffective treatments, and improve general and oral health and quality of life [1,2,8,9,10,11].

Interdisciplinary management for patients with specific needs is particularly crucial [1,2,8]. Immuno-compromised patients are among such category of patients [10, 11,12,13,14,15] (Table 1) due to the presence of bleeding and adverse reactions from medications [1,2,3,10,11,12,16,17,18], susceptibility for infection [2,11,12,16,19,20,21,22], the need of aggressive diagnostic investigations for blunted signs of infections [16], the potential of the oral cavity to serve as a port of entry for infections [4,10,11,23], and the frequency and diversity of systemic and/or oral complications [1, 2, 3,10,11,12,13,15,16,17,18,20,24,25,26]. As the number of patients living with immune-compromised medical status increase, they are expected to have more demand for oral health care [15,27] (Table 2).

Table 1. Major immunocompromised patient groups [12,15]

• Solid organ transplant recipients
• Hematopoietic cell transplant patients
• HIV-infected patients
• Patients with autoimmune diseases receiving immunosuppressive care
• Patients with malignant diseases of the leukopoietic system

Table 1. (Continued)

• Neutropenic patients
• Cancer patients receiving chemotherapy and/or radiotherapy
• Untreated diabetes mellitus cases

Table 2. Main reasons for increasing demand of immunocompromised patients for oral health care

• Increase in HIV-infected patients/survival of AIDS patients [2,12,14,15]
• More patients receiving immunosuppressive treatment for various autoimmune diseases [15,18]
• More patients developing end-stage diseases (ESD) [19,28,29]
• Increased number of candidates for transplantation [16,28,29]
• Wider use of transplantation therapy [2,12,16,24,27,29,30,31]
• Advent of newer and potent immunosuppressive regimens [17,19]
• Decreased surgical complications with transplantation [16,32]
• Increased graft survival rates [16,19,25]
• Prolonged life of transplant recipients [12]
• Broader definition of oral health including all aspects of dental, oral, and craniofacial complex [3]
• Clarification of the bidirectional linkages between oral and systemic health [1,2,4,7]
• Profound effect of oral diseases on general health, quality of life, and economic well-being [4,7,9,10,11,17]

Immunocompromised Patients: Common Oral Features and Impact of Oral Care

Any disorder that impairs host resistance has a subsequent impact on oral cavity due to immunosuppression and/or the inability of the immune system to defend against opportunistic pathogens [1,2,12,15] (Table 3). Oral complications are experenced in almost all patients receiving radiation for head and neck malignancies, in more than 75% of bone marrow transplant (BMT) recipients and in nearly 40% of patients receiving chemotherapy [10]. Oral lesions are often non-specific and may be either localized or a part of a more disseminated disease [15]. Oral mucosal cells are more susceptible to chemotherapeutic regimens and mucosal thinning, mucositis, salivary gland dysfunction, severe pain, loss of taste, and edema are frequently observed [11,20]. Oral mucosa is involved in 60% of patients with leukemia and 40% of patients with heart transplant (HT) [15]. Myelosuppressed patients present with more ulcerative mucositis, bleeding, and leukopenia [10,11] and are at higher risk for secondary infections [11,20], particularly in the presence of mucositis [20]. Radiotherapy increases the risk for xerestomia, caries, periodontal disease, osteoradionecrosis, and candidiasis [10,11], while xerestomia in cancer patients may interfere with eating habits and nutritional status [10,11,13]. Leukemia, sickle cell anemia, aplastic anemia, and neutropenia may manifest increased gingival inflammation, bleeding, and alveolar bone loss [1,12,26].

Oral signs (e.g. gingival bleeding, aphtous ulcers [15]) may lead to the diagnosis of leukemia [12]. Erythematous candidiasis (EC), hairy leukoplakia (HL), conventional gingivitis and periodontitis forms, necrotizing ulcerative periodontitis, deep mycoses, cancers, Kaposi's sarcoma, and necrotizing stomatitis may associate HIV disease [1,2,12,14,25], and such lesions may be markers for disease progression, while painful oral changes may interfere with mastication and thus may result in unintentional weight loss [14].

Table 3. Common oral lesions in immunocompromised patients

• Mucositis
• Candidiasis
• Hairy leukoplakia
• Conventional gingivitis and periodontitis forms
• Necrotizing ulcerative gingivitis and periodontitis
• Necrotizing stomatitis
• Gingival bleeding
• Alveolar bone loss
• Aphtous ulcers
• Lymphoproliferative disorders
• Angular cheilitis
• Deep mycoses
• Kaposi's sarcoma
• Geographic tongue
• Herpes lesions
• Cancers
• Traumatic ulcerations

Iatrogenic immunosuppression affects the oral status [12,15,30] and HL is related to immunosuppression in general [25]. As a result of long-term iatrogenic immunosuppression, development of lymphoproliferative disorders or cancers [12,25,30], (e.g. reactive lymphoid hyperplasia, aggressive malignant lymphomas, carcinomas of the skin and lips [12,16,25,30]), EC, and HL are frequent in solid organ transplant (SOT) patients [15,25]. Renal transplant (RT) recipients may present with HL, intraoral leukoplakia, canidiasis, angular cheilitis, fibroepithelial polyps, traumatic ulcerations, geographic tongue, papillomas, pyogenic granuloma, and acute necrotizing ulcerative gingivitis [25]. Some malignancies may be related to viral infections [16].

Various dental procedures (e.g. periodontal surgery, scaling and root planning), tooth brushing, and irrigation may lead to dissemination of oral bacteria to the bloodstream [12,23]. Under unique circumstances, oral flora may be associated with an increased incidence of morbidity (even mortality) [12]. However, it is difficult to assess the morbidity and mortality from oral foci of infections [12]. In individuals with a lowered immune response, the probability of a systemic disorder occurring from oral foci of infection increases [6], and the amount of plaque and gingival inflammation may relate directly to the degree of bacteremia-associated morbidity [12]. Intensive care unit patients may be at further risk of developing dental plaque colonization because of the difficulties in oral hygiene practices, changes in salivary properties, and reduction of anaerobic flora by antibiotherapy [23]. Poor oral health in SOT recipients may lead to bacterial and fungal infections [27]. Due to gastrointestinal disturbances and loss of appetite emerging from chemotherapeutic regimens, more ingestion of refined carbohydrates may contribute to development of caries [33]. Side effects from immunosuppressive medication can influence the oral status [12,30] and more SOT recipients present with gingival signs and tooth loss [15,30,34].

Since oral health care of immunocompromised patients is integral to their overall health, dentists may contribute to both decreased morbidity and improved quality of life. A good working relationship of dentists with other health care workers helps to improve the efficiency of care for all immunocompromised patients [12,14]. Neglecting oral hygiene in neutropenic patients may worsen oral status while regular care and professional treatment can prevent progression of periodontal breakdown [26]. Reduction of plaque through chemical plaque control and mechanical debridement seems to be efficient for most leukemic patients [12]. With the diagnosis of HIV-infection, easy access to intensive oral care programs and follow-up care (e.g. for necrotizing periodontal diseases) is required [12]. Dentist is often the most appropriate person to treat such problems [14]. Comprehensive oral care is essential for prevention of oral complications associated with cancer therapies [8,10,11]. In immunocompromised patients dental and nutritional services also need to be coordinated [13]. Despite compromised health, well-controlled immunocompromised patients may experience no periodontal problems [15,24]. The benefit of oral care/management is not confined to the oral cavity and can improve the quality of life of patients [11,12].

Transplantation Therapy, Candidates for Transplantation and Transplant Recipients

Bone marrow transplantation (BMT): Hematopoiteic cell transplant is widely used for various malignancies and disorders of the blood and blood-forming organs and for other malignancies and disorders including acute myeloid leukemia, acute lymphocytic leukemia, chronic myeloid leukemia, myelodysplasia, severe aplastic anemia, myeloma, or non-Hodginks lymphoma [12,20,24,35]. Due to immunosuppressive regimens and the subsequent depressed cell-mediated immunity, allogeneic BMT patients manifest immune dysregulation and T-cell dysfunction [35], increased susceptibility to intracellular pathogens and herpes viruses [12,33], and ulcerative, hemorrhagic, or infectious complications that potentially lead to increased morbidity and mortality [20]. Graft-versus-host-disease (GVHD) is one of the most serious complications [12]. High dose chemotherapy is included in pre-BMT conditioning regimens and to prevent or treat GVHD long-term immunosuppressive drugs are prescribed after BMT [35]. Besides other side effects [36,37], this iatrogenic immunosuppression may be associated with the development of secondary malignancies such as leukemia or lymphoma [35].

Degree of stomatotoxicity and myelosuppressive nature of the therapy determines the incidence and severity of associated oral complications [8,10]. Oral cavity and salivary glands are commonly involved and mucositis, ulcerations, hemorrhage, infection, and xerestomia are among acute complications [10]. Dryness of mucosal membranes [10,12,33,35] and oral lichenoid mucositis may develop as oral signs of chronic GVHD [35]. In some cases oral GVHD may be a predisposing factor for oral or gingival squamous cell carcinoma [35].

Higher caries risk, more missing teeth, increased plaque accumulation and gingival inflammation, and susceptibility to periodontal disease may occur [24,33]. In children, as gingival and mucosal health may be the poorest during intense immunosuppression period when the risk of odontogenic bacteriemia is high [33], implementation of strict oral hygiene may have a positive effect [24].

Infection and graft rejection are among common complications associated with transplantation [12] and the oral cavity may serve as a source of systemic infection [8,10,33]. Thus, eliminating oral foci of infection [12,33] and implementation of careful oral care is important to the overall health of BMT patients [10,33]. However, as a result of fear of causing hemorrhage, infection, and increased morbidity and mortality, therapies that involve mechanical manipulation (e.g. flossing) may be excluded [20]. For severe mucositis extra soft tooth brushes and non-drying or moisturizing agents may be advised [8]. When used for immunosuppressive/chemotherapy associated soft tissue inflammation and ulceration, chlorhexidine mouth rinse may reduce the incidence and severity of mucositis, allow shorter hospital stays, and decrease the risk of morbidity and mortality [20].

Solid organ transplantation (SOT): The increase in patients with ESD [19,28,29] creates significant medical, social, and economic problems for patients and their families [28]. SOT is a widely accepted treatment modality for many ESD and is an important therapeutic option for multiple chronic diseases [19,27,29,31,37]. Quality of life and survival rates following SOT have greatly improved due to advances in surgical techniques, organ preservation, obtaining donor-patient tissue matches, transportation solutions, improved anti-rejection therapy, and more effective antibiotics [16,19,29,31,37,38,39]. Liver, kidney, heart, and lung transplantation have become a standard therapy to replace the failing organs and the pancreas and small bowel transplantation are also accomplished [4,16,27,29,31,32,37,40]. RT has become a cost-effective treatment that prolongs life and improves the quality of life of patients with end-stage renal diseases (ESRD) [16,19,22,28], while liver transplantation (LT) is an effective treatment for patients with end-stage liver disease (ESLD) [27,37]. Including children [37], each year more ESLD patients become candidates for this life-saving operation [27]. The most important evolution of pediatric transplants is the rapid expansion of the use of technical variants of reduced-size liver grafts and xenografts may provide unlimited access to donors [32]. Even HT has evolved from an experimental procedure [29] to an accepted treatment option for patients with end-stage heart disease and congenital cardiac malformations [29,31]. Patients who would not have been candidates in the past are being accepted for HT today [29]. Advances in immunosuppressive therapy after HT reduce the susceptibility of patients toward life-threatening oral and systemic infections. Thus, more patients receive HT and survive longer [29,31]. However, rejection, graft failure, donor shortage, clinical status before transplantation, and long transplantation waiting times still remain as relevant causes of morbidity [31]. Similarly, infection [19,22] and allograft rejection stay as major causes of morbidity and mortality in RT and LT [22,27.].

Transplantation treatment often includes life-long use of immuosuppressive agents [12,15,16,41]. Cyclosporin is a powerful immunosuppressive agent with the potential of inhibiting the production of suppressor T lymphocytes and inducing T helper functions without any direct effect on mature lymphocytes [18,38]. It is also used for the treatment of various immunoregulatory disorders (e.g. Behcet's disease, uveitis, rheumatoid arthritis) [18]. It prolongs survival of allogeneic transplants and is the major choice of drug to prevent rejection [18,42]. Some newer immunosuppressive agents (e.g. tacrolimus - a macrolide that potently inhibits the expression of interleukin-2 by T-lymphocytes) present major advances in the management of graft rejection [27,37]. Tacrolimus provides more significant reduction in the acute rejection than cyclosporin [37] and it may be the choice of drug for children undergoing LT [37].

Despite surgical advances nephrotoxicity, hepatotoxicity, hypertension, gastrointestinal disorders, hirsutism, cardiovascular events, malignancies, tremor, paresthesia, leukopenia, hypertrichosis, gingival overgrowth (GO), neurological and gastrointestinal effects, renal dysfunction, diabetes, bone disorders, hepatic dysfunction, susceptibility to infection, and malignancies still remain as serious consequences of immunosuppression [16,17,18,19,22,27,32,36,37]. In RT recipients, malignancies are the 3rd most common cause of death after cardiovascular diseases and infection, while post-transplantation diabetes due to immunosuppressive agents is increasing [16]. Cyclosporin-related lymphoproliferative disorders, which may also present oral symptoms, can be life threatening [12,30] and an increase in oral cancer may be expected due to long-term immunosuppression [25]. New and potent immunosuppressive agents provide improved graft survival, but this is at the expense of an increased risk of development of infection [16,19,22,28].

Oral Cavity as a Port of Entry for Infection

Immunosuppresion lowers immune status and increases the risk of developing superimposed infections with opportunistic organisms [28]. Infection in SOT patients may evolve differently based on the state of immunosuppression, type of transplanted organ, degree of exposure to possible infecting organisms, surgical techniques, and environmental exposure of each transplant center. There are time frames during which infection of specific types most frequently occur [16,19,21,27]. Opportunistic infections usually occur in the first few months (1-6 months) after transplantation primarily due to immuosuppressive drugs [16,21] and the primary sites of infection are abdomen, bloodstream, surgical wounds, and lungs [21]. Cytomegalovirus infections, urinary tract infections, and chronic hepatitis are late-transplant infections [16]. Although deaths are usually caused by viral (cytomegalovirus-most common [19]) and bacterial infections [19,32], bacterial (most common [21]), viral, fungal, and parasitic infections all may occur [21]. Since infection in SOT is closely related to rejection [19] prevention decreases morbidity and mortality from infectious complications and is more cost-effective [19]. However, the usual signs/symptoms of infection is usually difficult to detect and aggressive diagnostic approaches are frequently required [16,27].

Oral infections have a profound effect on oral health, general health, quality of life, and economic well-being and the linkages between oral and systemic health/diseases are bidirectional [4]. The oral cavity is exposed to many microbial, physical, and chemical irritations, and can be a primary source of systemic infections in an immunosuppressive status [20]. Hundreds of oral bacterial, fungal and viral spieces [4,43], some of which are capable of disrupting the integrity of the oral cavity and causing diseases such as candidiasis, herpes, mumps, squamous papilloma, streptococcal tonsillitis, and HIV infection [4] are available and oral cavity serves as an entry point of infection [1,2,4,6,8,10,11,23,43]. 'Focal infection theory proposes that bacteria or their toxins arising from a circumscribed infection within a tissue may disseminate systemically, resulting in the initiation or exacerbation of a systemic illness or a damage of a distant tissue site' [2,6]. Oral infection has a negative impact on systemic health as a result of the entry of oral bacteria or their products into the bloodstream, leading to a transient bacteremia from the oral cavity [12,43]. Transient bacteremia may be triggered by dental procedures, tooth brushing, flossing, tooth picking, and even by mastication [2]. During swallowing, repeated bacterial translocation that may occur from dental site of colonization may explain some occult bacteremias and colonization of dental plaque is highly predictive of subsequent nosocomial infections in intensive care unit patients [23]. There is a potential for hematogenic spread of oral infections to the brain, heart, lungs, liver, kidney, hip, and knee joints [43]. Oral bacteria are implicated in the pathogenesis of gastrointestinal colonization, sepsis, and hematogenic pneumonia. Dental plaque may be a reservoir of respiratory pathogens [2,23,43], and poor oral hygiene and periodontitis may generate more risk [2].

Opportunistic oral lesions, lesions related to medical care, and their changes as markers for systemic changes need to be recognized [12]. Dentists may be the first health care providers to diagnose immunocompromised patients [14] and dental care for transplantation patients lies within the concept of medically-necessary dental care [5,8]. Oral cavity is a common anatomical site where initial symptoms of immunodeficiency could be observed [15] and oral infections can have severe consequences [4,9,39,43]. Untreated caries provides a reservoir of contagion for abscesses, cellulites, and the systemic spread of disease [9]. Bacteria from the root canal may be recovered from peripheral blood during root canal treatment and bacteremia or the associated bacterial endotoxins may cause potential systemic complications [6]. Periodontal disease is infectious in nature and the associated microbiota may act as a focus of infection that influence the morbidity and mortality of systemic diseases [2]. It is likely that in addition to the ulcers of mucositis, an important site of systemic entry for bacteria into the bloodstream is through the inflamed gingival tissue [33]. During invasive dental procedures, infected oral tissues may give rise to transient bacteremias which can result in endocarditis in at-risk patients [4,43]. Immunodeficient conditions and adverse reactions from medications lead to impaired homeostasis and development of opportunistic oral lesions [12]. During intense immunosuppression and profound neutropenia infections are most likely to originate from the oral cavity [33]. Untreated dental disease in medically compromised patients can significantly affect general health and quality of life as acute dental infection can be life-threatening [41,43,44]. In leukemia death may result from infection or bleeding associated with neutropenia/thrombocytopenia and there is greater risk for developing infections by oral commensal pathogens [11]. Deterioration of gingival health may increase the risk of septicemia due to increased oral bacterial loading in BMT patients [33]. Due to xerestomia and decreased immunity, patients undergoing radiation therapy are at great risk for developing caries and periodontal infections which can lead to life-threatening osteonecrosis [10,11,24].

To prevent life threatening bacterial infections, patients with BMT are on antibiotic regimen [24]. Antimicrobial mouth rinses prior to intraoral procedures may be beneficial for immunocompromised patients [12]. Oral infections in these patients tend to be recurrent and progressive and are sometimes resistant to local and systemic treatment [15]. To prevent bacteremia from the oral cavity maintenance of oral health [43] and performance of good oral hygiene on daily basis is crucial [43]. In patients undergoing BMT, removal all possible oral foci of infection before conditioning regimen and preventive care which includes effective tooth brushing to reduce oral bacterial loading is essential, while fluoride supplements may reduce caries incidence [8,33]. Taking into account the potential role of tooth brushing in occult bacteremia, antiseptic dental paste may be used to reduce the bacterial inoculum and avoid the risk of blood translocation from the dental site in intensive care unit patients [23].

Transplantation and Gingival Overgrowth (GO)

Higher predisposition to GO [15,37] is associated with HT [15,34, LT 17,37] and RT [16,25,36,45] (Table 4). In fact, cyclosporin-related GO is recognized as the most common oral/gingival lesion (22%-63% [25,36,37,45]) in all transplant recipients [16,17,30 ,34,36,38,42]. GO with cyclosporin resembles other drug-induced GO and usually occurs within 3-6 months after transplantation [36,37,38]. The precise cellular and molecular mechanisms are not fully understood [4,36,37,38,41,42,46]. Increased number of fibroblasts and volume of extra cellular matrix, and perturbation of collagenase activity [46], increased gingival extra cellular matrix proteins infiltrated with inflammatory cells [37], enhanced inflammatory process in the presence of large numbers of gram (-) rods and anaerobic bacteria [41], sensitivity of periodontium to the drug 34 and genetic factors either in the expression of HLA frequency or in the determination of the fibroblast phenotype [42] may play a role. Severity does not seem to be related to the type of transplanted organ [42] and sex does not have any influence [36]. However, GO is seen more in younger patients [36,42]. The impact of cyclosporin dose, blood concentration, or duration of therapy is controversial [25,36,42,45]. As improved plaque control and reduced gingival inflammation inhibit GO development and recurrence [17,41] inadequate oral hygiene, bacterial plaque accumulation, and gingival inflammation are risk factors [2,26,36,38,42]. Defective restorations, iatrogenic conditions, calculus, ill-fitting prosthesis, and orthodontic appliances may favor the appearance of GO [17].

Cyclosporin has significant interactions with other drugs, including calcium channel blocker agents [17,18,25,38,45]. This combination, being higher with nifedipine [18,25,37,38], increases the risk of GO [25,38,42] and doubles the surgical need [42]. (Tacrolimus, unlike cyclosporine, it is not associated with GO [17,37]). Clinical appearance depends on local inflammation [17]. In severe cases it may affect the function and/or esthetic appearance [20,31] and may interfere with plaque control [36]. As a result of recurrence GO may require repeated surgery [16,17,38,42] and may not always be benign [12].

Table 4. Main features of gingival overgrowth in transplant recipients [12,25,36,37,41,45,46]

• Most common oral/gingival problem in transplant recipients
• Multifactorial etiology
• Association (mainly) with immunosuppressive regimen (cyclosporin)
• Increased incidence with drug combinations
• Development within 3-6 months after transplantation
• Interference with plaque control
• Association with periodontal problems

Table 4. (Continued)

• Interference with mastication
• Association with esthetic problems
• Risk for malignancy
• Frequent need for surgical interventions
• Tendency for recurrence
• Positive impact of plaque control and oral care on GO

Maintenance of a strict oral hygiene, professional tooth brushing instructions, calculus removal, root planning, and removal of iatrogenic or defective restorations comprise the first treatment step, followed by surgery to improve the masticatory function and esthetic appearance [17,27]. For long-term success, patients need to be encouraged towards meticulous oral hygiene and frequent dental visits for professional assistance [27,36]. Severity of post-transplantation complications may be reduced or prevented with proper management with a priority for standard dental prophylaxis [16,27,36]. As patients are naturally concerned with their gingival condition [42], eliminating or minimizing GO may bring esthetic and oral comfort [17].

Impact of Oral Health on the Quality of Life

Oro-facial tissues have functions that we often take for granted, even though they represent the very essence of our humanity because they allow us to chew, swallow, speak, touch, taste, kiss and smile [3]. The term "quality of life" is being increasingly used in evaluating health care [2,4,5,31]. The impact of oral conditions on an individual's quality of life may seem to be underscored [2], however, when measured in functional, psychological and economic dimensions [3] there is a crucial and extensive relationship between oral health and lifelong well-being and quality of life [3,4,13,48]. However, oral health means more than healthy teeth [3] and there is a complex interaction among teeth, jaws, muscles, tongue and salivary glands 1,4. Maintenance of the integrity of the oral complex is essential to overall heath [3,4.]

Diet and nutritional factors can play important roles in oral health and disease and oral health contributes to good nutrition and general health [13]. Oral health allows for food choice and selection of optimum nutrition [1,4]. Poor oral health and tooth loss result in reduction in chewing efficiency and dietary preferences to foods that require less mastication leading to marked changes in dietary intake [48]. Since the mouth is a portal for nutrition and source of communication, it affects the growth and development of children [1]. Oral disorders are mostly painful [3,48] and may create facial pain, chewing and speech problems that restrict daily activities of people [48]. Severe dysfunction that limits choice of food, ability to chew, smile, and talk, and comfortable social interaction or causes pain may have a negative impact on the quality of life, and psychological and social well-being [3,4,48]. Since oral conditions are important determinants of social, psychological, and physical health and functioning [2], oral health can be a source of psychological and physical comfort. On the contrary, functional, infectious, and esthetic difficulties can result in considerable physical and psychological distress [4]. Morale and life satisfaction affects the quality of life and oral disorders may result in low self-image and low self-esteem [48]. Oral diseases, though not conventionally considered serious, are now accepted to undermine the well-being and more emphasis is put on the way in which diseases and disorders affecting various body systems compromise the quality of life [48]. 'What "oral health" rather than "oral disease" means for the public is difficult to assess but peoples' perception of oral health changes. Tooth loss is no longer considered as an inevitable consequence of aging and life-time retention of teeth has become more possible while for some segments of the public oral health has become synonymous with esthetics' [4].

Benefit of Further Collaboration between Dental and Medical Professionals (Table 5)

- The mouth reflects general health/disease status, medication, harmful habits, and nutritional status. Oral cells, tissues, and fluids can be used as diagnostic tools [3].
- Due to the growing number of patients with immunodeficiencies [,12,14,15,18], the increase in ESD/candidates for SOT and wider use of transplantation therapy [2,16,19,24,27,28,29,30,31], more immunocompromised patients have demand for dental care [15,27]. Dentists may be the first health care providers to diagnose oral lesions in these patients. They may encourage them to seek medical advice and refer patients with lesions beyond their expertise [14].
- Patients with ESD, who are in fact long-term candidates for transplant procedures [27,28,29], need interdisciplinary management (e.g. ESRD patients may present uremia stomatitis, bleeding, xerestomia, bad taste, oral malodor, painful teeth to mastication, tumours, metastatic calcifications, and are prone to a variety of infections [28,39]). The importance of good oral health may not often be fully realized [9,44] and patients may not acknowledge the impact of oral hygiene on the prevention of various oral and systemic problems related to ESD [27]. Oral hygiene prior to transplantation is a preventive measure [36] and increased awareness of candidates/SOT recipients on oral hygiene may reduce the risk of complications [2,27,40].
- Routine evaluation for active oral infection prior to transplantation is essential for all candidates [8,12,27,33]. Through comprehensive examination, oral foci of infection can be identified and oral infections with the potential for exacerbation or dissemination can be eliminated [8,12,27,33]. Within the concept of medically-necessary dental care [49], all patients undergoing immunosuppressive care need to have a dentist involved in the overall management prior to therapy [12] and to provide continuing care for all patients with immunodeficient conditions [12]. Meticulous dental care needs to be an integral part of these patients' life-time care [8,27].
- Dental management of an immunodeficient patient requires understanding of the patient's medical status and knowledge of oral/systemic complications. For provision of safe oral care, a dentist needs to consult with the patient's physician the stability and stage of the disease [12,27], systemic adverse reactions from the

immunosupressive medications [12,27], multi-drug resistant pathogens, medication toxicity, drug-drug interactions [12,19,27] and necessity/ appropriateness of antibiotic prophylaxis prior to and after dental care with effective antimicrobials [12,19,27].

- As dentistry's oral disease prevention/health promotion armamentarium can be used by all health care professionals, they may play significant roles in oral health promotion [3,50]. Oral hygiene programs supplemented by professional care may prevent future oral infections [12].
- Physicians can play important roles in the maintenance of oral health [13]. With increased awareness of the risk for dental complications among their patients, they may monitor for them and refer at risk patients for dental care to improve the patient's overall well-being [7].
- Despite profound immunosuppression, strict oral care can provide optimal plaque control and periodontal health [24]. Physicians may advise on tooth brushing, use fluoride mouth rinses, and antiseptic dental pastes for immunocompromised patients [13,23]. Children and families may also receive advice on dietary modifications for prevention of dental diseases. Furthermore, fluoride supplements may be prescribed and oral cleaning may be demonstrated [50].
- For patients with a reduced number of platelets, treating/preventing gingival inflammation and alternative methods of tooth brushing may reduce the bleeding tendency [12]. Intraoral leukoplakia and erythematous candidiasis may require modification of denture design and advice in denture hygiene [25]. Dentists may carefully and regularly screen lips and oral mucosa for cancer [25].
- GO may cause periodontal, functional, and esthetic problems [12,17,37,38], interfere with plaque control [36], and require surgical intervention [12,30]. Plaque control and alternative tooth brushing methods may minimize GO and it's recurrence [12,36]. Initial periodontal therapy and curettage may reduce the need for stressful surgery. Gingival biopsies may reveal the first signs of post transplantation lymphoproliferative disorders [30].
- The medical community may not be less familiar with drug-induced GO. More medical concern for drug-associated GO and referral to dentists for control of local causal factors may reduce the frequency of this entity [38]. A change from nifedipine to verapamil [38,45] and a change from cyclosporine to tacrolimus may also be considered [17,37].
- To provide comprehensive care for patients with oral health risks/dental problems, physicians may further review the relationship between nutrition and oral health, routinely screen patients for dental risks, consider oral factors/oral health needs, and further cooperate with dentists [1,13,50]. Oral health and dental care is likely to be underscored [9,39,49] and may be considered superfluous and time consuming by medical staff [23]. Oral hygiene measures need to be implemented within the primary goal of preventing plaque colonization in patients with medical problems [23]. More awareness of the medical community [9,38] and a change in health care providers' perceptions about oral health may increase the approval of oral health as a component of general health [3].
- Especially in medically compromised children [9,44], childhood oral diseases have significant consequences for health and well-being [9]. This may not be recognized

as a result of the historic separation of medicine and dentistry 9, or because of the primary attention of families usually focusing on medical treatment [44]. A system integrating medical and dental care [3,9,44], including routine specialized dental care, needs to be part of medical re-evaluation protocol for medically compromised children [44].

- Indirect cost of oral disorders - work or school loss days, or reduced activity days - may become significant when the whole population is considered. 'Currently, we are not sure of economic and social impact of oral contributions as a portal of entry to respiratory disease, otitis media, gastrointestinal diseases, sexually transmitted diseases and the economical implications of linkages of oral infections to diabetes, cardio-vascular diseases, stroke and low-birth-weight babies' [4].
- People's perception of oral health is changing [4]. Although oral diseases were not considered to be serious in the past, they are now accepted to undermine the well-being to a surprising degree [48] but the public still may need more emphasis on the impact of oral health on general health.
- Instead of functioning in relative isolation, dental profession need to become a more integrated component of the overall health care system [9,51]. Dentists may improve general health/quality of life of patients via their advice on nutrition and healthy life-styles, tobacco-use prevention, behavior modification programs, and provision of necessary oral care for the preservation of teeth [3,51]. Education of HIV-infected patients and the community by dentists is an example of their potential in serving the public [14]. 'Instead of the traditional tooth-doctor, dentistry may need to commit to an oral physician concept and play a more active role in public health policy' [51].
- SOT patients are under the risk of developing oral complications [10,12,15,16,25,29,30,33,34, 35,37,45] and in need of interdisciplinary management [31,34]. As no firm protocols seem to exist for provision of safe dental care for these patients [12,19,22,27,39,40], improved collaboration can ensure proper dental care and the team approach to become a routine part of the transplantation protocol [8,22,39,40].
- 'In future, further integration of dentistry and medicine will bring up new opportunities for collaboration across many specialties. A greater interaction will likely require the dentist to take more responsibility for the management of their patient's systemic health, and the physician to assume a more active role in their patient's oral health' [2].
- Further integration of dental and medical education may improve professional relationships, collaborative working practices, standards of care, and the team approach [9,51,52]. Team-based learning exercises may increase the personal and professional confidence, and respect and honesty, and may reduce professional antagonism [52].
- Most oral health problems are not solely dental in nature and fall into overlapping educational and patient care environments of both health care providers [51]. Many conditions that affect the oral, dental, and craniofacial complex which require a team approach may provide a challenge and opportunity of more job satisfaction for all health care providers [3].
- Improved cooperation between dentists and physicians leads to more effective care and better treatment outcome and improves the quality of care and quality of life of

the patients [8,9,49,51,52].'A team composed of various types and degrees of skill and knowledge is more efficient and the team as a whole has an impact greater than the sum of the contribution of it's members' [52].

Table 5. Major factors increasing the need of interdisciplinary management for transplant recipients

• Improved prognosis of transplantation [16,25,32,39]
• Increasing transplant recipients visiting dental clinics [16,27,37,39]
• Oral complications of ESD and transplantation [2,16,24,30,33,39]
• Increased susceptibility to infection [,11,12,16,19,20,21,22]
• The potential of oral cavity to serve as a port for bacteria [1,2,6,39,43]
• Serious consequences of untreated oral infection [12,39,43] and the impact of oral infection on quality of life [4,13,48]
• Lack of firm protocols for provision of safe and appropriate oral health care [22,39,40]
• Need of cooperation with physicians for provision of safe oral care [12,27]
• High frequency of GO 2,38,42 and the impact of drug combinations on GO [17,25,38,42]
• Frequent need of surgical interventions for treatment of GO [38,42]
• Correlation between GO development and poor oral hygiene [2,37,38,42] and the positive impact of oral care in reducing GO and oral complications [12,17,36,39,41]
• Need of more concern for oral health and further awareness of medical community [38,39,49]

ACKNOWLEDGMENTS

The authors are grateful to Professor Henry Magloire for kindly reviewing the manuscript. The authors also wish to thank Mrs.Jenny Syratchev for her kind assistance during the preparation of the manuscript.

REFERENCES

[1] Casamassimo PS. Relationship between oral and systemic health. *Pediatr. Clin. North Am* 2000 47: 1149-1157.

[2] Garcia RI, Henshaw MM, Krall EA. Relationship between periodontal disease and systemic health. *Periodontol. 2000* 2001 25: 21-35.

[3] Evans CA, Kleinman DV. The Surgeon's General Report on America's oral health. Opportunities for the dental profession. *J. Am. Dent. Assoc* 2000 131: 1721-1728.

[4] Mandel ID. Oral infections: Impact on human health, well-being, and healthcare costs. *Compend. Contin. Dent. Educ.* 2002 23: 403-413.

[5] Patton LL, White BA, Field MJ. State of the evidence base for medically necessary oral health care. *Oral Surg. Oral Med. Oral Pathol. Oral Radiol. Endod* 2001 92: 272-275.

[6] Murray CA, Saunders WP. Root canal treatment and general health: a review of the literature. *Int. Endod J.* 2000 33: 1-18.

[7] Rose LF, Steinberg BJ, Minsk L. The relationship between periodontal disease and systemic conditions. *Compend. Contin. Educ. Dent.* 2000 21: 870-877.

[8] Barker GJ. Current practices in the oral management of the patient undergoing chemotherapy or bone marrow transplantation. *Support Care Cancer* 1999 7: 17-20.

[9] Mouradian WE, Wehr E, Crall JJ. Disparities in children's oral health and access to dental care. *JAMA* 2000 284: 2625-2631.

[10] Oral complications of cancer treatment. What the oncology team can do. U.S. Department of Health and Human Services. National Institutes of Health, publication no. 99-4630.

[11] Oral complications of cancer treatment. What the oral health team can do. U.S. Department of Health and Human Services. National Institutes of Health, publication no. 99-4630.

[12] Holmstrup P, Glick M. Treatment of periodontal disease in the immunodeficient patient. *Periodontol. 2000* 2002 28: 190-205.

[13] Palmer CA. Important relationships between diet, nutrition, and oral health. *Nutr. Clin. Care* 2001 4:4-14.

[14] Glick M. The role of dentist in the era of AIDS. *Dent. Clin. North Am.* 1996 40: 343-357.

[15] Meyer U, Kleinhanz J, Handschel J, *et al.* Oral findings in three different groups of immunocompromised patients. *J. Oral Pathol. Med.* 2000 29: 153-158.

[16] Cohen D, Galbraith C. General health management and long-term care of renal transplant recipients. *Am. J. Kidney Dis.* 2001 38 (6 Suppl 6): S10-24.

[17] Bader G, Lejeune S, Messner M. Reduction of cyclosporine-induced gingival overgrowth following a change to tacrolimus. A case history involving a liver transplant patient. *J. Periodontol.* 1998 69: 729-732.

[18] Faluds D, Goa KL. Cyclosporin. A review of it's pharmacodynamic and pharmacokinetic properties and therapeutic use in immunoregulatory disorders. *Drugs* 1993 45: 953-1041.

[19] Villacian JS, Paya CV. Prevention of infections in solid organ transplant recipients. *Transplant Inf Dis* 1999 1: 50-64.

[20] Rutkauskas JS, Davis JW. Effect of chlorhexidine during immunosuppressive chemotherapy. *Oral Surg. Oral Med. Oral Pathol.* 1993 76: 441-448.

[21] Shhehy EC, Beighton D, Roberts GJ. The oral microbiota of children undergoing liver transplantation. *Oral Microbiol. Immunol.* 2000 15: 203-210.

[22] Batiuk TD, Bozdiak KA, Goldman M. Infectious disease prophylaxis in renal transplant patients: a survey of US transplant centers. *Clin. Transplant* 2002 16: 1-11.

[23] Fourrier F, Duvivier B, Boutinghy H, *et al.* Colonization of dental plaque. A source of nosocomial infections in intensive care unit patients. *Crit. Care Med.* 1998 26: 301-308.

[24] Pattni R, Walsh LJ, Marshall RI, *et al.* Changes in periodontal status of patients undergoing bone marrow transplantation. *J. Periodontol.* 2000 71: 394-402.

[25] King GN, Healy CM, Glover MT, *et al.* Prevalence and risk factors associated with leukopenia, hairy leukoplakia, erythematosus candidiasis, and gingival hyperplasia in renal transplant recipients. *Oral Surg. Oral Med. Oral Pathol.* 1994 78: 718-726.

[26] Pernu HE, Pajari UH, Lanning M. The importance of regular dental treatment in patients with cyclic neutropenia. *J Periodontol* 1996 67: 454-459.

[27] Douglas LR, Douglas JB, Sieck JO, *et al.* Oral management of the patient with end-stage liver disease. *Oral Surg. Oral Med. Oral Pathol. Oral Radiol. Endod* 1998 86: 55-64.

[28] Kher V. End-stage renal disease in developing countries. *Kidney Int.* 2002 62: 350-362.

[29] Cimato TR, Jessup M. Recipient selection in cardiac transplantation: contraindications and risk factors for mortality. *J. Heart Lung Transpl* 2002 21: 1161-1173.

[30] Oda D, Persson GR, Haigh WG, *et al.* Oral presentations of post transplantation lymphoprolypherative disorders. *Transplantation* 1996 61: 435- 440.

[31] Bauer J, Thul J, Kramer U, *et al.* Heart transplantation in children and infants: Short-term outcome and long-term follow-up. *Pediatr. Transpl.* 2001 5: 457- 462.

[32] Kuang AA. Decreased mortality from technical failure improves results in pediatric liver transplantation. *Arch. Surg.* 1996 131: 887-893.

[33] Lucas VS, Robets GJ, Beighton D. Oral health of children undergoing allogeneic bone marrow transplantation. *Bone Marrow Transpl.* 1990 22: 801-808.

[34] Montebugnoli L, Servidio D, Barnardi F. The role of time in reducing overgrowth in heart transplant patients following cyclosporin therapy. *J. Clin. Periodontol.* 2000 27: 611-614.

[35] Otsuba H, Yokoe H, Miya T, *et al.* Gingival squamous cell carcinoma in a patient with chronic graft-versus-host disease. *Oral Surg. Oral Med. Oral Pathol. Oral Radiol. Endod* 1997 84: 171-174.

[36] Somacarrera ML, Hernandez G, Acero J, *et al.* Factors related to the incidence and severity of cyclosporin-induced gingival overgrowth in transplant patients. *J. Periodontol.* 1994 65: 671-675.

[37] McKaig SJ. Investigation of the effect of FK 506 (tacrolimus) and cyclosporin on gingival overgrowth following pediatric liver transplantation. *Int. J. Pediatr. Dent.* 2002 12: 398-403.

[38] Hallmon WW, Rossmann JA. The role of drugs in the pathogenesis of gingival overgrowth. A collective review of current concepts. *Periodontol 2000* 1999 21: 176-196.

[39] Klassen J T, Krasko B M. The dental status of dialysis patients. *J. Can. Dent. Assoc.* 2002 68: 34-38.

[40] Yamalik N, Avcıkurt UF, Caglayan F, *et al.* The importance of oral foci of infection in renal transplantation. *Aust. Dent. J.* 1993 38: 108-113.

[41] Fisher RG. The effect of cyclosporin-A on the oral microflora at gingival sulcus of the ferret. *J. Clin. Periodontol.* 1996 23: 853-860.

[42] Thomason JM, Seymour RA, Ellis JS, *et al.* Determinants of gingival overgrowth severity in organ transplant patients. An examination of the role of HLA phenotype. *J Clin. Periodontol.* 1996 23: 628-634.

[43] Muerman JH. Dental infections and general health. *Quintessence Int.* 1997 28: 807-811.

[44] Parry JA, Khan FA. Provision of dental care for medically compromised children in the UK by general dental practitioners. *Int. J. Pediatr. Dent* 2000 10: 322-327.

[45] Cebeci I, Kantarcı A, Fıratlı E, *et al.* The effect of verapamil on the prevalence and severity of cyclosporin-induced gingival overgrowth in renal allograft recipients. *J Periodontol.* 1996 67: 1201-1205.

[46] Thomason MJ, Sloan P, Seymour RA. Immunolocalization of collagenase (MMP-1) and stromelysin (MMP-3) in the gingival tissue of organ transplant patients medicated with cysclosporin. *J. Clin. Periodontol.* 1998 25: 554-560.

[47] James JA, Jamal S, Hull PS, *et al.* Tacrolimus is not associated with gingival overgrowth in renal transplant patients. *J. Clin. Periodontol.* 2001 28: 848-852.

[48] Locker D, Matear D. Oral disorders, systemic health, and well-being and quality of life. A summary of recent research evidence. Guidelines/database - Patient-Quality of Life. Canadian Public Health Association. http://www.fdiworldental.org

[49] Patton LL, White BA, Field MJ. Extending Medicare coverage to medically necessary dental care. *J. Am. Dent. Assoc.* 2001 132: 1294-1299.

[50] Schafer TE, Adair SM. Prevention of dental disease: The role of the pediatrician. *Pediatr. Clin. North. Am.* 2000 47: 1021-1042.

[51] Hendricson WD, Cohen WA. Oral health care in the 21st century: Implications for dental and medical education. *Acad. Med.* 2001 76: 1181-1206.

[52] Munro N, Felton A, Mc Intosh C. Is multidisciplinary learning effective among those caring for people with diabetes? *Diabet. Med.* 2002 19: 799-803.

INDEX

A

D

E

F

G

N

Q

R

S

T

U

V

W

X

Z